Veterinary Practice Management

Veterinary Practice □ Management

Edited by

Dennis M. McCurnin, D.V.M., M.S.

Diplomate, American College of Veterinary
Surgeons; Professor of Clinical Sciences; Director,
Veterinary Teaching Hospital, College of Veterinary
Medicine and Biomedical Sciences, Colorado State
University, Fort Collins, Colorado

With 29 Contributors

J.B. Lippincott Company

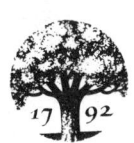

Philadelphia
London
Mexico City
New York
St. Louis
São Paulo
Sydney

Acquisitions Editor: Susan M. Gay
Sponsoring Editor: Delois Patterson
Manuscript Editor: Margaret E. Maxwell
Indexer: Catherine Battaglia
Design Coordinator: Michelle Gerdes
Production Manager: Carol A. Florence
Production Coordinator: Kathryn Rule
Compositor: Digitype
Printer/Binder: R.R. Donnelley & Sons

6   5   4   3   2   1

Library of Congress Cataloging-in-Publication Data

Veterinary practice management.

  Bibliography: p.
  Includes index.
  1. Veterinary medicine — Practice.   I. McCurnin, Dennis M.
SF756.4.V47   1988   636.089′068   87-21400
ISBN 0-397-50782-8

The authors and publisher have exerted every effort to ensure that
drug selection and dosage set forth in this text are in accord with
current recommendations and practice at the time of publication.
However, in view of ongoing research, changes in government
regulations, and the constant flow of information relating to drug
therapy and drug reactions, the reader is urged to check the package
insert for each drug for any change in indications and dosage and for
added warnings and precautions. This is particularly important when
the recommended agent is a new or infrequently employed drug.

Contributors

☐

George M. Angleton, Ph.D.
Professor of Biometry and Radiation Biology;
Director of Veterinary Teaching Hospital
  Computer Center
Colorado State University
Fort Collins, Colorado

Suzanne Arguello, M.S.
Department of Zoology
Director of CHANGES: Support for People and Pets
Colorado State University
Veterinary Teaching Hospital
Fort Collins, Colorado

Joseph Barton-Dobenin, Ph.D.
Professor of Management
Director of Small Business Development Center
Kansas State University
Manhattan, Kansas

Ronald L. Burk, D.V.M., M.B.A.
Assistant Chief of Staff
The Animal Medical Center
New York, New York

Ross D. Clark, D.V.M.
Co-owner and Managing Partner
Woodland Animal Hospital;
Owner of Veterinary Management Concepts
Tulsa, Oklahoma

Jack R. Dinsmore, D.V.M.
Glenview, Illinois

Donald R. Dooley
Veterinary Practice Management Consultant
Los Gatos, California

Stuart D. Forney, R.Ph., M.S.
Director of Pharmacy
Colorado State University
Veterinary Teaching Hospital
Fort Collins, Colorado

Walter R. Gillespie, D.V.M.
Phoenix, Arizona

Harold W. Hannah, J.D.
Professor Emeritus of Agricultural and Veterinary
Medical Law
University of Illinois;
Adjunct Professor of Law
Southern Illinois University
Carbondale, Illinois

Jack D. Henry, Jr., D.V.M., M.S.
Diplomate, American College of Veterinary
Surgeons;
Veterinary Surgical Referral Service, P.C.
Moon Valley Animal Hospital
Phoenix, Arizona

John W. Judy, Jr., D.V.M., Ph.D.
Professor and Associate Dean
College of Veterinary Medicine
Michigan State University;
Director of Veterinary Clinical Center
Okemos, Michigan

David R. Kauss, Ph.D.
Assistant Clinical Professor
University of California at Los Angeles
Los Angeles, California

William J. Kay, D.V.M.
Chief of Staff
The Animal Medical Center
New York, New York

Eugenia G. Kelman, Ph.D.
Supervising Psychologist
Kaiser–Permanente
Westminster, Colorado;
Formerly Assistant Dean of College of Veterinary
Medicine and Biomedical Sciences
Colorado State University
Fort Collins, Colorado

Edward P. Kerrigan, C.P.A.
Comptroller and Chief Financial Officer
The Animal Medical Center
New York, New York

Laurel S. Lagoni, M.S.
Extension Specialist in Human Development and
Family Studies
Colorado State University
Fort Collins, Colorado

Robert E. Lewis, D.V.M., M.S.
Diplomate, American College of Veterinary
Radiologists;
Professor
College of Veterinary Medicine
University of Georgia Teaching Hospital
Athens, Georgia

Dennis M. McCurnin, D.V.M., M.S.
Diplomate, American College of Veterinary
Surgeons;
Professor of Clinical Sciences;
Director, Veterinary Teaching Hospital
College of Veterinary Medicine and Biomedical
Sciences
Colorado State University
Fort Collins, Colorado

Ronald K. Patrick, C.P.A., M.B.A.
Tulsa, Oklahoma

Connee Pike
Human Development and Family Studies
Colorado State University
Fort Collins, Colorado

Frederick H. Rice
Director of Small Business Development Center
Kansas State University
Manhattan, Kansas

Carmen Rodriguez
Manager of Client Financial Operations
The Animal Medical Center
New York, New York

Ray L. Russell, D.V.M., M.A.M.
Special Assistant to the Governor of Arizona
Mesa, Arizona

Marvin L. Samuelson, D.V.M.

Associate Professor
Kansas State University
Veterinary Medical Hospital
Manhattan, Kansas

Joe H. Schwarz, M.Ed.

Assistant to the Dean
College of Veterinary Medicine and Biomedical
Sciences
Colorado State University
Veterinary Teaching Hospital
Fort Collins, Colorado

Bradford F. Spencer, Ph.D., M.B.A.

President
Spencer/Shenk & Associates, Inc.
Gardena, California

Robert A. Taylor, D.V.M., M.S.

Diplomate, American College of Veterinary
Surgeons;
Co-director of Del Rea Institute;
Co-director of Alameda East Veterinary Hospital;
Adjunct Associate Professor
Denver University
Denver, Colorado

Stephen J. Withrow, D.V.M.

Professor of Surgery;
Chief of Clinical Oncology
College of Veterinary Medicine and Biomedical
Sciences
Colorado State University
Fort Collins, Colorado

Preface

□

The veterinary medical profession has undergone numerous crisis situations during its evolution. Each critical period has been followed by the formation of a more dedicated and caring health-care profession. Veterinary medicine has made tremendous strides in the science and art of prevention, diagnosis, and therapy during the past 50 years. However, the profession has been remiss in the attention given to managing a successful practice.

The management of a veterinary practice is as much a specialized skill as are making a diagnosis, performing surgery, or evaluating a radiograph. Moreover, the success or failure of the entire practice may well depend on the knowledge and skill of the veterinary practice manager. Some larger practices are now managed by nonveterinarian managers with the support of the veterinarian owner.

Most practice case loads and gross incomes have stabilized because of the increased numbers of new veterinarians during the past decade. Attention has now been directed toward improving the effectiveness of managing clients, patients, staff, and practice. Practitioners are requesting and attending continuing education courses directed at improving practice management skills. Colleges and schools of veterinary medicine are now offering basic and applied practice management courses to veterinary students.

The profession is now in need of scientific research and reference material in the areas of management to provide the most current information, as is found in the traditional medical areas of veterinary medicine. To build and to improve today's practice, the practice team must possess skills in personnel management, client management, veterinary marketing, computer management, and financial management.

The purpose of *Veterinary Practice Management* is to provide the veterinarian, veterinary student, veterinary technician, veterinary technology student, and practice manager with a general management reference text. Practice management has become such a large field that this book required multiple contrib-

utors. Each chapter has been authored by a specialist actively involved in his or her field.

This book is dedicated to the people who work tirelessly behind the scenes of all successful practices to ensure the highest level of care for patients and clients. Practice management has evolved into a specialized area of veterinary medicine.

Dennis M. McCurnin, D.V.M.

Contents

☐

*Veterinary Practice
Management*

Chapter 1

☐

Leadership makes a difference

Bradford F. Spencer
David R. Kauss

As business consultants we were a bit surprised (but also pleased) to be asked to contribute a chapter for what, in essence, is a management text for veterinarians, veterinary students, and veterinary technicians. We were reminded of a recent meeting involving the heads of several organizations in the service field. Attending were the head of a moderate-sized law firm, the heads of two engineering firms, three veterinarians, one chiropractor, and the head of a small accounting firm. The average number of employees in the firms was 12.5. The average age of the men and women attending the meeting was 35. Each of them in their own right would be considered both prosperous and successful, yet each was extremely worried about issues in their companies or practices. For several hours they bemoaned their problems. Each of them wanted to believe they faced a unique situation. Finally, one of us broke in with an observation that none of them particularly liked and each of them fought. In fact, the lawyer's problem was very much the same as the accountant's problem, which was very much the same as the chiropractor's and veterinarian's.

The problems they were describing boiled down to one word—*people.* They had the wrong people in the wrong jobs, "demotivated" employees, poor performers who were not meeting standards, underqualified people, and so forth. We had seen this before in large and small companies, but the thing that jumped out at us was the commonality of this group. In each case, these individuals had been highly trained in a very specific field. Their training had consisted of years of highly technical specialization to allow them to perform with a high degree of competence and skill. Yet nowhere along this route of training had they been exposed to the two essentials that would make them successful in organization: management and leadership skills. It was clear to us that the problems they were facing and the opportunities that would allow them to grow were related to the effective direction and management of their staffs. Without the ability to lead, they were condemned to prosper only when they themselves were doing almost all of the tasks. And while they were willing to give 200% to their clients, they were left with the worry that those who were working for them fell painfully short of such motivated dedication.

Organizational problems are people problems. The financial management problems veterinarians eventually run into start with the people problem issues. The success of sales and marketing strategies depends on people. Staff turnover is a function of leadership. Competent bookkeeping, collections, and so forth are functions of management. Each begins with effective selection, requires effective initial orientation, and finally, depends on ongoing staff development and training. Surrounding this is what we refer to as the organizational climate, which makes for effective or ineffective output in a service organization, *regardless of what the service is!* There are some fundamentals that must be learned in every business. Veterinarians who hope to prosper in the coming years of increased competition have already started learning them.

☐
Leadership and management

There are numerous definitions of leadership. At last count, no less than 353 different ones dotted the literature in the field. Although we do not feel it is that complex a topic, it is clear after years in the field of business consulting that, whatever it is, leadership makes a significant difference in the effectiveness, growth, and success of an organization.

Not to add a definition to the field, but to clarify what we are talking about when we discuss *leadership,* we will segregate it from the concept that much of this book addresses — *management.* We offer this working definition of leadership: the effective leader is an individual with a vision and a direction who is *consistently working to do the right things.* A leader is differentiated from a manager: a manager is an individual who does things right or causes others to do them right.

In his recent book on leadership, Dr. Warren Bennis points out that the major cause of stagnation in American industry is the fact that most mature companies are not underled but overmanaged.[1] Too many people are paying attention to the bureaucratic processes of how to do things right and are not paying enough attention to determining the right things to do. Our experience with veterinarians bears out this observation. Frustrations coincident with practice growth inevitably manifest themselves as concerns about how to get people to do things right consistently, which is a managerial question. Our experience is that before this managerial question can be addressed, the significant issues related to leadership must be settled first. The operative question is: What are the right things to do in terms of motivation, communication, and ensuring a consistent message that aligns one's staff toward effective service and high-quality client care?

Clearly, a fundamental understanding of leadership and its execution is a major need of the veterinarian who is just entering practice or is looking to work effectively inside a larger practice. The veterinary practitioner who is highly skilled at diagnosing and treating animal problems oftentimes suffers a severe turnover of staff and is not able to optimize the situation to perform profitably either for his clients or for his personnel. This chapter, in its all too brief form, is designed to outline a model that is simple and accessible and enables practitioners to better understand the drives of leadership, including how to apply them on a day-to-day basis with their staff.

There is a significant body of research in this field that begins with World War II when the American army was forced either to languish without leadership or to challenge the historical assumption that "leaders are born, not made." In the attempts to produce second lieutenants in the quantity needed (at the time labeled "6-week wonders") and in the postwar 1950s when the leadership needs of the nation seemed unquenchable because of dramatic growth in American industry, it was indeed proved that leadership qualities and skills can be learned by each of us.

When we use the word *leader,* people tend to think of specific role models. Too many of us base our idea of a leader on the Hollywood archetype of an individual (usually male) with significant power and drive who causes people to behave in the way he chooses simply because he has tremendous authority and a title. Visions of the movie *Patton* or of the submarine captain that we saw in our youth come to mind: men snapping orders, with subordinates obeying immediately or being chastised for not being entirely and unquestionably cooperative.

A second and certainly opposite image of a leader is the "nice guy." This is the person who, because of his or her ability to establish rapport very quickly and create significant friendships and loyalties, actually makes people want to serve under them. The image of the best father in the world (remember Robert Young in *Father Knows Best?*) comes to mind, a man who led his family in such a way that no conflict called for raised voices. Instead, everyone wanted to be cooperative in a very caring setting. Squabbles were small and inconsequential, especially in view of the dominant theme: "Let us avoid conflict."

A third common type of leader is the individual who, through sheer expertise and focus on accomplishing the task, is able to rally the troops to move in the "correct" direction. The person's overwhelming insights into the problems at hand and quick grasp of solutions and technical expertise are reasons for immediate deferral and compliance. This person leads through reason and example.

Undoubtedly, we could think of other common leader types, but research in the field paints a different picture. While each of these leaders comes to the fore periodically, there is no one best leadership style, and certainly different styles are appropriate in different situations. It is especially useful to understand the context of these situations and where your own leadership style tends to fit. People often tend to model themselves after (consciously or unconsciously) a particular leader. In understanding how you lead, a good starting point is to identify which leaders you respect and which leaders you would try to emulate. Those of us without effective role models in leadership need to develop them to be more effective leaders. A classic problem we have found in the veterinary medical field is that the role models for veterinarians tend to be the technically competent individuals, not highly effective leaders or managers. Certainly the universities are filled with highly competent professors who are effective role models in developing confidence for performing tasks they are paid to perform, but these models are often not helpful in developing the leadership skills needed to grow and to become a leader in practice.

With so much written about the essentials of leadership, one might wonder how the subject can be covered in a hands-on, practical fashion in a brief chapter such as this. We will attempt no such task; instead we are going to focus our discussion on two fundamental objectives that our experience says you will be able to achieve and apply effectively on a day-to-day basis. The first is the ability to assess the situation, the employee's capabilities, and the appropriate leadership response for this combination of factors. We will provide the necessary tools to recognize the situation and the appropriate response to a given employee. The other objective is to understand what "motivated behavior" really is and to be able to cause others to exhibit it. Some veterinarians will hire only people with personalities and drives to excel that are similar to their own. However, some veterinarians hire very effectively and then systematically demotivate employees in a fairly short period of time. This is certainly avoidable. We will outline what research tells us are the key elements in developing and maintaining leadership patterns that are satisfying to the veterinarian and that help their employees to set and to meet high standards of performance.

To do this we are going to use two extremely well-researched models that have relatively easy practical application. The first is the research of Drs. Hersey and Blanchard, commonly called *situational leadership.*[2] The second is the motivation theory work of Dr. David McClelland of Harvard.[3] Our efforts will be to explain briefly these models and the implications for leaders in using them, both in small and in large practices.

☐
Situational leadership: a practical approach to leadership in your practice

Over the past few decades, people in the field of management have been involved in a search for the "best" style of leadership. Yet the evidence from their studies clearly indicates there is no single, all-purpose leadership style. Successful leaders are those who can adapt their behavior to meet the demands of their own unique situations.

The situational leadership model is a well-researched, powerful tool that acts as a common sense guide for managers. Situational leadership theory is based on an interplay among (1) the amount of direction (task behavior) a leader gives, (2) the amount of socioemotive support (relationship behavior) a leader provides, and (3) the "readiness" level a subordinate exhibits on a specific task.

Recently we were working with a veterinarian who had brought into the practice a second veterinarian who was very experienced and who was a potential partner. The second veterinarian had been out of school for 7 years and was very skillful, particularly in surgery. Four days after this new veterinarian joined the practice, the owner went on a 10-day ski vacation. When he returned, the practice was in a shambles. He was both amazed and distraught. What had happened?

Situational leadership theory[2] can help us understand this occurrence. The head of this practice made a common error. He assumed that the second veterinarian's fully developed competence in running one practice could be easily transferred to his practice. He assumed that the individual taking control did not need specific instructions and ongoing support to integrate his old knowledge into a new situation. This assumption is almost always false. With 2 or 3 more weeks of both veterinarians being on the job, the transition would have been, in all probability, very smooth.

The Situational Leadership model (Fig. 1-1) needs some clarification before it can be understood. It is made up of two parts. The first part focuses on the *subordinate,* the second on the *leader.* As you will note in the bottom portion of Figure 1-1, the model includes a concept labeled *follower readiness.* This simply refers to two fundamental variables. The first we call the *maturity level* the individual brings to the function; that is, how able is this person to do the job? To what extent do they have the necessary *ability,* experience, and skills to perform the task competently. The second, is the degree of *willingness.* Willing-

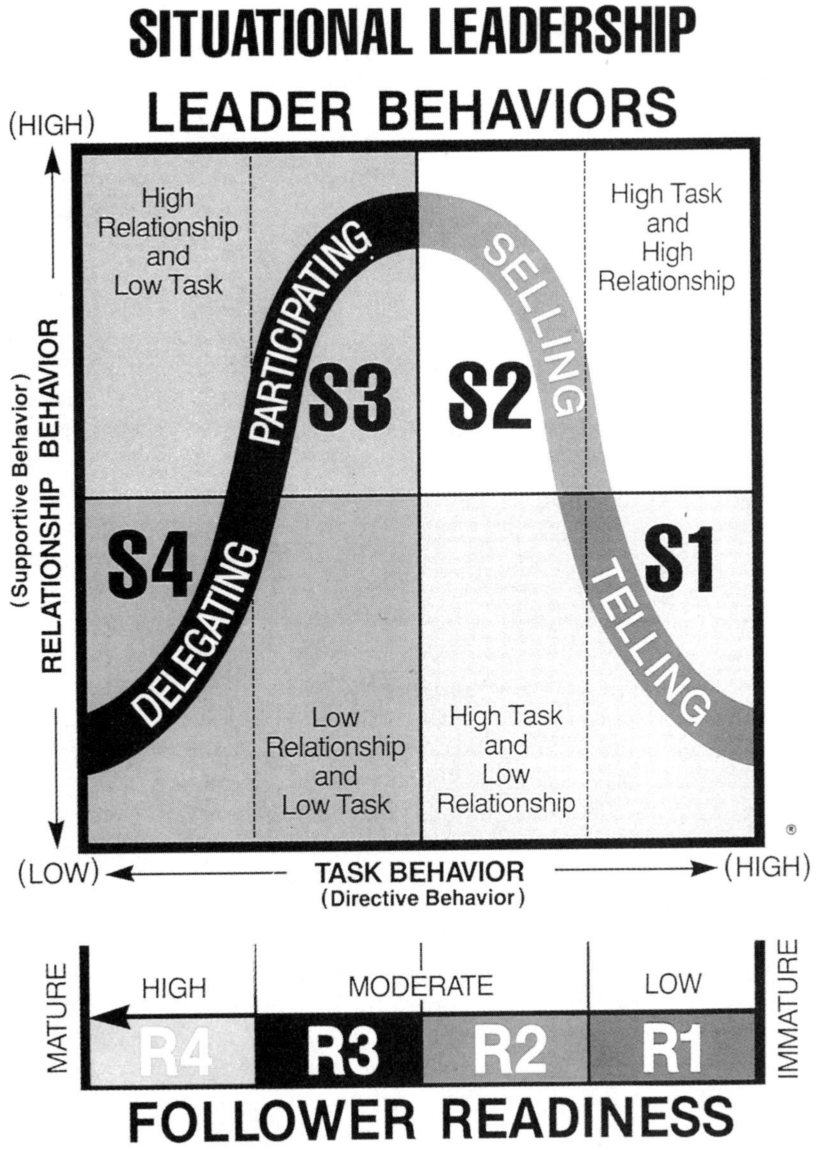

SITUATIONAL LEADERSHIP
LEADER BEHAVIORS

(HIGH)

RELATIONSHIP BEHAVIOR
(Supportive Behavior)

S3 PARTICIPATING — High Relationship and Low Task

S2 SELLING — High Task and High Relationship

S4 DELEGATING — Low Relationship and Low Task

S1 TELLING — High Task and Low Relationship

(LOW) ◀——— **TASK BEHAVIOR** ———▶ (HIGH)
(Directive Behavior)

MATURE ◀ HIGH | MODERATE | LOW ▶ IMMATURE

R4 | **R3** | **R2** | **R1**

FOLLOWER READINESS

Developed by Paul Hersey
© Copyright 1984 by Center for Leadership Studies. All rights reserved.

Figure 1-1. Situational leadership model (Reprinted with permission of Leadership Studies, Inc. All rights reserved.)

ness, as defined here, is the motivation, confidence, and commitment to perform. What we find is that almost any newly hired person lacks the necessary confidence and sense of security necessary to perform at a high level. By the model's definition of willingness (being highly committed and confident), such a person is unwilling to perform at a superior level and therefore must be managed in a fairly directive style.

What usually then occurs is that the individual moves (sometimes rapidly and sometimes gradually) through a series of steps from what we call a readiness level of 1 (R-1), which is a low degree of ability to work without supervision, to a readiness level of 4 (R-4), which denotes high ability and willingness to work without supervision. More specifically, the R-2 level is characterized by individuals who are still not capable of performing on their own but who are more willing to try because they have now gained a relatively higher degree of confidence, commitment, and motivation to perform the task. An individual at this readiness level, of course, should be dealt with differently than the individual who is unable but also very insecure. The major difference, of course, is the degree to which they are instructed what to do and how to do it. The R-3 level individual is now competent to a relatively high degree to perform a task but, for whatever reason, may have become unwilling or insecure again. This is often because at this point they do not feel the confidence that you feel in their abilities and therefore they need a fairly high amount of supportive direction to reinforce their mastery of the area. The R-4 individual is someone who is highly confident and highly capable. In our terms, such individuals are both able and willing to perform. R-4 individuals need very little in the way of direction and support and in fact, if given significant amounts of direction and support, feel they are being overmanaged.

The most important first step in using the Situation Leadership model is to assess where the individual lies on the scale of R-1 to R-4. A very interesting point that perhaps complicates this, however, is that individual veterinary technicians may be superb at anesthetizing animals and thus appear to be R-4s in this area but they may not be competent at dealing with clients on a one-to-one basis. For this reason, clients may be turned off to them, which results in a significant amount of evidence that the technicians are not doing a good job. Consequently, such technicians need to be supervised in two different ways. Supervision will necessarily vary depending on whether the technician is working with a client or is working on his or her own to anesthetize an animal. People generally tend toward a given readiness level, but some tasks are more easily mastered, and some people will be at different stages of readiness with respect to different parts of their jobs.

The key concept here is *task-relevant maturity*. We hesitate to use the term *maturity* because it is so encumbered with psychological connotations. We are not referring to age or to mental state readiness as much as we are to the ability to perform a given task without supervision. Think, for example, about being asked to perform a new procedure; initially you were probably very uncertain and had very little skill. As you performed this new procedure under encouragement, you gradually became much more confident. With the confidence came the competence until at some point the task became enjoyable, allowing it to be done relatively easily and without much direction. Initially (as an R-1) you may have seen the task as difficult but you also may have felt at a loss if someone was not at your elbow giving directions; now (as an R-4) you would resent such supervision. Thus, the leadership style used by a professor when teaching skills needs to vary with the task level of maturity of the student. This is no less true in the business world than it is in the classroom. As we think about the process of effective teaching, one can see there is a correlation with effective leadership in the practice.

We have referred, without explanation, to a couple of concepts that should be thoroughly understood. One is the concept of *task behavior;* the second is the concept of *relationship behavior.* Task behavior is defined by this model as the extent to which the leader engages in finding roles, telling what, how, when, where, and who is to do something. At the extreme, task behavior can be very directive, involving telling individuals everything they must do, when they must do it, and so forth. Relationship behavior, on the other hand, is the extent to which the leader engages in two-way communication, listening, and facilitating behaviors giving socioemotive support. Simply put, this is the degree to which the individual supports a subordinate by providing positive strokes when they perform effectively and negative strokes when they are ineffective. The individual with a low task-relevant maturity needs much more task behavior from the supervisor than the individual with a high task-relevant maturity. Thus, it is extremely important to understand accurately where an individual is on given tasks. To do this, one must again understand the level of ability and confidence or willingness the individual brings to the job.

If we focus on the top part of the model that suggests Leader Behavior in Figure 1-1, we see four leadership styles (S1 through S4) that correspond to the four task-relevant maturity levels. Drawing a line straight upward from the assessed maturity level of the individual leads one to the quadrant that identifies the leadership style appropriate to produce the optimum productivity from the individual subordinate. These styles are made up by determining the quantity of relationship behaviors versus task behaviors that will be appropriate for the leader to use.

Style 1 is labeled the *telling style.* When a new employee starts, they usually have very little knowledge of how the practice works. Confidence is often low. Thus, the appropriate style is style 1, telling. In this case, the leader will make all decisions. Adjectives that characterize this style include *telling, guiding, directing,* and *establishing* methods. It is clear at this point that the followers are simply being asked to do what they are specifically told to do. An individual in the R-1 mode will be very receptive to this style and will appreciate it. R-1s usually feel such a lack of confidence that the telling style of leadership (S-1) allows them to know they will not make serious errors. Most of us who have gone up the maturity scale ourselves tend to believe others treated in this more controlled, directed manner will resent it; in fact, for beginners at anything (R-1s) the opposite is true.

The next leadership style (S-2) is labeled a *selling style.* In the decision-making process, the major difference here is that the leader, instead of simply telling the individual what to do, oftentimes gives an explanation or has some dialogue with the subordinate, thus in a way "selling" the decision to the subordinate. Whereas the telling style is characterized by high task and low relationship behaviors, the selling style is characterized by high task and high relationship behaviors. There is a lot of interaction but, nevertheless, the leader makes the decision and gives the direction. In this style one will find that decisions must be explained and an opportunity provided for clarification, but not as many directions will have to be given as were given to an R-1. Again, R-2s are motivated because they are getting more confidence, but at this point they are not capable of performing on their own. Adjectives describing the behaviors of the leader in this style are *selling, persuading, clarifying,* and *explaining.*

The third leadership style, which is appropriate to use with people in the R-3 level of task-relevant maturity, is the *participating style* (S-3). At this point, there is a major shift. Decisions tend to be made together, with the leader and follower sharing information and working to come up with the optimum solution. Facts are discussed, and the subordinate at this point has a higher degree of ability and confidence. However, the subordinate still does not have the necessary sense of security in his or her ability to perform entirely independently. Therefore, the leader in the S-3 mode uses a fairly low amount of task behavior but a significant amount of supportive, relationship behavior designed to reinforce the subordinate's knowledge. When watching the leader who is dealing in this participating style, we observe a leader/subordinate dialogue characterized by collaboration and encouragement. The leader's primary task is to help the subordinate to recognize when he or she has made correct decisions; then the leader reinforces such successes.

When the subordinate has reached the R-4 level of maturity (see Fig. 1-1), he or she is at the highest level on this scale. The individual has all the knowledge, experience, and skills necessary to perform the job, and he or she knows it. Subordinates are willing and confident, have a high degree of commitment to do a good job, and are motivated to do so. At this point, the leader can engage in what we call the *delegating style* (S-4), that is, he or she can turn over responsibility for decisions and the implementation of such decisions to the R-4 subordinate. The delegating leader uses a low amount of task and a low amount of relationship behavior with the R-4 follower. In this nondirective atmosphere the subordinate will be motivated to work effectively and competently. S-4 leadership can be characterized as delegating and literally allowing followers to make decisions themselves, simply observing and periodically monitoring subordinate activities, and providing periodic discussions of a purely supportive nature, not necessarily to check on performance.

Let us look at an example of Situational Leadership applications that are directly relevant to the veterinarian. Consider new veterinary technicians who come into a new practice. Initially, despite schooling, they do not know what to do. Although anxious to please in the first several weeks on the job, they are very insecure and are not terribly competent in this specific situation. Depending upon the individual, they will remain at the R-1 level for anywhere from 2 hours to 2 months. It is important to realize that, even if new employees come to the practice competent at performing several tasks, they will need a great deal of feedback because they recognize that the way things are "done around here" leaves them situationally incompetent. In our experience the largest single mistake veterinarians or supervisors make is to assume too quickly that a subordinate is at a higher level of readiness than is actually the case. Thus, the people who will get the highest degree of productivity out of these new, R-1 technicians will simply tell them what they want done, when to do it, and how to do it. The R-1 individual will very quickly and productively carry out these tasks because of the increased assurance that clear direction brings.

After some time, as a technician becomes more secure and more able, simply being told in detail what to do yields not productivity but resentment. The R-2 technician expects to have some degree of dialogue and explanation. The supervisor is now in the S-2, selling, mode of leadership. When the technician first arrived, explanations resulted in imprecision and confusion, slowing the technician's learning process. Now, in the R-2 mode, the technician thrives on such interaction with the supervisor — a combination of direction and discussion.

After a short while, the technician is ready for an even more participative (S-3) style of leadership. The time comes to discuss and to share concepts, to allow the technician to make several decisions under the guidance of the supervisor. This will give the technician (as an R-3) a greater sense of satisfaction because the supervisor now recognizes his or her increased abililties. This is the point at which maintaining a relationship is essential.

Once a technician has been an R-3 for some significant period of time, the supervisor will have license simply to back off and to allow the technician to perform tasks as he or she sees fit. This is the delegating style of leadership (S-4).

When you think about it, when you were first asked to diagnose an animal under the supervision of a veterinarian, despite all the "book learning," you were an R-1. You were insecure and not able to work very effectively. Thus, the professors looked over your shoulder carefully and told you what to do. As time went on they explained why you were told how to do it, and as more time elapsed they asked for your input and decisions because you were capable of making the right decisions and implementing them effectively, but still without total confidence. Finally, as you progressed in maturity to perform the function, they simply left you alone to take care of the animals.

What is interesting about this model is that productivity increases significantly when the leader uses the leadership style appropriate to the readiness level. As a rule of thumb, if productivity goes down somewhat, then the leadership style–follower readiness match is off by one quadrant; that is, if a follower is really at the R-2 level and the leader is using either the participating (S-3) or telling style (S-1), productivity will not be as high as it should be. If the match is off by two quadrants (say, an R-4 level follower dealing with a leader using an S-2, or selling, style), confusion and anger will result. This, of course, leads to relatively low productivity. Last, if the match is off by three quadrants (new subordinate needs a telling style but the boss is using a delegating style), chaos and almost no productivity will be the result. Individual growth will be hindered, and total confusion will follow.

Before concluding our discussion of the Situational Leadership model, which is so appropriate to managing a service organization such as a veterinary practice, there are several other key points that need to be covered. First, recognize the simplicity of the model. There are only two main categories of follower characteristics to focus on: task-relevant ability and willingness (security). All four leadership styles are common communication patterns that are easily accessible to almost all leaders, and there is a direct, one-to-one correlation between categories of follower readiness (R-1 through R-4) and leadership style (S-1 through S-4). The model is concise and practical.

Second, accurate diagnosis of follower task-relevant maturity is essential for the model to work. Emphasis is placed here not on general, overall follower readiness but on task-specific readiness—a vital point.

Third, although accurate assessment of the readiness level of the follower will determine the success in choosing the correct leadership style, one's own ability then to implement the correct style may vary significantly. Our experience is that each individual has a preferred style. It seems that some people are always using the telling style regardless of its appropriateness. They do very well with R-1s, but their R-4s tend to be very disgruntled and to leave. Others tend to prefer the S-3 style and very easily get seduced into assessing subordinates as R-3s regardless of where they actually are.

It is appropriate to determine what one's preferred style is and then to avoid the seduction of seeing all subordinates as needing that style. It is also appropriate to recognize that there is no good or bad R level. The model seems to indicate that we would prefer to have all R-4s with whom we can use a delegating style for optimum effectiveness. This does not mean, however, that the individual who is an

R-4 is a better person or even a better employee. It simply means that they require a different style that will allow the leader more freedom to spend time on other tasks.

The goal may be to move people through the model as quickly as possible, but again we want to reiterate that the issue is the appropriate fit of style to readiness level, not which is the best readiness level. Do not forget that an airline pilot who has been flying for 20 years is still required to use the preflight checklist every single time. The reason is clear: there are some tasks that are better done if the leader assumes the telling style. As long as the individual subordinate fully understands why and is accepting of this, there is usually very little problem.

We are often asked, "What is the best way to find the style for a given individual?" There are some key indicators (presented below), but in the end, you will find yourself using trial and error as much as the indicators. When you have your antennae up, you will find yourself very perceptive to the nuances of change in the subordinate. This will tell you immediately whether your style selection was correct or incorrect for the readiness level of the follower. No matter what style you are using, if it yields less than smashing success with a given follower, a different style should be used. Personal experimentation is the best teacher of this model.

One indicator of the R-1 level is the degree of ability the person demonstrates. R-1 individuals are very rarely willing or confident enough to undertake the task on their own. They will have very little experience to apply to the job and very little specific job knowledge. Their independent ability to solve problems will be low, and one will find that they need and, in fact, invite frequent close supervision. They will not know how to follow up, and they will ask questions like *when, where,* and *how.* With these individuals, if one delegates a task or even explains a task, the level

will be far enough off the mark to ensure less than optimum productivity. Instead the supervisor must give specific directions telling them what, when, where, and how to do the job.

R-2 individuals possess greater ability and they are occasionally willing to undertake the task independently. They have some relevant experience at this point and some job knowledge. Their ability to solve problems independently has gone up, but they still need a significant amount of information and support from the supervisor. They will invite close supervision frequently and will occasionally follow up on a problem or issue. They will ask, in addition to the how, where, and when questions, questions that lead to the whys of things. If the supervisor only responds to the R-2 individuals by telling them what to do, this will dull their motivation. It now satisfies them to know why they are performing a task and how it fits in with other parts of the job. They are growing in the job! They will tend to become discouraged and feel overcontrolled by an S-1 telling style. If one simply delegates (S-4) to these people, they will feel lost and, though maybe not saying so, will be very fearful that the job they are doing is not adequate.

R-3 individuals have quite a bit of ability. They will at times be somewhat more insecure than is expected. They may try to hide this insecurity, but it will be shown by their unwillingness to attempt a new task. At this point they will have gained experience and knowledge related to the task, and they have a good ability to solve problems independently. Close supervision will seldom be needed, and they will do their own follow-up independently. They will also offer new ideas for the supervisor. They will be very interested in participating in decision-making and problem-solving processes and will be competent to do so. They will look to the supervisor to support them so their sense of insecurity diminishes as rapidly as possible. They can do anything as long as it is in cooperation with the supervisor; true independence, with no supervision, scares them.

Delegating complete responsibility to these individuals will, therefore, create a problem. At this point you need to be on the lookout for this insecurity because it may be masked. It is very easy to mistake readiness level 3 for readiness level 4 because of personal confidence in the person's ability. However, to continue to treat such individuals as R-1s would, of course, be very frustrating to them. They will see this as pedantic and in some cases as insulting to their ability. It will be very easy for the supervisor to sense the tension when an individual at the R-3 level is being treated in a telling style.

When individuals reach the R-4 level, they have a significant background of experience and ability, and they recognize this. They are willing to undertake new tasks and are very secure in their ability to accomplish them well. The R-4 individual will have significant background knowledge and specifically related experience and will be aware of the applications of their knowledge. They will have an excellent ability to solve problems independently and will rarely need any close supervision. They will almost always follow up and offer independent solutions, and they will take significant amounts of initiative. Again, one will know when this person is inappropriately handled.

One more important point about the application of situational leadership styles is that when first starting with the model, veterinarians tend to see the extremes. They may easily recognize an R-1 and easily recognize an R-4 and may, depending on their preferred style, be fairly adept with the appropriate telling or delegating style. It is the nuances in levels between these two that cause difficulties. Thus, the problem of bringing R-1 employees on board and then expecting them after a period of days to be R-4 is unrealistic. It is very impor-

tant to step new employees through the model and treat them at the appropriate level, time period by time period, rather than trying to move them too quickly or hold them back when they have jumped ahead. Again, there are four stages to the readiness level, and they will fall in sequence despite the fact that some stages will take less time than others for different people. Do not be seduced into looking at this as a two-stage model.

The model is called Situational Leadership for a very good reason. The environment has a tremendous amount to do with task-relevant maturity. Thus, technicians who have reached an R-4 level working directly under their supervisor may be temporarily thrown back to an R-1 level when forced to work under a different supervisor or when faced with a new procedure. This in no way means they are poor employees but rather reflects the reality of how situations affect each of us. Thus, when individuals move from the security of the school into their first practice or move from one practice to another, it is important to be alert. This applies equally to a new receptionist and a new veterinarian. Every job, every person, every day is a new "situation"—hence, the model's name. For the veterinarian running a practice, we suggest these watchwords: when low productivity or poor communication with staff develops, consider the *situations* as defined here. This model provides strong clues as to what is wrong as well as four alternative styles in which to lead the staff into a happier, better-functioning practice.

□
Motivation—the key to effectiveness

Although the Situational Leadership model is a fundamental first step toward providing the leadership and direction employees need, there is a second conceptual area we have found extremely valuable in helping veterinarians to manage staffs well—the area of *mo-*

tivation. The ideas described here come out of the seminal work of David McClelland, for many years head of the Department of Social Psychology at Harvard University.[3] In order to understand McClelland's work, one must first understand what we refer to as a *Needs Satisfaction Model.* The best example of a need we can all relate to is hunger. When we are hungry we will act to satisfy that need; that is, we will eat. When we are extremely hungry, we can be pushed into unanticipated behaviors. When our hunger is satisfied, we are capable, ready, and willing to do many, many different things, but when hunger is not satisfied, we automatically focus exclusively on that one area, to the detriment of any other activity.

Paralleling our physical needs are our psychological needs. Just as with physical needs, psychological needs must be met. It is not a matter of choice. What David McClelland has done is help us to understand some of those psychological needs. The three we will focus on are the needs for *achievement, affiliation,* and *power*. All of us have each need to some degree. A very useful example of motivation is an individual looking to satisfy his needs. We cannot make this point too strongly: when we have a psychological need that is unmet, we will behave so that we meet that need just as surely as we will seek food when we are hungry. It is very important to understand, however, that the type of "food" that will satisfy our achievement need will not necessarily satisfy our affiliation need. So the behavior patterns that will satisfy each need are different and important for each one of us to understand. If we have an extremely high need for achievement, it will take much more "food" ingested at more frequent intervals to satisfy that need. An individual with high affiliation needs cannot "eat" achievement "food," but instead must have affiliation "food."

Dr. McClelland was concerned with the question of whether there might be a personality variable in the male population that would affect economic performance. An important study was performed in the two Indian cities of Rajmundi (R) and Kinkinada (K). From an academic testing perspective, these two cities historically had the same economic ups and downs, weather conditions, crop structure, and religion (an important factor in India). They were located approximately 300 miles apart on two sides of a mountain. The cities shared the same river. R was the test city, with 50 businessmen in a test group and 50 in a control group. In K there was a control group of 100 people.

The test group in R was put through a program to arouse the level of the motive we call the achievement motive. The intent of the experiment was to see whether this would have any effect on their economic performance and perhaps have some ripple effect on the city.

Over the years an amazing thing has happened. The economic base of R has grown considerably compared with that of K. The economic performance, and literally the personalities of the people trained in achievement arousal, were changed. The conclusion is that, as measured by traditional western values of success, achievement arousal made a considerable difference in the economic performance of the people who were trained. This experiment was repeated in several small towns in Mexico with similar results.

Why would a veterinarian want to know about these experiments? The reason is that motivation variables are so important in the change process in the people with whom we work. The same variables affect their success or failure, their ability to take advantage of opportunities and to be motivated to do a job. Motivation is the key in terms of people accepting responsibility and wanting to do a job.

Hundreds and hundreds of studies have been done and have backed up the initial findings of McClelland that the majority of all motivation and behavior patterns stem from three thought processes or needs. These are (1) the *achievement motive,* or the need to perform better; (2) the *affiliation motive,* or the desire for close, friendly relations; and (3) the *power motive,* or a desire to feel (and be perceived as) strong and influential.

Of these three, the achievement motive is by far the most researched. It is the variable McClelland sought to change in India and the variable we look to change or to arouse in individual contributors in our organizations. Top salespeople, for example, have a naturally high achievement motive; that is, they have a drive to do things faster, better, and more effectively than other people.

The affiliation motive is the least researched of the three, and the power motive has started to be researched more fully over the past 10 years. If McClelland could rename the motives, he would call the power motive the *need for influence* because of the negative connotation that the word *power* currently holds. Actually, a motive is neither good nor bad. The important point is to realize that people are motivated differently and will respond differently to the same situation or treatment.

We can define the thoughts that identify and help us recognize the motive operating in an individual. The achievement motive is present in individuals when they think about

1. Outperforming others. These people get very excited in contests and need a lot of feedback on how they and others are doing.
2. Performing against self-imposed standards of excellence. These people want to do well regardless of how others are doing.
3. Contributing a unique and innovative accomplishment. These individuals are always striving to find new ways to do things. They are great contributors but must be managed so there can be an end to the project. One could imagine a problem with engineers motivated in this

way: they would always want to change their design.
4. Setting long-term career goals. A young person who decides to become a veterinarian and then works to accomplish that goal exemplifies this type of individual.

The affiliation motive is a key variable in terms of keeping the fabric of the organization together. The thoughts that signal the presence of this motive are

1. Concern about warmth and maintenance of relationships. This person would rather work with friends than experts.
2. Concern with disruption of relationships. This can be a problem for supervisors who are motivated to preserve relationships at all costs. The necessity of firing an employee could prove to be a paralyzing experience.
3. Desire to join group activities. These people are organizers of communal activities. They can be motivated by putting them in a place where they can talk with other people and not be disruptive. It is important not to isolate affiliative people: in such conditions their needs will not be met.

The power motive is the key to managerial performance because central to it is the need to influence others. There is a statistical correlation between effective managerial performance and an above-average power motive. Individuals with such a motive are more likely to delegate, follow up, and get people to work more effectively than are those with other motives. These individuals want to

1. Exercise strong, forceful actions that affect others. They might move a desk in an office just for the effect.
2. Give unsolicited support or advice. People will often reject that advice because it is unsolicited.
3. Try to influence, persuade, or make a

point when the concern is not to reach agreement. They like to argue for the sake of arguing.

4. Try to impress people. They want people to feel they are important; thus, they will surround themselves with evidence of their standing — a bigger desk, nicer furnishings, and so forth. They want to be recognized as someone special. Their motivation to win a contest would be to impress other people.

5. Generate strong positive or negative emotions in others. They want to see the effect of their actions. Failing to react to their attempts to arouse anger will frustrate such people. They are looking for emotional response. If emotion can be aroused, their need will be satisfied.

6. Express concern for their reputation or position. Physicians, lawyers, dentists, and other professionals typically have this sort of concern with status.

The way to recognize these thoughts is to see the behaviors that arise from them. Those with achievement motivation

1. Set challenging goals
2. Take moderate risks
3. Take personal responsibility
4. Seek a lot of feedback — and use it to do a better job and to optimize their performance. They get frustrated when they are unable to get truthful feedback.

Those with affiliation motivation

1. Stay in touch with people — they write long letters and make long phone calls. Because their needs generate behavior different from someone with other motives, some people they call may not understand a call "just to say hello."
2. Do not like to be alone — they do not like to live alone.
3. Put people before tasks — they choose to work with friends rather than experts.

4. Avoid confrontation — they try to maintain relationships and are nurturing, consoling, and supportive.

5. Communicate with others more from feeling than from logic. Because of the desire to enhance communications and acceptance, an affiliate manager could be a good balance in managing a group of achievers.

Those with power motivation

1. Seek positions of leadership
2. Enjoy influencing others to perform tasks
3. Delegate
4. Collect prestigious objects
5. Are good mentors — they train and instruct others
6. Are active in organizational politics
7. Tend to seek, withhold, and use information to control others

In summation, we might think of the children's game, King of the Mountain.

Children with achievement motivation will bite, scratch, and kick to *get to the top for the purpose of achieving the climb.* Affiliation-motivated children will do the same, but *to join their friends.* If their friends do not go, they will not want to either. Power-motivated children *want to be on top of everyone else.* They will step on others' fingers if anyone tries to pull them off.

We can recognize these behaviors in the individuals with whom we work. If we understand their motivation, we can work with them more effectively. In thinking about your own staff, try to understand the individuals in terms of these behaviors and the three motives underlying them. Remember that no one is a purely achievement-, affiliation-, or power-motivated person: we all have varying proportions of each motivation. Dominant motives do show in our behaviors, however.

Remember that until individuals' highest needs are met, they will do little besides trying to meet them. Affiliative people will achieve very little until they feel "connected" to others at work. Once the dominant need is met, however, other activities can take place, even at a very high level. An example we all have seen is the veterinary technician who must chat with everyone upon coming to work—meeting affiliation needs—but who then does a fine job—meeting achievement needs. Leaders who encourage their staff members to recognize and meet their needs remove a powerful obstacle from the path of task completion.

□
Organizational climates

Farsighted leaders can do more than just recognize motives: they can actually establish what we call an *organizational climate* that will elicit achievement-oriented activities in the practice. Once again, Dr. David McClelland's research is central to this concept, with the early labeling of this aspect of motive arousal. The organizational climate has much to do with whether it is pleasant in the organization, terrible, or uncomfortable or whether people want to work, play, fight, or whatever.

Six major dimensions of organizational climate have been identified as related to motivation, behavior, and, thus, performance. These climate variables are conformity, responsibility, standards, rewards, clarity, and team spirit (Fig. 1-2). An understanding of these variables is vital to arousing and depressing the key social motives of individuals in the organization.

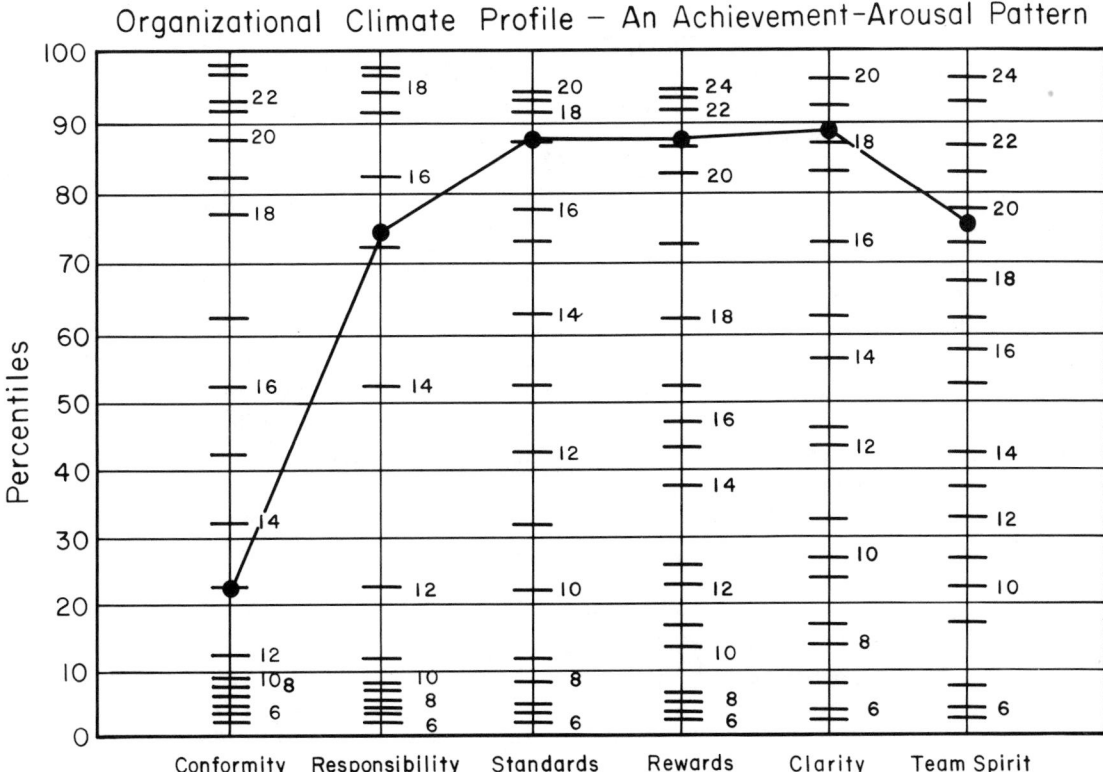

Figure 1-2. *Organizational climate profile—An achievement-arousal pattern*

Why is this so important? As managers, we literally have the ability to control which of these needs we want to be at the forefront of a person's mind and thus what they are driven to do in performance. Managers always have an effect on the key organizational variables.

Indeed, when individuals accept the managerial, supervisory, or executive role (and this certainly applies to veterinarians running a practice), they are accepting the responsibility to influence the people under them to perform to the best of their ability. The key is to consciously influence the six organizational climate variables that research has shown make the biggest difference.

Given this background on the importance of climate variables, let us look at brief definitions of the dimensions before we delve into each in more detail.

1. *Conformity*—the feeling employees have about constraints in the work organization and the degree to which they feel there are many rules, procedures, policies, and practices to which they have to conform rather than being able to carry out their tasks as they see fit
2. *Responsibility*—the feeling that employees have a lot of responsibility delegated to them; the degree with which they can run their jobs on their own; the feeling they are "their own boss," not having to double-check all decisions
3. *Standards*—the emphasis employees perceive management to be placing on doing a good job, including the degree to which people feel challenging goals are set
4. *Rewards*—the feeling of being rewarded for a job well done, both through criticism and punishment and through a more tangible reward system
5. *Clarity*—the feeling goals, roles, tasks, and so forth are clear and well organized rather than being chaotic and confused
6. *Team spirit*—the feeling that good rela-

tionships prevail, that people in the organization are warm and trusting, and that people are proud to belong to the team

Now with this overview of categories, let us look at the specifics of each dimension.

Conformity

The first variable that we look at in doing an organizational climate survey test is *conformity*. With this variable, as with the others, we can measure clearly and concisely in surveys its actual level and where employees would like it to be. In this way, we can look at discrepancies and shifts over time.

Conformity is a fascinating variable and quite different for people who grew up at different time periods and in different cultures. We see this in comparing people who grew up in the mid-to-late 1960s and early 1970s with those who grew up during the Depression. It is certainly a different variable as seen through the eyes of someone from Japan.

Conformity is the degree to which people perceive their roles, regulations, policies, and procedures in the organization as requirements they must adhere to but which prevent them from doing their best job. Often these rules and procedures are not even seen as relating to the job but only as limits confining the degrees of individual freedom. Conformity is really a statement of how one behaves and how one will perform. Individual perception is absolutely the key to the definition of conformity.

When an individual comes out of school and begins work at a large corporation and is told that he must wear a white shirt and conservative suit, he will often perceive this as a high degree of conformity. One will find however, that after the same individual has been with the corporation 10 years or so, he will wake up in the morning, go to his wardrobe, which is filled mainly with white shirts and gray suits, and not really feel that there is a great deal of restraint in the way he is asked to dress.

It is clear that when people first go into the army and are told to follow many rules and regulations, they see that as high conformity. When people have been in the military for 5 years, they are so used to saluting that the act is no longer perceived as high conformity.

High conformity tends to produce, in some people, a response that we have come to call "reactance"—a need to rebel against the conformity. Reactance is often a reflection of anger because high conformity for many people causes anger and a need to act. This results in inefficiency. It is necessary to have some degree of conformity, but when people perceive that the demand for conformity is higher than the situation requires, major problems in the organization can result.

We have a client who had several procedures that were felt to be unnecessary. When asked about the procedures, the employees got red in the face and talked about them with anger, but they assured us they were "following them to the T." What they were engaging in was a series of steps termed *malicious obedience.* They were conforming absolutely, knowing that following through to the letter of the law would create tremendous problems in the organization, which indeed it did.

The boss in this case had threatened to fire anyone who did not follow his regulations exactly. The employees did so in anger, and it brought the company to its knees. Remember that what pilots do when they want to cause a slowdown is simply follow rules and regulations. Following rigid taxiing rules would slow down a busy airport considerably. In fact, most rules are policies and guidelines; they are not set in concrete.

Responsibility

The next climate variable over which managers have considerable control is *responsibility.* People who show a high degree of responsibility in discussions or surveys are saying they feel they have a high degree of control over what is supposed to happen in the workplace. They feel they are their own bosses and that they are expected to behave as if they are the president of the company. The desirability of such an attitude is obvious.

If you look at a parking lot, the people who are there early and leave late are those who are psychologically invested in their work and believe the work would not get done properly if they were not there. They feel a tremendous sense of responsibility. Ideally, we want all employees to feel this. The way to do this is to imbed in people a tremendous sense of responsibility.

Historically there has been a theory that people are innately lazy and do not want to accept responsibility, that the manager has to stand over them with a stick to cause them to perform effectively. We now know that the vast majority of people who end up in positions of any consequence in private industry are individuals who desire to take tremendous responsibility. It can be at the lowest levels in the organization. To deprive them of this is to make them feel less than adequate.

Lack of opportunity for responsibility is terribly demotivating and deprives employees of an essential part of their psychological need —show the manager they can help. People who have a high sense of responsibility often feel like they are helping, and meeting this need within themselves goes far beyond any motivation you can extrinsically create. Why not allow them to feel they are contributing; that is, why not say, "I am delegating this to you, and you have significant responsibility"? With that comes authority and accountability.

We have a client who recently went through a leveraged buy-out with his firm and had to rename the company. He had a very interesting idea that is still talked about in the company. He asked every employee, including the union people on the floor, to submit prospective names to the company. The employees got very interested, and he had several hundred names submitted. He then submitted the names to the lawyers to determine which ones were legitimately available in the state of California. An employee panel pared this list down to seven. They then sent the names through the mail to all of their clients and asked them to vote on what they thought the company should be named. Everyone, therefore, got a chance to take some responsibility and to become vested in the company's success.

One of the best ways to increase employee perceptions of responsibility is to *listen* to people. Really listening makes people feel like they have tremendous amounts of responsibility for doing the job and making sure it is done well. In addition, recognize that these climate variables are not independent. Let us relate responsibility and conformity. If one has a very high level of conformity in the organization—that is, if people must do things the way they are told to do them—it is almost impossible to have a high level of responsibility at the same time. People who have a high degree of responsibility believe they have the right to figure out how they are going to get their jobs done.

Standards

Standards is the next organizational climate variable. When people say they have high standards, they mean that they are challenged to use their energies, both mental and physical, to accomplish the task. However, a score of 100% on a standards survey means that people believe the job is simply not doable, that standards are too high. No longer is the job seen as having a high degree of challenge, requiring a moderate degree of risk to accomplish it; rather it is seen as a gamble, a job that in all probability cannot be done. This becomes terribly demotivating.

Someone who thinks standards are very low has also been demotivated. They are saying: "I could do this job with my hands tied behind my back. It is very simple, not important, and anyone could do this job." The manager loses a significant amount of energy and effort from this person—energy they will direct elsewhere in life. If they felt challenged on the job, they would bring this energy to the job, and the practice would benefit. When people believe they do not need to work hard to accomplish a task, they probably will not, and even though they believe the task to be simple, it may not be accomplished at all. Because they see it as so simple, they will put it off to the last minute to make it more of a challenge. The probability of the task getting done well goes down significantly. Thus, giving people a series of simple tasks tends not to be in their or the manager's best interest. It does not motivate the employees to do their best work.

There is another factor that comes in here as well. When people believe they are not being challenged, they also tend to feel "put down." They feel the organization does not see them as worthwhile. If individuals feel the organization believes they are not good and they think otherwise, then these people have to deny the organization and turn their energies to another place where they can get their self-image reinforced.

One must find a way to set challenging objectives. It is difficult to have challenging standards without having prewritten goals and objectives that are measurable, time phased, concrete, meaningful, and moderately risky (65% to 85%). Good employees need to feel they are good and competent and that they must stretch a little to do their jobs really well.

A major problem with veterinarians is that of getting standards mixed up with conformity. High standards of medical practice are common concerns of veterinarians; thus they establish methodologies by which they expect their staff to perform to be sure these standards are met. The "how-to's" in terms of procedures, however, need to be understood as the conformance required to accomplish a certain goal and should not be mistaken for the standard itself. *How to* (conformity) does not equal *how well* (standards).

Rewards

The next variable in the climate survey is *rewards*. When people think about rewards, they think about compensation; this is an incorrect interpretation of what we are discussing here. If people feel they are ill paid in the marketplace or compared with others in the company, this is a different issue that results in other problems.

What we are looking at here is the degree to which people feel there is positive reinforcement for doing a good job and criticism or punishment for doing a bad job. Individuals who feel they are receiving more positives than negatives in the workplace score above 50% on that measure. A key variable to look at is the extent to which the organization has systems to reinforce the desired behavior patterns. If one is looking to change and to direct behavior toward specific actions or patterns, positive reinforcement is a much more powerful tool than punishment. The "negative stroking" profile is essential to understand.

The issue of rewards is critical. Punishment will cause a given behavior pattern to go away; however, one is not just trying to get a specific behavior pattern to stop but rather is trying to get a specific new one to start. The only way to have any success at getting a new behavior to start, and to maintain it, is through the use of "positive stroking" patterns.

Thus, when people have low reward scores or very large discrepancy scores on the rewards dimension of the climate survey, not only are they feeling underappreciated and underthanked but they are very unlikely to begin acting in the way the manager wants them to behave. When they feel their bosses do not believe they are trying their hardest when they themselves believe they are, they

are in fact underappreciated. Someone who feels this way for a while comes to feel that the other person owes them: they owe them a large number of positive strokes. Once an employee feels that the manager owes them, rather than that they owe the manager, management is on the wrong side of the ledger. Management always wants employees to believe that management is owed a favor. This is accomplished by having employees believe that the manager has given them more positive than negative strokes. The manager can then ask them to work overtime or longer on a project without receiving resistance or having employees ask for a raise. An employee who asks for a raise in that situation is saying, "I am not getting my psychological appreciation, so you will have to bribe me to do this."

The manager has control over whether employees feel they are getting more positive or negative strokes on the job. Make sure they are getting more positives. One can always find something to genuinely compliment them on, and then corrections can also be made. Beware of thinking, "He is paid to do that; I should not have to say thank you."

Clarity

Clarity is the next climate survey variable. Organizational clarity is the single most important of all the variables; it is what gives people the "big picture."

Individuals who do not have the big picture of what the organization is all about just go to work and do a "job." People who have the big picture feel they are on a mission; they are excited to perform and want to contribute. Those who score their organizations high in clarity understand where the organization is going and what they have to do to help it get there. They want to make sure their department pulls its weight to get the practice where it is going. It is essential to motivation to have the big picture; otherwise, people only doing a job really do need a carrot and a stick.

It is very difficult for employees to have high responsibility or high standards if it is not really clear what the organization is trying to accomplish. Many times supervisors and managers must create organizational clarity for an individual department without having it for a whole group. To say, "I cannot create clarity for my department because I do not have it personally," is, in our experience, a cop-out.

What is organization clarity? It is the degree to which management understands what the practice is all about, the degree to which the managers understand what they are expected to contribute to get the practice from point A to point B.

Research in industrial psychology has focused on the relationship between the variables in the organization climate survey and turnover in white-collar workers. The only variable statistically tied to turnover in white-collar workers in one study was the clarity variable. Findings show individuals leave jobs when the actual organizational clarity drops and when their expectations for clarity increase; that is, the discrepancy between what they feel it is and what they feel it ought to be shifts, dramatically. The study showed that compared with reliable measures of job satisfaction, the only individual variable on the survey that correlated with these measures was organizational clarity.

When people say that the organizational clarity is very high and should be, they are generally very challenged, motivated, and satisfied by the job. It is extremely important that supervisors, managers, and executives cause their organizations to have very high organizational clarity.

About 10 years ago we worked with an organization that spent quite a bit of money toward achieving organizational clarity. This effort was headed by the vice president of research and development of this Fortune 500 company. The VP set a goal that within 6 months the organizational clarity would be remeasured and would go up significantly. At the end of 6 months, the survey was readministered. He had met with employees at least two times each month in the previous months to go over the programs he was implementing to improve organizational clarity. At the end of the 6 months, the clarity had not moved a bit. In frustration he swore, "If those sons of guns want to know what color tie to wear in the morning, I will tell them!" It dawned on us that he had been working on conformity, not clarity. He had been telling them how to do the job, not what their role was and what to do. As a general rule of thumb, conformity is telling someone how to do it, and clarity is what to do and how it matters. At that point we were able to make some significant changes in clarity, but we also had to work on reducing conformity.

The lesson of this company should not be lost on veterinarians who tend to confuse conformity and organizational clarity. Organizational clarity has to do with what business the practice is in and what the individual is expected to do to play a role to support that business. Again, conformity has to do with how one goes about doing that. When role clarity in veterinary practice becomes fuzzy, oftentimes things will fall through the cracks, or people will have to fill in where they are not accustomed. The result is that they often feel underappreciated for all the extra work they are doing to cover for someone else. In many cases the head of the practice does not feel this is "covering" but rather is part of the expectation. These expectations are best clarified early to avoid problems.

Team spirit

The last climate variable is *team spirit;* the degree to which people feel loyal to the organization to which they want to belong and the degree to which they feel the organization is warm and supportive. It is an extremely important part of an organization, and indeed, individuals who believe they are part of a highly productive team want team spirit to be high.

There are data, however, suggesting that if we understand someone's motives, and if we are trying to arouse achievement motivation in individuals, team spirit is a secondary variable. If we know the first five variables, we can effectively tell how motivated the individual is, and we do not need team spirit as a variable. During the 1950s consultants in our field were espousing what we call the *human relations school of thought*. Its manifestation was a great concern that people feel good and have high morale and that there be significant team spirit in the organization. In fact, the consultants thought team spirit was the only thing that was important. There were recommendations to remember your secretary's birthday, bring flowers, get people involved in the company softball league, and so forth. What we know now is that team spirit is only a small part of the puzzle and, in and of itself, team spirit does not lead to productivity. High team spirit is usually an offshoot of the other variables being in the right place, and it is very hard to develop in a vacuum, as in fact is each of the variables that have been discussed.

In summation, the six variables — conformity, responsibility, standards, rewards, organizational clarity, and team spirit — are each individually in the control of the supervisor. The manager or supervisor has a great deal to do with whether these variables are perceived where they ought to be by subordinates. One has much less control over whether they really are where they should be. The practice manager has direct control over the perception of the employees in the organization.

In the beginning of this section we mentioned that an understanding of these climate variables is vital to arousing and depressing the key social motives. Let us look briefly at the relationship between these variables and the three motives.

How can an achievement-oriented climate be created and what would be its value?

An achievement-arousal organization pattern would be low conformity, mid-to-high responsibility, high standards and rewards, high clarity, mid-to-high team spirit (see Fig. 1-2). Achievement motivation seems to be stimulated or aroused by climates that (1) emphasize personal responsibility, (2) allow calculated risks and innovation, (3) give recognition and reward for excellent performance, and (4) create the impression that the individual is part of an outstanding and successful team. It is also important that there not be a high degree of structure and constraint (in the form of rules, procedures, or formal communication channels). A moderate degree of structure, however, is accepted by achievement-motivated people and is preferred by younger achievers.

Achievement-oriented climates appear to be appropriate in areas that demand individual initiative and calculated risk taking (as in many sales organizations and some applied engineering departments). Such climates would also be appropriate in any organization seeking to grow rapidly in a changing environment where individual responsibility and risk taking are inevitably required.

One of the keys to establishing and maintaining high achievement motivation is feedback systems. What we find is that it is almost impossible to have superb feedback without objectives. Without the targets one has very little feedback about progress toward goals. This implies that goal setting is essential to any achievement-oriented practice. Our experience is that this is true. It is also something most people avoid fastidiously. Our recommendation over the years to practitioners has been to establish both personal and organizational goals and to chart progress toward such goals.

A word about goal setting is in order, however. It is clearly understood through research that if a goal is set in such a way as to meet five criteria, the probability of accomplishing that goal will be statistically increased. The criteria are

1. Make goals *specific* and *clear.*
2. Tie goals to definite *time limits.* Include subgoals at short intervals with feedback (especially early on).
3. Make sure success or failure in reaching goals is *measurable.*
4. Goals must be *realistic.*
   a. Do not have any 110% goals.
   b. Take moderate but challenging risks.
   c. Set up goals to win initially, then stretch for more.
5. Make goals *meaningful* to all concerned but especially to the goal seeker. To ensure this set goals in a *participative* manner.

Good goal setting takes some work, but following the crtieria listed can make a world of difference to the manager and staff. In particular, high achievers need goals that are clear, receive regular feedback on how they are doing, and perceive that the goal is challenging but entails moderate risk. Goals that are easily reached or are impossible to reach soon become meaningless.

How can an affiliation-oriented climate be created and what would be its value?

Low conformity, moderate responsibility, moderate standards, high rewards, moderate clarity, and high team spirit characterize an affiliation-oriented climate.

Affiliation motivation seems to be stimulated or aroused by climates that (1) allow the development of close, warm relationships; (2)

provide considerable support and encouragement for individuals; (3) provide considerable freedom and very little structure or constraint; and (4) give individuals the feeling they are an accepted member of a family group.

Affiliation-oriented climates appear to be appropriate in areas where work requires building close relationships (as in counseling centers or industrial departments charged with responsibility for coordinating the efforts of others). Affiliation orientation is a must in the client contact aspects of your practice. Affiliative climates might also be appropriate in situations where highly competent and motivated people are working on very specialized tasks and some noncoercive means for generating organizational cohesion and team spirit seems required (as in many scientific research laboratories). Generally, some degree of affiliation orientation would seem to be appropriate in large, complex organizations where close coordination and integration of different functions is required.

How can a power-oriented climate be created and what would be its value?

High conformity, low responsibility, very high standards, low rewards, high clarity, and low team spirit characterize a power-oriented climate. Power motivation seems to be stimulated or aroused by climates that (1) provide considerable structure (in the form of rules, procedures, and so forth); (2) allow individuals to obtain positions of responsibility, authority, and high status; and (3) encourage the use of formal authority as a basis for resolving conflict and disagreement.

We have been rather hard on power-oriented climates, but it does appear that such climates are reasonably appropriate for very hierarchical organizations (such as military organizations) and for organizations where the work is highly routine and repetitive (as in many manufacturing operations).

Recently we started work in a major referral

practice where the major symptoms of problems were high turnover, significant employee dissatisfaction, and feelings of under-appreciation. After reviewing the organizational climate data, it became apparent that the power motive was being aroused. People felt conformity was far too high. Standards were far lower than the veterinarian had perceived them to be. Responsibility was far lower than the individuals felt it should be — that is, individuals felt they were not required to accept responsibility and that the only person who took it on his shoulders was the boss.

When we worked with the owner to alter his style to affect the organizational climate perceptions of the employees, very dramatic changes came about. Not only did the case load per employee go up significantly, but job satisfaction changed, and turnover "for the wrong reasons" has disappeared. Everyone is indeed happier and more productive, and the organizational climate is reflecting an achievement arousal profile with room for affiliative tendencies.

A word of caution needs to be stated in terms of the application of this material. In our western society, the word *achievement* takes on natural, positive meanings; the word *affiliation* has some positive meanings despite fears that its use is not appropriate in a business setting, and the word *power* is usually perceived as bad. Here, these are meant to be neutral words and need to be interpreted in the context of this chapter; however, it is very apparent through much of our research that one is generally better off with a staff that is achievement-aroused toward the task, with specific feedback on how they are doing. This will make a major difference in the efficiency and flow of work.

This does not mean that every person hired needs to have as their dominant drive the achievement drive. Oftentimes it is best to have a receptionist who has achievement drive but is a highly affiliative individual. This means that the receptionist and others meeting your public will most likely be very caring about both employees and clients. They will attempt to establish and maintain relationships and will be very concerned about the "rough" relationships (clients leaving). The fact that there are motives that may be more appropriate than others for specific jobs in no way implies that any motive makes for good or bad people.

Summary

As this chapter's title suggests, we have learned through experience and research that leadership does indeed make a significant difference. There is much that can be overcome by good leadership, whereas bad leadership can take the best practice into bankruptcy. It is apparent that leadership is not a trait one is born with but rather a skill that one can develop.

This chapter hardly covers the entirety of the issue of leadership in your practice. It does, however, introduce two practical frameworks in which individuals can begin to mold their own style of leadership. Experience tells us that chapters and seminars only spur thoughts of change; it is practice over time that results in change. If you would like to lead your employees toward a better-functioning, happier future, try some of the approaches suggested here. They work.

References

1. Bennis AW: Organizational Development. Reading, MA, Addison-Wesley Publishing Co., 1985
2. Hersey P, Blanchard K: Management of Organizational Behavior, 3rd ed. Englewood Cliffs, NJ, Prentice-Hall, 1982
3. McClelland D: The Achieving Society. New York, Irvington, 1961

Chapter 2
☐
Client management

Dennis M. McCurnin

Clients are one of the most important assets to a successful veterinary practice. Every animal we care for has an owner. Some owners are sentimentally attached to the animal (pets), whereas others are economically motivated (food animals). Regardless of the relationship between owner and animal, the owner will make the final decision about the economic value of the care to be received. Veterinary medicine today is truly a *people business.*

Even though our primary motivation is caring for our patients, permission to proceed with treatment can only be obtained through effective communication and concurrence with the client. The establishment of a primary diagnosis is often client dependent through a detailed history-taking process. This dependence on the client and effective client communication and management puts us in a position of being unable to exercise our medical expertise unless we gain client confidence.

We deal with a cross-section of people in practice. Some people are enjoyable to work with whereas others are difficult. Our clients, in general, are no worse or no better than those in any other service profession. If you enjoy working with people and animals, private practice will be both personally and financially rewarding. Your personal attitude about your work and life will be reflected in your attitude toward the client and patient. This deep-down attitude toward the client and patient will have a positive or negative effect on the final decision (go or no go) made by the animal's owner.

Public opinion about the veterinary medical profession has changed during the past 20 years at a much more rapid pace than previously. We have moved from the "horse doctor'' to the ''vetnary'' and finally to the veterinarian who is a respected health care specialist. This change has been painfully slow but continues through the combined efforts of organized veterinary medicine and each one of us. During the same time that our profession was changing, so were our clients. The general public has become better educated and informed. High-quality service that is high tech and economical has become the expected standard. Today's client demands space-age technology *and* economy delivered by a personalized approach. Each of us must strive to retain the professional status we have worked so hard to gain.

☐ Practice area, people, and animals

Where to live

The selection of a practice area will become an exercise in personal preference, practice opportunity, and career timing. Practice opportunities can be found in any location that contains both animals and people. The success of a practice will be dependent on the concentration of animals, the number of practitioners, and the quality of care given to both client and patient.

For example, if you want to live in a rural environment but practice high-volume small-animal medicine, you probably will not move to Mitchellville, Iowa. On the other hand, if you want to live in an urban area but have a swine confinement practice, you probably will not live in New York City. The site you select is very personal but must reflect your life-style as closely as possible. If you are not happy with the recreational and free time activities, your work time will suffer. The bottom line becomes one of compromise, balancing life-style with practice opportunity. Few people are able to have both the life-style and exact practice type they have dreamed. See Chapters

7 and 9 for additional information on practice location.

Type of client

In addition to the area you want to live in you must consider the type of clients you want to serve. Some large-animal veterinarians want a few large producers in a small concentrated area, whereas others prefer the small, family operation or ''backyard'' client. Knowledge of the potential practice area demographics will be helpful, but animal population density would provide more useful information for the large-animal practitioner. The State Department of Agriculture can serve as a resource for estimating animal density in a given area.

Client type is more closely defined in small-animal practice. If one chooses to become associated with an existing practice in an old, established neighborhood, the clients are more often older and have older pets. Retirement communities in the Sunbelt cities have older clients with older pets, and most of these communities tend to be newer, rapidly growing areas. The general attitude of these older clients is one of genuine concern for the proper care of a long-time family member.

The demographic features of the small-animal practice area can be very helpful. This information can be obtained from the local chamber of commerce and could include income levels, occupations, family size, age, and area growth rates. In general, the very poorest or richest areas of a community may not make the best practice sites. Exceptions to the aforementioned exist, but both wealthy people and poor people can be difficult to collect fees from after services. The wealthy sometimes invest all available money until payment is forced, whereas the poor are waiting for their next income opportunity to develop. There are ways to deal effectively with collection problems, so this one point should not prevent service from being available to any income group.

In young family communities the pets tend also to be younger. The young family tends to want more vaccinations, elective surgery, and trauma care. The pet's role in the young family may not be as firmly developed as in the older family; however, the medical problems tend to have a better long-term prognosis in the young animal than in the older patient. The type of services requested (i.e., cancer therapy or euthanasia) depends somewhat on the income level of pet owners in the practice area. The middle- to upper-income family tends to make a good solid client base.

The type of community you practice in will help dictate your practice hours. If your clients are farm and ranch related, most of their large-animal contact will be early morning and late afternoon. Thus your practice hours should be developed around the hours of greatest need.

In small-animal practice, working couples will find it difficult to meet office hours between 9:00 A.M. and 5:00 P.M. Opening the office from 7:00 A.M. to 7:00 P.M. four days per week might be the answer. Having evening hours two nights per week and opening a half day on Saturday might also meet the needs. If you practice in a retirement community, 9:00 A.M. to 5:00 P.M. five days per week could be very adequate.

New vs. established clients

New clients must be handled with some extra attention to ensure that they will return to become established clients. New clients will make some preliminary conclusions about the staff and practice within the first 4 minutes of contact. The contact may start directly with the veterinarian (in some large-animal practices) or receptionist (small-animal practice) during the first visit. Our clients are consumers like us and as such require the same courtesy and pampering we would like to receive when we purchase services or goods.

During our first visit to a hotel, restaurant, airport, physician's office, and so forth, we are somewhat apprehensive about doing or saying the correct thing. Our clients feel the same way, in addition to having genuine concern about the health status of the animal and the potential costs. Everyone in the practice should recognize the potential apprehension of the new client and provide additional general information about the procedures and hospital policies that might be applicable. A warm smile and a helpful, professional attitude by the veterinarian and staff will go a long way toward reducing this tension. Again, remember the importance of the first 4 minutes with the new client.

The established client has returned to the practice presumably due to acceptable previous services. The first 4 minutes are not as critical with returning clients as with the new clients. However, returning clients cannot be ignored. Making some brief personal notes on new clients' records will ensure some personal remarks when they return. These notes may be made by either staff or veterinarian. Attention should be paid to these notes when the clients return, thereby ensuring client satisfaction by recall of specific personal information.

Well-established clients should be given special attention by being thanked for their

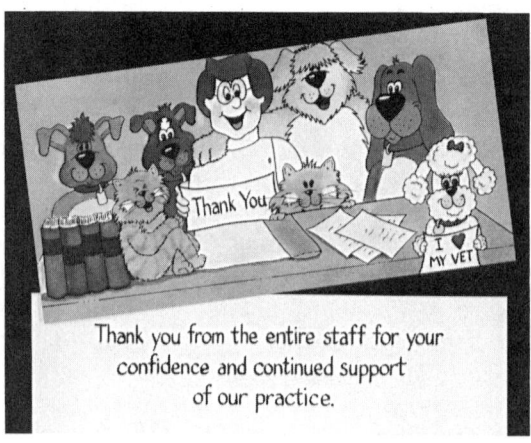

Figure 2-1. *Thank-you card (Courtesy of Apple Creations, Lutherville, Maryland)*

loyalty or new client referrals. At times, Christmas holiday gifts may be appropriate for very special clients. Thank-you cards (Fig. 2-1) to clients who have referred new clients to the practice are also very helpful. One of the best ways to clearly express client concern is by sending a letter or a sympathy card (Fig. 2-2) to the client after the death of a pet. Veterinarians who use cards or letters receive positive feedback from their clients as well as continued support.

□
Staff – client relations

People orientation

The support staff of a practice, clinic, or hospital must be *both* people and animal oriented. Everyone in a healthy and growing practice who has public contact must be acutely aware of the importance of the client. Clients should not be an unpleasant interruption during the day. If it were not for clients requesting service, the practice would cease to exist. If the truth were known, the practice is more dependent on the client than the client on the practice. In most locations in the United States a veterinarian may be quickly found by driving down the street or going to the next listing in the phone book; therefore, it becomes easier for the client to find a practitioner than for the practitioner to find a client. We must treat each client as we expect to be treated when we are obtaining goods and services for ourselves.

To maximize the strongest staff – client relations, each employee must be *people oriented.* Each person must like themselves, their lifestyle, and working with client problems. If you do not like to solve problems and deal with people who have problem, you will not enjoy practice. A serious mistake is made when our employees believe they will be good in practice because they "really like animals." Practice personnel must be mature and professional and have a real desire to deal with both the client and animal problems.

The attitude of employees affects the quality and quantity of their work. Employees with numerous personal problems will usually not

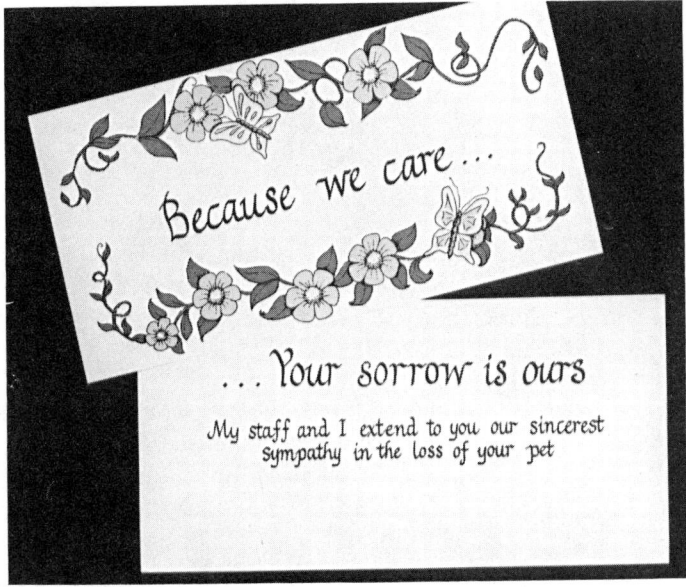

Figure 2-2. Sympathy card (Courtesy of Apple Creations, Lutherville, Maryland)

deal effectively with client problems. The attitude may become "my problems are much larger and more important that yours." A troubled person has difficulty in hiding this from clients and other staff members. New employees do not have to work very long in a practice before they will reflect the attitudes and values of the employer and other employees. This self-attitude can be positive or negative.

Enthusiasm is the second most contagious attitude in a practice. The most contagious and dangerous attitude is a negative outlook on yourself, the practice, clients, and life in general. It is necessary that everyone dealing with the public be enthusiastic about themselves and the services provided. To maintain enthusiasm one must be surrounded by enthusiastic people.

Unsatisfied clients may be the result of poor staff–client relations. Displeased clients will usually switch veterinarians rather than complain about staff members. It simply becomes easier for the client to pick another veterinarian rather than approach the problem of poor relationships. Clients most often leave practices due to poor human relations, not because of inadequate medical care.

Communication skills

Communication skills are developed and improved through constant attention to detail and personal commitment. Interpersonal communication is much more than good oral communication. In most veterinary practices our oral communication accounts only for 35% to 40% of our total communication efforts. As an example, facial expression is a powerful communication tool that can be interpreted to be very positive or negative.

A frown or sullen look can communicate an immediate negative message, whereas a smile says "I'm happy to see you." A ready smile and sense of humor are invaluable to anyone working with people. A bright, cheery smile in no way detracts from the professionalism of the hospital or the seriousness of the practice.

In addition to facial expression, communication results from body language, personal appearance, hospital cleanliness, building repair, room odor control, interior decorating, exterior landscaping, hospital signs, and cleanliness of the parking lot. In the large-animal practice, cleanliness and repair of the mobile clinic (car or truck) are extremely important and send a message loud and clear, well before one foot is placed on the client's property. When a client enters the parking lot of a clinic or hospital, the unconscious mental examination of the practice begins. Is the parking lot clean, well striped, and marked to designate the proper place for the client to park? Employees' cars should not be parked near the entrance of the building but in a remote location to allow clients ready access. The landscape should be well maintained and neat in appearance. Dead and dying plants (outside or inside the building) send a negative message to the client. As a rule of thumb, never go to a physician whose plants have died.

The exterior of the building should be in good repair, with the entrance plainly marked. These small, seemingly unimportant exterior points collectively add up in clients' minds as positive or negative impressions even before they actually enter the building.

Upon entering the building most people become immediately aware of sounds (barking dogs or crying kids) and odors (pleasant or offensive). Loud noises and offensive odors increase client anxiety. It is hoped that people will enter a quiet, clean, odor-free environment and be greeted with a pleasant smile from a helpful and caring receptionist. If clients are not acknowledged by the receptionist, they will immediately wonder how important they are to the practice. Will they have to wait and, if so, how long? Again some of these feelings are negative, and no one (client or receptionist) has spoken one word.

Oral communication begins when the receptionist greets the client and starts the problem-solving process. The appearance of the receptionist is especially important because he or she is usually the first staff member seen by the client. Especially because we are in a health care profession, cleanliness of employees and facilities is extremely important. Clothing, hair, and hands must receive special attention. Professional, clean uniforms will help reinforce the professional image. The type of clothing, however, may not be as important as its being in good taste, clean, and neat.

Nonverbal communication with the client continues during time spent in the reception room and examination room through the aesthetics of the facility. The surroundings should be clean, quiet, odor free, and warm feeling. The use of woods, pastels, and wallpaper will help avoid the cold, sterile appearance of some hospitals. Indirect lighting will also soften the environment.

Communication is always a two-way street, and to become fully effective, listening modes must be developed. To be an effective listener requires concentration and acceptance of information from the other person. Listening skills must be developed and are critical to both staff and veterinarian in obtaining information required to make a diagnosis or manage a patient. Care should be taken to employ *active listening* as often as possible. Active listening involves listening to the clients and then verbally rephrasing their thoughts back to them. As an example, Mrs. Jones may state, "Barney just can't seem to get up and down stairs anymore." You may respond by saying, "It must be difficult for you to see Barney becoming restricted to one floor of your home. Our examination may reveal the source of the problem to enable us to help Barney move around more easily." The client will have little doubt that you have heard her statement concerning the inability to climb stairs.

Professional, helpful attitude

Both professional and support staff need to maintain a positive, friendly, helpful attitude. Veterinary medicine is a service profession that deals directly with the animal's owner. Most of our clients call or come to the hospital somewhat reluctantly. The client has a problem that must be solved, and the solution usually involves spending money. Our clients would much rather spend their money on a vacation, clothes, and so forth rather than veterinary care. Therefore, we must make the veterinary experience as positive and pleasant as possible.

All members of the practice have an obligation to all others to maintain a positive outlook of themselves and their work. If everyone has a positive outlook within the practice, this internal reinforcement will effectively penetrate to the client. The client should have the feeling that "we care." On the other hand, if the attitude internally is negative, even the positive client will become negative.

To maintain a positive attitude requires personal commitment and effort on a consistent basis. You must enjoy what you are doing. If you receive satisfaction from your work most of the time, you can maintain a positive attitude during your "down days" by consciously trying to overcome these negative feelings. However, if you are down more days than "up," the extra effort will not always mask your true feelings. A new career direction should be given consideration when work becomes a "job." If you do not want to start your job at 8:00 A.M., you cannot wait until 5:00 P.M. when your job is over, or you wait all morning for the noon hour, you need a change. Veterinary practice should not become a job. Practice should be the opportunity to help owners solve the medical problems of their animals. If you enjoy people, animals, and problem solving, practice will be very rewarding.

The overall practice attitude should be one

of providing a quality service in a professional and friendly manner. Each person in the practice should be willing to take the necessary "extra step" to provide quality service even to the difficult client. A few clients have very negative feelings about themselves and veterinary medicine, and we need to meet that challenge. The message each person in the practice should convey to each client is "I care."

Attire

One of the most effective means of communication is personal appearance. Attention to personal hygiene and appropriate attire produces a message that says "I care." Lack of attention to attire and personal hygiene sends an "I don't care" message well before a word is spoken. If you care about your work and yourself, spend a little extra time on yourself each day. Proper attire for a practice setting depends on the type of practice and clientele. In the large-animal setting, clean coveralls and washable boots are appropriate for the farm or ranch. This same attire might not be appropriate for making a stop at the bank or treating a small-animal patient in the clinic.

Most small-animal practices allow both veterinarian and staff to be more formally dressed than a mixed or large-animal practice. Professional smocks, jackets, or coats allow comfortable clothing to be worn underneath as well as protect that clothing from soilage. Untidy or soiled outer garments should never be worn in the public areas of the practice.

People will act and feel more professional if they are attired in neat, clean clothing. The kennel or stable person should feel as much a part of the professsional team as the veterinarian or technician. Therefore it is vitally important that all staff members be professionally attired and that each practice meticulous personal hygiene.

Receptionist

The receptionist is the most important person in the practice in dealing with public relations.

The receptionist is usually the first and last contact each client has with the practice (large animal or small animal). Only a few people will become outstanding receptionists. It takes a special person to be able to effectively perform the variety of tasks required while constantly being in the public eye. A talented receptionist may be required to perform several duties simultaneously. Frequently, for example, the receptionist will be required to answer the phone, greet a new client, and fill out a dismissal form, all at the same time (Fig. 2-3). These requirements mandate a *people person* who really enjoys the challenges of client problem solving.

The receptionist must be able to speak easily and confidently with clients about their concerns. The ability to project concern, interest, enthusiasm, professionalism, and competence is a must. In addition to possessing excellent verbal communication skills, the receptionist must be fastidious about appearance and work environment. A quality receptionist will anticipate the needs of clients and staff.

Since the client normally makes the first contact with the receptionist, the reception room must be maintained in a clean, neat, and odor-free condition. As was discussed earlier, the client starts the practice evaluation process

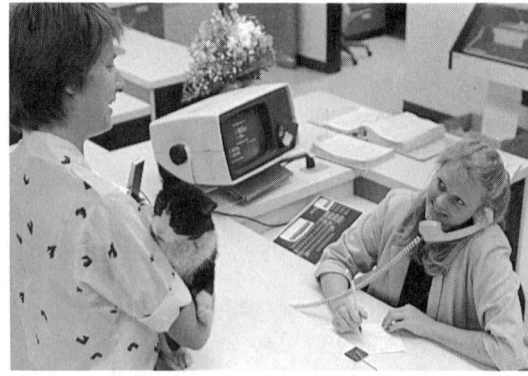

Figure 2-3.   *Receptionist greeting client, answering phone, and completing record*

during the first phone contact or during the first 4 minutes in the reception area. Consequently, the reception area must be under the direct control of the receptionist, who should have full responsibility for its organization and maintenance.

In addition to the receptionist being a "superperson," a quality receptionist must also know hospital procedure and be able to market the profession and practice. When asked basic questions about animal care or activity, the receptionist must have competent answers. If questions become more involved, they should be referred to the technician or veterinarian for an in-depth answer. A deep understanding of the human–animal bond (see Chapter 16 for more information) is necessary in a pet practice to allow proper concern to be expressed during life-threatening situations or at euthanasia. The actions and responses of the receptionist are critical to good client relations during these more stressful situations.

An understanding of good accounting practice is required of most receptionists to handle financial transactions. Hospital procedure will dictate client credit policies, but these policies must be explained and enforced. Special skills are necessary to allow the receptionist to be understanding yet collect the account. Financial management information is found in Chapter 19.

Having good marketing skills is a must for the quality receptionist. As Robert Louis Stevenson said, "Everyone lives by selling something." The basic mood and feeling about veterinary medicine and the practice will be established by the receptionist. We are selling professional service, and the scope of those services can be greatly expanded by the receptionist. Much of the preventive medicine (i.e., immunizations, nutritional needs, dentistry, elective surgery, prepurchase examinations, pregnancy examinations, and so forth) can be queried by the receptionist and this information given to the veterinarian or technician for appropriate follow-up. For additional information on marketing, see Chapter 6.

Veterinary technician

The professional relationship between client and technician is an extension of the veterinarian–client relationship. These relationships should supplement and strengthen one another. Often the client will relay information more freely to the technician than to anyone else in the practice. When the client has made a poor decision about the seriousness of an animal's condition, he or she may be reluctant to express this to the veterinarian but will confide in the technician.

Complete utilization of the veterinary technician will enhance both the practice and the profession. The level of patient care and cost to the client can be greatly affected through the proper use of technical support staff. Many client–patient duties can be accomplished by the well-trained technician. During the past 15 years the dental profession has improved the level of service while being cost conscious through more-efficient use of dental technicians. Veterinarians are now beginning to more fully use the potential of the technician.

The veterinary technician must possess the same communication, marketing, public relations, and personal appearance skills as the receptionist. In addition, the technician must also have professional care skills, animal handling skills, and client bereavement counseling skills. The cleanliness of the examination room should be the responsibility of the technician. Just as the receptionist is responsible for the reception area, the technician should assume the responsibility for the examination areas.

The veterinarian, technician, and receptionist personality match must be right for everyone to act and function as a team. No one individual has all the necessary skills to provide a complete service for all clients, but by combining all staff skills the needs of the client, patient, and practice are met. Additional information on utilization of the veterinary technician can be found in Chapter 12.

☐
Veterinarian – client relations

One of the key factors in a successful practice is the interpersonal relationship that develops between veterinarian and client. This positive client relationship begins with the receptionist and is further developed by the technician, but the final act of competence and trust must be executed by the veterinarian.

Many small factors go into the formation of the client's decision about the veterinarian and the practice. Most of these factors are what would appear to be "little things" that in themselves are not important. When we collectively assemble these little things, they produce an opinion about the practice. Examples of these isolated items are professional sign, clean parking lot, building in good repair, clean windows in the reception room, odor-free reception room, new magazines in the reception room, a smiling receptionist, professional and clean uniforms or coveralls, the "I care" attitude of staff and veterinarian, ability to quickly locate the medical record, calling the client by name, answering the phone before the third ring, providing handout material, dispensing medication with typed labels, dismissing clean and dry patients from the hospital, and so forth. Most of these little things we know about and probably believe are important. Why then are some of these things neglected? Most of the reasons (excuses) relate back to personal attitude about oneself and the practice. Because clients are usually unable to judge the veterinarian's technical competence in performing major medical procedures, they often make decisions based on relatively unimportant things.

Attitude and confidence

The self-concept of each member of the practice is extremely important. Often the attitude a person has in their private life carries over into their professional life. If a person is basically fulfilled in their private life and has a positive attitude and outlook on the future, he or she will become confident in that feeling and position. This positive attitude and confidence carries over into their professional life through the feeling of enthusiasm. The opposite is also true in that a negative attitude and lack of self-confidence will usually result in the client detecting a lack of enthusiasm and feeling of "I don't care." When "I care" enthusiasm is found in the practice, this attitude is felt in both the staff and the client. The positive behavior of the client reinforces these feelings. Few people can maintain total enthusiasm all the time. If you know a person who is on a constant "high," they probably need professional counseling! Most people have down days and during these periods must work to make their responses appear positive. This self-motivation will work for short periods of time, but if this becomes the rule rather than the exception, a new or altered career objective should be considered. Life is too short not to be enjoying our work.

When the veterinarian and staff have confidence and enthusiasm, the objective of client confidence and enthusiasm is more easily met. Demonstration of competence and attention to the little things are client confidence builders. Being able to call a client by name, find the medical record quickly, and relate to the animal's problem produces permanent positive feelings in the client.

Clients need to feel that they have made the correct decision to call the veterinarian or come into the clinic. The client wants to be recognized as a responsible and intelligent owner. Even when the animal's problem appears to be of minor concern to the veterinarian, the client should be assured that he or she has made a good decision in bringing the animal to the clinic or calling the veterinarian to the farm. No one wants to feel that they have made an obvious error.

On the other hand, the client should not be criticized harshly for waiting too long to contact the veterinarian. When obvious neglect has occurred, this should be handled professionally because most times clients are unaware of the seriousness of the condition. Only through careful communication with the client can the veterinarian educate without being intimidating.

Client confidence can be strengthened if the veterinarian is thorough in performing a complete physical examination and takes time to explain the findings. Most clients expect the following five things during a consultation: (1) examination of the patient, (2) diagnosis (cause if possible), (3) prognosis, (4) treatment, and (5) fee estimate. Communication of prognosis and fee estimate is difficult for some veterinarians. Clients feel ill prepared to make judgments without this information and often complain if complications occur. Malpractice concerns (see Chapter 8) can be virtually eliminated if these areas are discussed with the client.

Client communication

The majority of complaints against veterinarians are the result of improper or misunderstood communication between veterinarian or practice personnel and client. For communication to be complete there must be concern for both client and animal. Additionally, one must learn to *listen* to the client and then communicate in a spirit of conveying information that is understandable and effective. Most people *hear* other people talk, but few people have developed the art of effective listening.

Not only should veterinarians and staff listen to what the client is saying but also listen to how it is being expressed. The client may be concerned with payment or concerned about the pain the animal is experiencing. Effective communication is a two-way process many of us violate by failing to listen. If we sense the client's concern, we may be able to alleviate the problem by suggesting a fee payment plan or expressing our concern with eliminating the pain.

To ensure effective communication, consider these three points: (1) Use terminology the client will understand; too many scientific terms can be confusing to the nonprofessional listener. (2) Do not rush through the information just because it appears to be "common knowledge" to you, or the client will feel "brushed off." The veterinarian should never assume the client is knowledgeable about a medical problem or the medical procedures available. (3) Do not assume a superior manner or tone to the extent that the listener feels "put down."

In short, be honest and courteous, show concern, and attempt to treat everyone as if they were special. If you treat each client as you would like to be treated when you are selecting or securing a service, the result will be clients that experience courtesy, concern, and the "I care" attitude. When the communication is open, honest, and effective, most problems can be prevented.

Only about 40% of all communication is verbal. Sight, touch, smell, sounds, and body language are all important communication factors. Client experiences upon entry into the parking lot or reception room, odors, sounds, and body language (e.g., nod of the head, raised eyebrow, frown, smile) are all evaluated by the client to form a total impression (positive or negative) of the practice.

The client can also be observed for information from body language. By watching how the client handles the pet, important clues can be obtained concerning the client–pet bond. When the client holds the pet close and talks a great deal to the pet, a strong bond between the two is evident; however, if the client appears disinterested in the pet or can provide little information about the activity of the animal, a very shallow bond probably exists.

When speaking to the client the veterinarian should face the client and make good eye contact. By observing the client's eye contact the veterinarian can often perceive that the client is "lost" and can transmit the information in simpler terms or in more detail. To reinforce the information given to the client verbally, a variety of informative pamphlets are available from commercial sources and professional organizations or can be internally generated to give to the client. Handout material (Fig. 2-4*A* and 2-4*B*) is an excellent follow-up or rein-

forcement to the office or farm visit. This printed information also serves as a marketing tool for your practice. Additional information on marketing can be found in Chapter 6.

The difficult client

Some clients are just plain difficult to deal with regardless of the efforts of everyone in the practice. The attitude of the difficult client

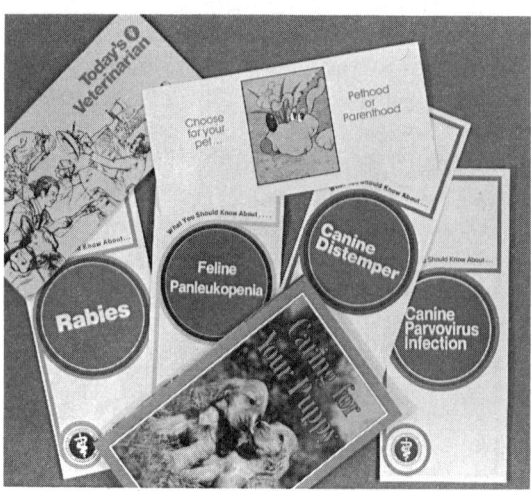

Figure 2-4. (A) *Handout material for use in client education.* (B) *Client handout material provided by commercial source (Courtesy of American Veterinary Medical Association and Hill's Pet Products, Inc, Topeka, Kansas)*

A

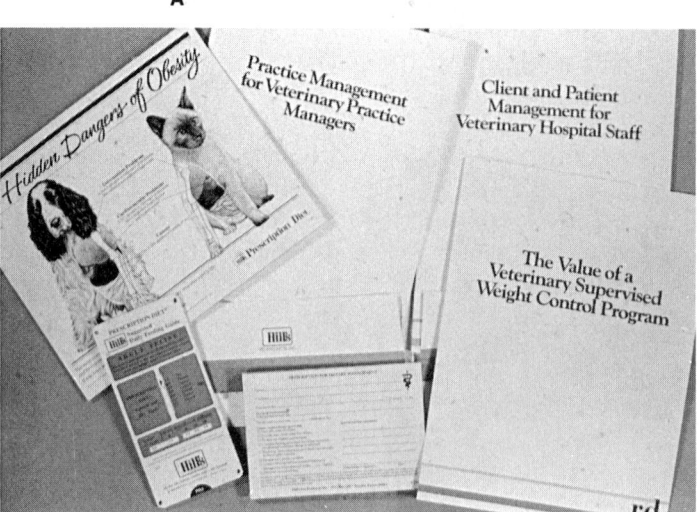

B

toward the staff may be completely different from the attitude toward the veterinarian. A very arrogant, demanding person can suddenly become quite reasonable when the veterinarian enters the room. Veterinarians should defend and support their staffs in these unusual situations and communicate the displeasure in such actions.

When dealing with someone who is politely complaining, listen and attempt to convey that you understand the problem (you will appear to be agreeing, and this will help reduce the level of the confrontation). A good example would be the common complaint that fees are too high. "Yes, fees are high! Everything seems to be too expensive these days. Let's talk about the fees and services rendered."

In situations in which the client appears to be unreasonable about the complaint, you must establish the exact nature of the complaint. Discussion with the unreasonable client should occur in the privacy of an examination room or private office, not in the reception room. In most unreasonable client situations, however, the confrontation is initiated in the reception room where the area is full of people. Once the client and problem have been identified, the solution should be sought as quickly as possible and the client sent home before additional clients are involved.

Never argue with a dissatisfied client. The client is always right, even when wrong. If a client leaves angry, ten other people are told how awful you, your staff, and your hospital are. Sometimes we must "eat a little crow" to keep the client's good will. In the long run this will benefit all concerned. Only on rare occasions should a client be asked not to return.

The most difficult people to reason with are people who have been drinking or are abusing drugs. Be careful how substance abusers are handled because they can become violent and uncontrollable. In situations in which drugs or alcohol have been taken to excess, law enforcement officials should be contacted to

handle the situation. Do not attempt to physically control the situation because you may endanger yourself, the staff, and the client. Call for professional help from the local police.

Personal touch

Our world has become one of high technology and impersonal service. People really want both high technology and highly personal service. The entire practice staff must function as a team to be able to deliver personalized service. The frequent use of the client's name, the use of the pet's name, and recall of specific information about the client, all lead to the client feeling important. We all want to feel important, and impersonal service reinforces to us that we are not important. This feeling of unimportance is provided to people daily in the food store, gas station, bank, and so forth. In many department stores, mail order departments, and ice cream shops, service is provided by taking a number. When your number is called, you get your chance—now serving number 208. We have now been reduced to just a number.

When everyone on the practice team works together to provide quality personal service, people really take notice. Some people will not become appreciative of the extra effort and personal touch. Try to make clients feel important, it works!

☐ Client selection of a veterinarian

How does a client choose a veterinarian or veterinary practice? The profession would like to think veterinarians are chosen for knowledge and skill. Unfortunately this is not true. Many veterinarians and veterinary practices are chosen because of location. Most veterinarians who have established practices know the most important three factors in the selection of practice real estate are (1) location, (2) location, and (3) location. Practice location cannot be underestimated.

Beyond practice location people select their veterinarian based on (1) personality, (2) how they handle the animal, (3) how well they communicate, and (4) professional knowledge. The "world-of-mouth" recommendation is the best advertisement a practice can have. Most of the word-of-mouth–type recommendations are based on the personality of the veterinarian and the practice staff. Commonly you will be told "you are just great. You just did a great job for me." Most of the time this "great job" or "is just great" relates to personality not to professional competence or skill. If you have doubts about the previous statements, recall how you choose your attorney, accountant, physician, or dentist. Usually selection is based on the recommendation of a layperson who has no special skills to evaluate the professional competence of the person being recommended. In the selection process it becomes readily apparent that practice location, facility appearance, and recommendations from satisfied clients are extremely important to practice growth. Attitude and professionalism of the support staff are critically important in this whole process.

□
Use of support staff

The well-trained receptionist and veterinary technician are positive extensions of the veterinarian. Today's successful practice must fully utilize the support staff as an important part of the veterinary health care team. Some practices could be greatly improved with the addition of a veterinary technician rather than another veterinarian.

Once the practice functions as a team, everyone benefits. The veterinarian benefits through improved time utilization. The client benefits through more personalized and pro-

fessional service. The patient benefits by having an experienced health care team providing complete, consistent care. In addition, the practice benefits because of satisfied clients.

The profession must continue to increase the utilization of support staff to become increasingly efficient. The squeeze on net income during the past 10 years has forced the veterinarian to take a close look at practice personnel management, including both professional and support staff. The efficient practice cannot afford to have three veterinarians taking a radiograph when two technicians and a veterinarian can provide the service. The professional veterinarian must function in diagnosis, surgery, and prescribing, and the technician must function in the technical and professional support areas.

Practice efficiency may be improved through the utilization of technicians in the examination room to initiate the medical record, history, and preliminary physical examination (Fig. 2-5). In large-animal practice, medical records could be completed by the technician on the farm before leaving or driving the veterinarian to the next call, thereby allowing him to complete the records in route.

□
Clients and hospital procedures

Appointments

For the convenience of both practice and client, an appointment system should be developed. The receptionist is the key player in controlling the schedule. In a group practice the receptionist should determine whether the client prefers a certain veterinarian. This gives each veterinarian an opportunity to build and maintain a rapport with his clients.

The veterinarian's schedule must be fully known by the receptionist to allow appointments to be made during times when the veterinarian will be available. When a client

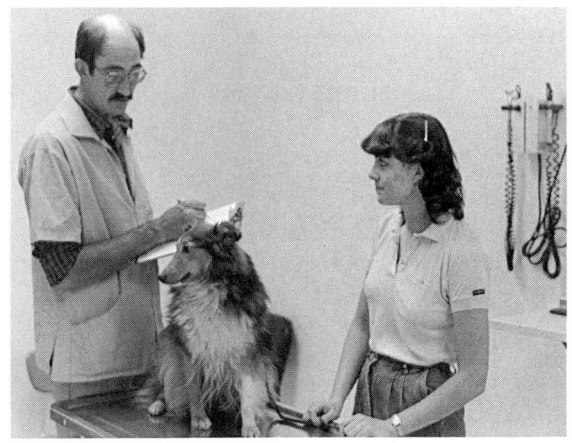

Figure 2-5. *Veterinary technician obtaining history from client*

schedules an appointment, it is assumed the veterinarian will be available at the appointed time. If, for some reason, this is not possible, the client should be contacted promptly. When the client cannot be contacted before an appointment cancellation, special attention should be given to the client immediately upon arrival at the clinic.

The most common reason for failure to keep an appointment is an emergency case. Emergencies should not become the standard answer for inefficient practice management. When an emergency occurs, the affected client should be informed of such immediately upon arrival and given the choice of waiting a prescribed length of time or rescheduling the appointment for a more convenient time. When the delay is only 15 or 20 minutes, one rescheduled appointment can put everyone back on schedule.

If appointment delays are common, scheduling more time for each appointment or leaving several open appointments should be considered. If unscheduled clients (walk-ins) become a problem, several open appointments may be left in the schedule to accommodate them. These clients should be reminded that making an appointment is desirable and to their benefit. When walk-ins occur during a completely booked schedule,

they should be worked into the schedule around the appointments and not taken in preference to the appointment. At times, the walk-in may have to wait until the office closes (noon or night) if the situation is not an emergency. The animal could also be hospitalized until an examination can be performed.

Emergency policy

What constitutes an emergency? The true and practical meaning of an emergency is anything the owners perceive as an emergency. If the owners did not think there was a serious problem, they would not have called or brought the animals to the clinic. The definition of the emergency call is put to the test at 2:00 A.M. when a client calls with a "wire cut" in the horse or an anal sac abscess in the dog. In a few cases it may be possible to determine over the phone that the condition is not a real emergency. Most of the time, however, an assessment of the patient is needed to make an accurate determination of the patient's true status.

When the determination over the phone is one of a nonemergency in the eyes of the veterinarian, a period of careful listening is required to determine how the owner feels. If the owner is still convinced it is an emergency situation, then the veterinarian should see the patient. Otherwise, the client will simply call another veterinarian if he or she is still concerned about the status of the animal.

In some large-animal situations, the client is more animal husbandry oriented and has a good idea about the seriousness of many conditions. Large-animal emergency calls will usually have to be worked into the schedule. In small-animal practice many of the so-called emergencies are really not emergencies in the true medical sense; however, the owner may be in an emergency state about the animal and simply rush it to the clinic. When this occurs, the owner should be considered and the animal examined and probably hospitalized for a short period of time. The hospital stay will allow the owner to calm down, and the animal can be cared for as the hospital schedule allows.

The true emergency (e.g., milk fever, equine colic, canine gastric-dilation-volvulus) must always be handled on a priority basis day or night. When the hospital schedule does not allow for emergency cases to be received, the receptionist should be given clear instructions as to where patients are to be referred. Referrals may be to an emergency clinic or another practice in the area. Nighttime emergencies in small-animal practice are more commonly being sent to full-service, full-staff emergency clinics. In some situations the client, patient, and referring veterinarian are all better off using a full-service emergency facility.

Telephone utilization

The telephone is the "life blood" and connection to the outside world for all practices. At times during very busy periods, one would like to rip the phone out of the wall. Yet without the phone the practice would quickly die.

The Charles, Charles and Associates Veterinary Services Market report prepared for the American Veterinary Medical Association in 1983 indicated that "even in the case of some light users, one visit to a veterinarian often made them comfortable enough to feel they could call for veterinary advice." It is important to note that considerable veterinary care is consumed over the phone—free. Improved use of the telephone will allow increased client numbers to be presented to the practice. Some practices do a very poor job of working the telephone. In most instances the client should be encouraged to bring the animal to the clinic or have the veterinarian come to the farm. All telephone calls should be answered by the third ring, and the caller should be greeted by "Good morning, this is XYZ Animal Hospital. Cindy speaking. May I help you?" This format will allow callers to immediately know they have reached the correct number and Cindy is there to help them. Since the telephone is often the first contact a client has with the practice, proper telephone manners and answers are essential.

It is interesting to note that a smile on one end of the phone line can be perceived by the caller on the other end (Fig. 2-6). The tightness of the facial muscles and tone of voice are received by the caller in addition to the words. It becomes difficult to hide your true feelings even over the phone.

When answering a multiline phone, the receptionist should always allow the caller to agree to being put "on hold." The caller should be asked "Can you please hold for a

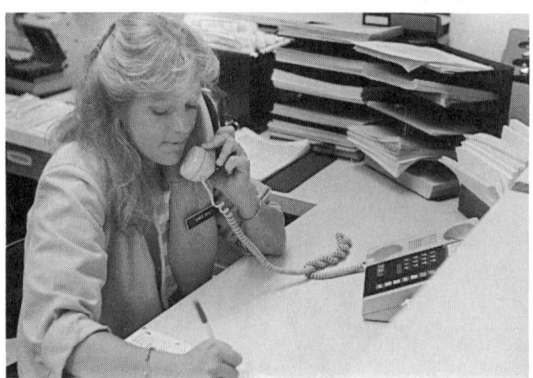

Figure 2-6. *Telephone communication should be done with a smile*

minute?" Too often the phone is answered by "Hold please!" No one should be kept on hold for longer than 1 minute without going back to the line and asking whether they can continue to hold or would they prefer to leave a message.

Telephone courtesy is just as important as personal courtesy because most clients have the initial contact via the phone. When the technical and veterinary staff treat each call with common courtesy, the feeling the client will receive is genuine concern and "I care."

The office phone of all practicing veterinarians should be answered 24 hours a day. If the practice does not provide on-site emergency care, then the caller should be directed by an answering service or phone recorder. To have a phone go unanswered is unprofessional.

The first visit

When a client first comes to the hospital or asks the veterinarian to come to the farm, the client is somewhat apprehensive. The veterinarian and staff should do everything possible to make the first visit as informative as possible. The client will be judging the practice, staff, and veterinarian during the entire visit but more acutely during the first 2 to 5 minutes of contact. Extra effort should be made during the first visit to explain the practice services, gain information about the client, get to know the animal(s), and discuss practice philosophy.

Continued interest and courtesy must be extended to the established client, but the practice is not being scrutinized as severely as during the very first visit. During subsequent visits the client should receive positive reinforcement with the "I care" practice attitude. Personal notes on the medical record will help recall information on the next visit. Handout materials are useful to explain practice philosophy and also serve the client as a reminder of the practice.

Office and farm visits should start and end on time. This enforces the priority placed on the call schedule and efficient practice management. Clients should not feel rushed but feel their needs and their animal's needs have been met. The veterinarian must assume the primary responsibility for time management. Chapter 13 provides more information on time management.

Hospital visiting policy

Each practice should establish a patient visiting policy and inform clients of the policy. In general, most patients are better off not being visited by the client. Oftentimes, the patient must again adjust to the hospital environment. In the past, some practices have had a no-visit policy that is certainly outdated today. Some consideration must be given to the client in that the client may have an emotional need to visit the animal.

As the human–animal bond (see Chapter 16) is more clearly understood, the visiting policies in veterinary hospitals will become modified. One major consideration on the part of the practice is the amount of staff time required with each visit. This staff investment is a true expense to the practice. Hospitalization fees must be adjusted to compensate for all overhead.

Certain patients will benefit from regular visits from the owner. The patient that is despondent, depressed, or anorexic will oftentimes improve in attitude after owner visits. The final decision on hospital visits should be made jointly between the client and attendant veterinarian. Visits with the patient may occur in the ward or in the examination or treatment room. The most appropriate location for the visit is in an area away from routine hospital activity so that other patients and staff activities are not disrupted. Often, the examination room may be the most appropriate place unless special monitoring equipment is needed. The veterinary technician can play a very useful role during client visits. They can provide the client with medical update information as well as console the client.

Patient dismissal

The dismissal of a hospitalized patient is similar to that of the outpatient except that dispensed medications, itemized fee statement, and patient cleanup must be completed *before* the owner's arrival. When dismissing a hospitalized patient the following points should be considered: (1) an itemized fee statement should be ready; (2) all medications should be prepared with proper labels; (3) the veterinarian should be available for consultation with the client; (4) the veterinary technician should be available to demonstrate treatment and home care techniques with handout instructions for home reference; (5) fee collection should take place after an explanation and review of the case; (6) the next appointment or recheck should be scheduled; and (6) the patient should be presented to the client, dry, clean, and odor free.

Some conditions dictate that the patient be presented before fee collection and scheduling of the next appointment. When this occurs, someone should be available to hold or control the animal until the client has completed the dismissal process. The technician can be extremely valuable during the dismissal process by explaining to the client what to do if specific events develop (through reinforcement of directions given by the veterinarian) and by ensuring the patient *always* is as clean or cleaner than when admitted. Most clients will judge the total care an animal has received by the condition and appearance of the animal at dismissal. When dismissing surgical patients, in addition to the animal itself being clean, the surgical incision, bandage, splint, or cast must be clean and dry. The surgical technique will be judged by the neatness of hair removal at the surgical site and the appearance of the incision.

After dismissal from the hospital, the client should receive a follow-up telephone call from the veterinary technician. This call is made to inquire about the progress and condition of the animal since dismissal. Most clients will be pleasantly surprised by this personal touch. To prompt the call, the technician should keep a log of all dismissals with the date, name, condition, and phone number of the client. Approximately 2 to 4 days after dismissal the call is made and patient's condition noted in the log. If any problems are detected during the initial call, the veterinarian is informed and requested to return the call.

Client referrals

Most practices are unable to provide all professional services needed or requested by the client. When services are needed that are not available in the practice, a referral to another practice or veterinarian should be considered. Clients are familiar with obtaining several consultations for their own medical care, so having another opinion on a case is not unusual.

When board-certified specialists are available, they should be used when possible. Some services that are required or requested are only available through the specialist. A list of specialists should be available for use by clients and veterinarians. Additional information on specialist and referral practices can be found in Chapter 20.

□
Summary

Effective client management involves attention to detail and personal service. Everyone in the practice must be enthusiastic about their team role and the quality of care delivered to both patient and client. Poor human relations result in client loss and negative staff attitudes. Veterinarians must set the example for client and patient care.

Chapter 3
☐
Personnel management

Joe H. Schwarz

This chapter is intended to provide the practitioner, veterinary student, supervisor, or practice manager with a commonsense approach to personnel management. Regardless of the practice size, effective personnel management skills are essential ingredients to meet the goals and objectives of the unit. Keep in mind that in the majority of veterinary practices the largest single expenditure is personnel. Personnel resources must be used to their maximum potential in the business world. The payoff for an effective personnel management approach will be increased productivity, improved organization, and saving of time and money.

Veterinarians and technical staff receive very little training or education in personnel management techniques. Success in the business world, however, is related to how effective individuals are in managing people. The personnel functions of organizational and job analysis, hiring, orientation training, evaluation, supervision, conflict resolution, and communications need to be mastered by individuals in managerial or supervisory roles. The information provided can be used as a basic guide for a personnel management program in any veterinary practice regardless of size or type. Combining a program that fits the manager's philosophy and style with practical experience will prepare the individual for the challenges inherent in human resources management. Additional information about the duties and function of the practice manager can be found in Chapter 14.

□
Philosophy and style

To create a personnel management program that will work, it is important that individual managers objectively analyze their strengths and weaknesses, willingness to delegate responsibility and authority, openness and approachability, and goals and objectives for the practice. An honest appraisal should influence how the practice is staffed and the types of people that are hired. The questions asked should include the following: Can I accept constructive criticism? Do I need to maintain control of all aspects of the practice? Do I enjoy working closely with people? Can I be open-minded about suggestions to improve the operation of the practice? Is it important to seek others' input before making decisions? Do I prefer a team approach, or do I feel comfortable working with a group of independent workers who know what to do in their own area of responsibility? There are no right or wrong answers to these questions. The purpose of questions like these is to assist individuals in sorting out their personal style of management and makeup of their personality.

Strong managers know their personality and tend to surround themselves with people they can manage effectively yet who complement their strengths and provide coverage for their weaknesses. There is no one right way to manage people. What is important is that individual goals and objectives be similar and that work habits and expectations do not clash. In working with supervisors and managers in discussing personal styles and philosophies, the topics of discussion tend to center on whether they are assertive or not assertive, look at the big picture or tend to get involved in the details, are open- or close-minded, tend to develop close working relationships or are removed from their employees. What is important is the willingness of individuals to adjust themselves to changing environments.

Managers should acknowledge their approaches and avoid trying to be what they cannot be. This statement does not imply that managers should avoid innovations or test different styles and methods. The test is whether the manager ultimately feels comfortable with the change and is effective using the new approach.

Leaders and managers are not born. They learn the necessary skills, take risks, and acknowledge their limitations as well as their assets. Adaptability is important in managing personnel. Each person is different and responds uniquely to a manager's style. It is important to acknowledge the individual difference in responses to the same rules or procedures and adapt the management style to become more effective. Some people need detailed instructions on a procedure; others require general guidelines and would prefer to have less direction. It is important to cultivate working relationships that build on mutual respect for individual differences. Flexibility in management style can save time and effort and can tap employees' resources to improve performance. Acknowledging the strengths of professional, technical, or support staff builds morale.

The manager must leave behind feelings of being personally threatened. It is good business to compensate for individual weaknesses by hiring people who have strong personal qualities, skills, and abilities that make the practice a profitable, enjoyable place to work. The people who work for an organization are a reflection of the practice that is viewed not only by clients but also by peers and the business community as a whole. Unless the practitioner runs a solo practice with no professional or technical support, the individual must rely heavily on employees' ability to perform. The staff is essentially the key to a successful practice. The success of a manager in a personnel function should be viewed in relation to how strong the staff working for the practice is. The personnel management skills to be developed include communications, coaching, listening, motivating, delegating, planning, organizing, coordinating, training, and supervising. The successful practice will be rewarded if the aforementioned skills are priorities and develop as do veterinary skills.

□
Analysis of personnel requirements

In developing a staffing plan, reorganizing, or making adjustments to current position assignments, it is important to consider all the pertinent factors possible. Considerations should include caseload, seasonal fluctuation in business, size and location of facilities, type of practice (small, large, mixed, or specialty), normal working hours, emergency services offered, and any special features that make the practice unique. The type of clientele and services provided coupled with the goals and objectives of the practice should provide a benchmark of the requirements for professional staff. By using the requirements for professional staff as a guide along with an analysis of the aforementioned factors, technical and support staff needs should be identified. It is helpful to list staffing needs on paper in relation to the work variables, responsibilities that must be covered, hours of staffing, and the interrelationships between positions. The general responsibilities to be covered will tend to be divided between business/administrative/record keeping and technical/animal care/laboratory. Depending on the size of the practice, decision points that will frequently arise include whether the staffing plan should use specialized staff positions, that is, surgical, laboratory, or anesthesia technicians, or veterinary technicians handling a broad range of responsibilities. The decision point requires that the manager have an overall plan and sight of ultimate goals. In analyzing the organization, objectivity and a firm hold of reality are

necessary to protect against miscalculations or overprojecting needs. A conservative approach in staffing usually will be in the best interest of the practice. During the analysis, it is also necessary to anticipate personnel issues that affect all businesses including coverage in case of illnesses, vacation, or terminations. *Cross-training* is an important tool in handling such occurrences as well as improving morale and the depth of a practice staff.

The individual positions' responsibilities will firm up when the staffing plan is sketched out. Consider the various types of employees needed to meet the requirements and objectives. The possibilities will include hiring full-time, permanent staff for key positions; part-time, permanent staff; full-time, short-term staff; and part-time, temporary or hourly staff. Again, the factors to be considered in the analysis include peak work loads, average work loads, fluctuations by seasons, clientele, training requirements, nature of work (specialized vs. nonspecialized), and overall real costs in terms of dollars. There are many formulas in staffing; each organization or business is unique and requires an approach that will work based on the work environment in the practice's locations.

□
Job analysis and development of job descriptions

The next step in the development of a staffing plan is to analyze each individual position and develop job descriptions. In the field of personnel management, a complete and accurate job description is a critical element in recruitment, selection, compensation, and evaluation. The description serves as a guide to job success by outlining objectives in relation to tasks assigned to the position. If the job description is well constructed, it can help the employee realize the high priorities in relation to the entire assignment. Highlighting the tasks of greater importance and assigning higher percentages of time allocated to certain areas of responsibility will assist the employer in communicating expectations when responsibilities conflict. The complete job description ensures the employee of a specific outline of accountable responsibilities.

Once the manager has analyzed personnel needs, the process of creating job descriptions for the practice has commenced. Compiling the component parts of the staffing pattern outline and combining these with observations of the position will enhance the manager's ability to write a complete description. If the practice currently has employees on staff, it is important to include their input in the process. The practitioner should interview the individual staff members or have them write their own version of their job description. By incorporating the employees' valuable input and information into the formal job description the supervisor will ensure completeness.

The complete job description includes the following: the title of the position, purpose of the job, relationship to other positions (i.e., supervisor, coworkers and, if applicable, subordinates), actual duties, normal working hours, equipment to be used and maintained, level of responsibility, and authority assigned to the position (Fig. 3-1). It is important to have percentages of responsibility assigned to

JOB DESCRIPTION
VETERINARY HOSPITAL

Name _____

Title of Position _____ Receptionist/Clerk _____

Purpose of the Position

Coordinate appointments, handle admissions, create records for the veterinary hospital. Act as general receptionist providing information, screening clients, taking messages, and greeting and directing the public. Coordinate work of veterinarians and staff. Handle discharge procedures and file records.

Position Reports to _____ Practice Manager _____

Position Supervises _____ (1) Full-time clerical assistant _____

_____ (2) Hourly clerical assistants _____

Percentage of Time Allocated	Specific Duties
40%	Responsible for admissions, including emergencies. Verify all client information, assign case numbers, and generate invoice and related paperwork. Enter data into computer via terminal. Page veterinarians assigned to case. Provide the staff all appropriate information. Direct the client to proper exam room. File all paperwork and work with medical records to ensure records are pulled, filed, and accounted for. At times, pull medical records as well as file.
15%	Set up appointments, rechecks, and consultations as requested by clients and veterinarians. Answer telephone; direct phone calls to

Figure 3-1. *Veterinary hospital job description*   (Continued)

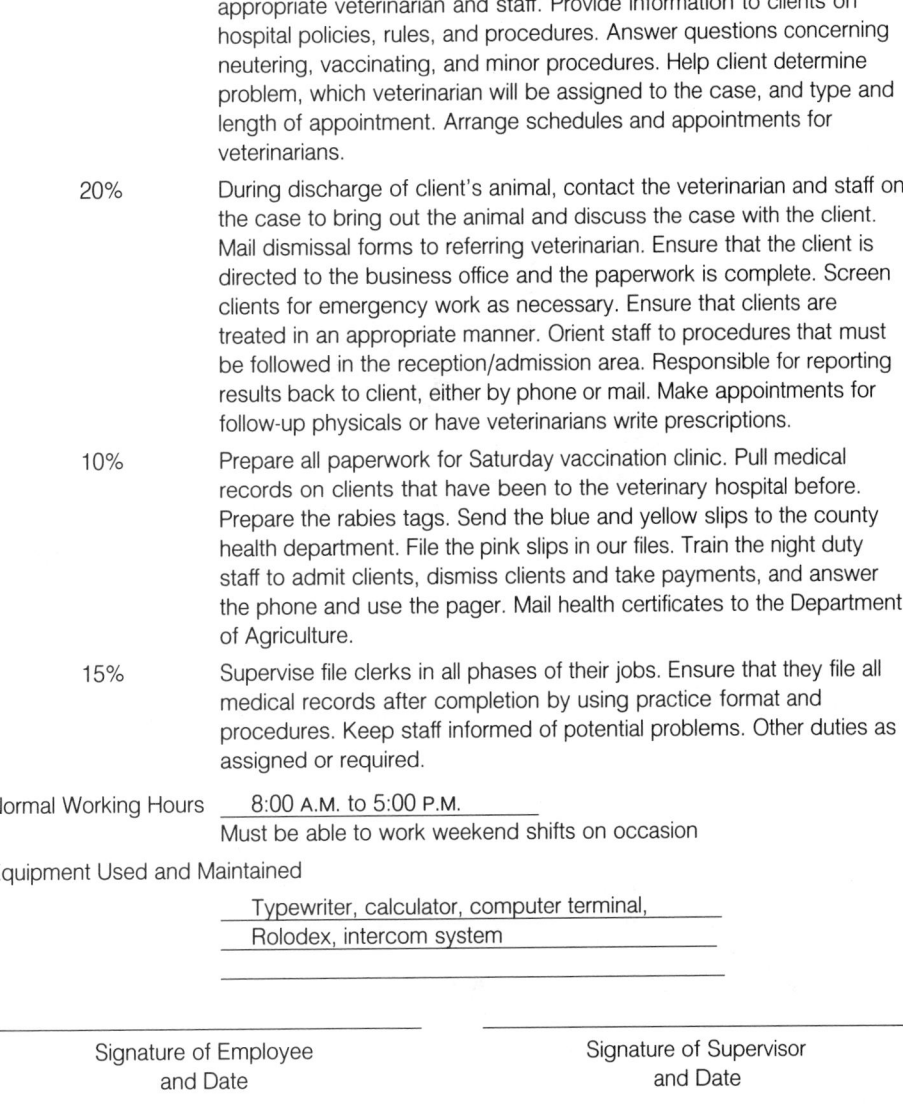

appropriate veterinarian and staff. Provide information to clients on hospital policies, rules, and procedures. Answer questions concerning neutering, vaccinating, and minor procedures. Help client determine problem, which veterinarian will be assigned to the case, and type and length of appointment. Arrange schedules and appointments for veterinarians.

20%   During discharge of client's animal, contact the veterinarian and staff on the case to bring out the animal and discuss the case with the client. Mail dismissal forms to referring veterinarian. Ensure that the client is directed to the business office and the paperwork is complete. Screen clients for emergency work as necessary. Ensure that clients are treated in an appropriate manner. Orient staff to procedures that must be followed in the reception/admission area. Responsible for reporting results back to client, either by phone or mail. Make appointments for follow-up physicals or have veterinarians write prescriptions.

10%   Prepare all paperwork for Saturday vaccination clinic. Pull medical records on clients that have been to the veterinary hospital before. Prepare the rabies tags. Send the blue and yellow slips to the county health department. File the pink slips in our files. Train the night duty staff to admit clients, dismiss clients and take payments, and answer the phone and use the pager. Mail health certificates to the Department of Agriculture.

15%   Supervise file clerks in all phases of their jobs. Ensure that they file all medical records after completion by using practice format and procedures. Keep staff informed of potential problems. Other duties as assigned or required.

Normal Working Hours   8:00 A.M. to 5:00 P.M.
                        Must be able to work weekend shifts on occasion

Equipment Used and Maintained

                        Typewriter, calculator, computer terminal,
                        Rolodex, intercom system

_____   _____
Signature of Employee   Signature of Supervisor
and Date   and Date

Figure 3-1. Veterinary hospital job description (Continued)

all duties or tasks. For example, if a technician should spend approximately 20% of the time maintaining treatment rooms in order, stocking supplies, or cleaning equipment, then the tasks and time allocated should be documented. Special conditions of employment including night, weekend, on-call, and shift work should also be listed in the description.

It is important to add the skills, abilities, and personal qualities necessary for success in the position. The overall job description should be clear, concise, and specific to eliminate confusion and provide direction. It is helpful to keep logs of activities for a period of time to assist in the writing process. For recruiting purposes and eventual compensation level, indicate on the description the minimum requirements for the work assignment including appropriate education and experience.

The process of developing job descriptions and creating a staffing pattern assists the practice manager in determining personnel requirements. The analysis will be complete when the components fit together. The manager should be able to take complete job descriptions (which, when combined, create a staffing pattern) and hours of coverage and establish clear outlines for personnel requirements. It is essential that the job analysis process continue through evaluation of results. If adjustments are necessary, update the job descriptions and staffing pattern. The creative manager will try new approaches and take calculated risks in assigning new duties, delegating responsibilities, and changing coverage plans to become more efficient and organized. The payoff for in-depth analysis and consistent review is improved productivity.

□
Recruitment and selection

Hiring the right individual is one of the most difficult tasks a manager will face. Making the wrong decision in the selection process can have ramifications for months, even years. Interviewing and selection, like any other skills, require training and experience. This section will attempt to provide the manager the basic requirements in the selection process outside of actual experience.

It is likely that the results of the selection process will be compromised when shortcuts are taken. Spend adequate time and attention in preparation and the actual interview process. Turnover among personnel is very time-consuming and expensive. Time spent up front can save countless hours in repairing the damage to the practice due to poor personnel decisions. The payoff will be evident in terms of reduced turnover, improved quality of employees, and in the long term, a savings in time spent dealing with problems.

Legal complications should be avoided by becoming knowledgeable in the labor laws of the U.S., state, and local governments. Although laws vary from location to location, it is important for the practice manager to know what practices are considered legal, illegal, or discriminatory. Equal Employment Opportunity legislation is specific and clearly outlines what is lawful in the selection process. Later in this chapter, a list of example questions that can be asked potential employees is provided. Good intention is a poor defense when breaking applicable laws in a specific locale. Diversity of the staff and equal opportunity are good business practices. Affirmative action programs are designed to go the extra step by expending more effort to hire and promote individuals in protected classes. It is important to be familiar with and have a working knowledge of all laws that apply to the practice. The practitioner can avoid discrimination problems by incorporating practices encouraged or legally required by governmental organizations. An overview of legal concerns of the practitioner can be found in Chapter 15.

Application forms and advertising

The collection of application forms and resumes in the application process is usually the first step leading to a screening of potential candidates for an open position. Application forms are, in broad terms, calling cards or work and education histories of individuals attempting to use their knowledge, skills, and abilities to find employment. They are tools that can provide basic information to screen out unacceptable candidates and provide a pool of individuals that will be worth the investment of time to interview or consider further for an open position. A well-constructed application form should also include space for personal information (i.e., name, address, home and work phones, social security number). The form should provide sections for education background, work history, reason for leaving past jobs, special skills and abilities, type of position individual is interested in, drivers license information, and any custom features unique to the needs of the practice (Fig. 3-2).

There are a number of methods that can be used to recruit new staff members. The easiest method is to have individuals looking for work fill out an application form when they drop by the practice inquiring about work opportunities. This method has its inherent problems but can suffice for certain positions. Advertising in local publications is a common method used by many businesses and organizations. If the practice advertises, the advertisement should be constructed to attract the type of individuals who would be successful candidates. The job title, minimum qualifications for the position, brief description of the job, rewards, and opportunities of the position should be clearly and concisely communicated. The advertisement should have eye appeal. It is important to be specific to save time by discouraging individuals who do not have acceptable qualifications from applying for the position.

Alternative methods to attract suitable candidates include contacting local professional organizations (e.g., the state veterinary medical association) or placement officials at institutions offering degree programs in veterinary technology or related fields for referrals. Trade journals and periodicals can be used to recruit professional staff. It is also a good strategy to list open positions for professional staff with colleges of veterinary medicine that have previously made contact with the practice. Circulating the word of an opening through the staff of the practice can lead to applicants worthy of consideration. In these situations, it is important to carefully screen individuals to avoid problems that could arise in the selection of an individual who might have conflicts of interest with existing staff. Employment and temporary agencies can be used in the right circumstances to help in recruitment. In certain circumstances they have merit; however, there are costs associated with this method, and the results typically vary significantly from one agency to another.

Interviewing

The next step in the selection process is to screen the applications or resumes that have been collected. It is then important to categorize the applications into three groups: (1) invite for an interview; (2) hold for future screening; or (3) reject.

Interviewing requires a structured approach to be effective. To prepare for the interview it is wise to have available or develop a list of questions for the open position. Examples of lawful questions that can be used or modified for use are provided in Table 3-1. If possible, it is wise to have assistance in the actual interview. Having two or three interviewers who can contribute their perceptions of the candidates will help in a final decision. The manager should make sure the interview team is composed of knowledgeable individuals who are mature, have good listening and communication skills, and represent various areas of the practice.

During the interview the candidate should be put at ease. It is appropriate to relax and relieve the tension by smiling and suggesting the individual make himself comfortable. Interviewers should decide in advance which questions they would like to ask and consistently ask the same questions with all candidates to create a basis to judge the responses to the same questions. Provide the applicant a period of time to verbally detail their work history, educational background, career aspirations, strengths, weaknesses, personal qualities, and specific interest in the position. One

EMPLOYMENT APPLICATION
VETERINARY HOSPITAL

Date _____

Name _____ Social Security No. _____
     (Last)   (First)   (M.I.)

Local Address _____

City _____ State _____ Zip _____

Telephone _____

Application for

_____ Full-Time, Permanent   _____ Weekend, Temporary

_____ Part-Time, Permanent   _____ Part-Time, Temporary

_____ Flexible Hours, On-Call

Employment Interests

_____ Clerical   _____ Maintenance   _____ Other,

_____ Animal Care   _____ Laboratory   Please List

_____ Accounting   _____ Technical   _____

Education   _____

High School _____ Graduated ____ Yes ____ No ____ GED
        (City)   (State)

College, Trade School, or Related Education

	Institution	Location	Dates	Major	Degree
1.					
2.					

Work History (List your most recent employer first)

1. Employer _____ From ____/____/____
                                           Mo.   Day   Yr.

   Address _____ To ____/____/____
                                           Mo.   Day   Yr.

   Your Title _____

   Duties _____ Hr/Wk _____

   _____ Salary _____

   Reason for Leaving or Seeking Other Employment

   _____ Supervisor _____

2. Employer _____ From ____/____/____
                                           Mo.   Day   Yr.

   Address _____ TO ____/____/____
                                           Mo.   Day   Yr.

   Your Title _____

   Duties _____ Hr/Wk _____

   _____ Salary _____

   Reason for Leaving or Seeking Other Employment

   _____ Supervisor _____

   _____

Figure 3-2. Veterinary hospital employment application

(Continued)

3. Employer _____   From _____/_____/_____
                                                        Mo.   Day   Yr.

Address _____   TO _____/_____/_____
                                                        Mo.   Day   Yr.

Your Title _____

Duties _____   Hr/Wk _____

_____   Salary _____

Reason for Leaving or Seeking Other Employment

_____   Supervisor _____

_____

Special Qualifications and Skills _____

Clerical Skills

Typing wmp _____   Shorthand wpm _____Other _____

References
    Full Name   Home or Business Address   Occupation

1. _____

2. _____

3. _____

Person to be notified in case of Emergency

Name _____   Address _____   Phone _____

Applicant Signature _____   Date _____

Figure 3-2.   Veterinary hospital employment application   (Continued)

question should be asked at a time, if an explanation or a request for additional information is necessary, then it should be provided without making the applicant feel uncomfortable.

Close-ended (yes or no) questions should not be asked. Interviewers need to hear the applicants' concepts, thoughts, and conclusions. It is important for the manager to sell the position and practice to the candidates during the process. If the candidate for the position is not provided a good impression of the practice and people who work there, a good potential employee could be lost due to lack of interest. Interview in a comfortable room away from distractions. Provide the applicant a copy of the job description before the actual interview begins. Sometime during the interview provide relevant information on the practice. Invite questions on the position, practice, or anything that the interviewee might have an interest in. Mention the strengths and weaknesses of the position. Give the applicant an honest view of the employment situation. Salary range and benefits should be discussed during the interview process.

The manager and staff involved in the employment interview process should be assessing the candidate for the position. They should remain objective, listening for key information to determine differences between the candidates. The interviewers should avoid premature decisions and keep an open mind about each candidate until the process is over. The interviewers should provide honest impressions of themselves to the candidate. It is important to avoid interrupting while the candidate is speaking. The interview team should read between the lines and ask questions that bring out the information needed to make an informed decision. The applicant's background, skills, abilities, employment record, communication skills, general intelligence, interest to learn, progress within their career, special interests, and personality should be

Table 3-1
Examples of interview questions

Would you please review your work history, including the jobs you have held, the duties and responsibilities, and why you left the positions?

Please review your educational background.

Describe your strengths in relation to the job description that was provided to you. Weaknesses?

Have you ever been discharged by an employer? If so what were the circumstances?

Why did you leave your previous job? Why are you considering leaving your current position?

What are the attractive features of the position we currently have open?

How does this position fit into your long-term career objectives?

Why should I select you for this particular opening?

Would have any problems lifting a 35-pound dog into a cage 4 feet off the ground?

How do you feel about working shift work, flextime, on call, overtime, weekends or split shift?

What kind of working relationship do you expect to have with a supervisor?

Do you have any allergies to animal hair, hay, straw, chemicals, and so forth?

Do you possess any special skills, abilities, or personal qualities that we should be aware of in relation to the position you are applying for?

How do you accept constructive criticisms during informal discussions?

What kind of working environment and interpersonal relationship do you desire in a new employment situation?

judged fairly. The interviewers should make notes on the candidates *between* interviews and spend a few minutes checking each other's individual perceptions. The applications and resumes should be available during the interviews to refer to and compare with the other candidates. Interviewers should be involved and in control of the process. It is important to have good eye contact and body posture. Interviewers should let the interviewee do most of the talking and must ensure that the meeting keeps moving by asking questions when the timing and flow of the inter-

view require it. At the end of the interview, indicate how long the selection process will continue and how the final decision will be communicated.

Making a selection decision

The next step in the selection process is to check references, study employment records, and contact past supervisors and employers. Some employers prefer to do this before the interview. It is the author's opinion that contact with past employers and references is more meaningful after meeting the candidates. Assessment of the individual and checking perceptions of the candidate with more informed people will provide for a reality check. When checking a candidate's background, inquiries should include questions on willingness to work, independence of action, follow-through, loyalty to the organization, job knowledge, personality traits, and reason for leaving. If there are inconsistencies in perceptions or in the account provided by the candidate, there is definite reason for concern. The interviewers will have to weigh the credibility of the sources against that of the applicants to decide which information will be used as a basis for making a selection decision.

With the notes taken during the interview, applications or resumes, information gathered from references and past employers, job description, and any other information available, the interviewers should size up each candidate. The individual offered the position must have the best *match* of qualifications for the position and does not necessarily have to be the individual with the highest level of experience. It is also important to select for compatibility by hiring the individual with the personality and qualities that will fit well with the existing staff. Other factors to consider are interest in the position and practice, communication skills, job intelligence, motivation, and professionalism. The individual with a realistic view of the position will have a higher likelihood of succeeding than a person who has an inflated picture of the job. Another important factor to consider is the degree of supervision the individual will require or how independently the person can work. The manager needs to know how much can be delegated and the requirements the individual will need for direction in relation to the personnel resources available.

The job offer

The final decision to offer the position to a particular candidate has been made. Now it is time to offer the job to the individual. The manager should indicate to the individual the reasons for selection and then offer the position. If a salary range was discussed during the interview, then a firm offer should now be tendered. The individual should be given adequate time to decide whether to accept or decline the offer. The individual may accept the position at the time the offer is made or may need time to think about the offer and to discuss it with family. The manager should be prepared for a rejection of the offer or a counteroffer. Managers should decide in advance whether they are willing to negotiate and who will be offered the position if the number one candidate declines. Once the offer is firm, the starting date should be established. It is proper to provide at least 2 weeks notice to the current employer of the individual. Letters of rejection should be sent to the interviewees who were not successful to thank them for their interest and indicate that their resumes or application forms will be retained for future consideration.

□
Salary and benefits

Determining a fair and equitable salary package the practice can afford is a process the manager should become familiar with establishing. In setting salary and benefits for em-
ployees, the concept of equal pay for equal work is the primary consideration in setting remuneration rates. For example, if the practice employs four animal care attendants, it is important that a structure be in place so all four individuals will be paid fairly. It is not necessary that all four be paid the same rate. It is appropriate to increase salary rates from the base pay for longevity, merit, level of responsibility, shift work, and so forth. Pay rates should be able to be defended and free of bias (i.e., not based on friendship, sex, race, or any other discriminatory practice).

The factors to consider in setting salary rates for the positions in a practice include skill level, educational requirements, degree of responsibility, independence from direct supervision, degree of supervision required of the position, numbers of subordinates that report to the position, and level of decision making required. In developing a salary plan, it is wise to have a tiered approach for comparable groups (i.e., veterinary technicians, animal attendants, and clerical/business staff). The tiers include entry level, full working level, and advanced skills/supervisory. The base rate for each tier should not include merit increases, longevity pay, shift differential, or other optional items.

To set actual rates it is suggested that a market survey for comparable positions be performed by using benchmark positions (i.e., journeyman veterinary technician). By contacting other willing veterinary practices and analyzing the prevailing wages, the manager can set rates that are affordable without over- or underpaying employees. The purpose of this approach is to keep good staff, maintain morale, limit turnover, which is costly, and improve employee relations. The rate paid for each category of position is still the manager's decision; however, it should be based on factual information rather than guessing. Another approach that can be used is to contact the local or state veterinary associations to assist in the process of collecting and analyzing the data. It is also possible to survey comparable types of positions outside of veterinary medicine for businesses that have similar positions (i.e., clerical, accounting, laboratory personnel). The important adage to remember is "you get what you pay for." Managers sometimes do not look beyond what a worker costs per hour and do not consider the full costs of turnover, training personnel constantly, continuity, and so forth. The practice should not overextend itself. The main point is that personnel should be paid fair salaries in order to obtain and keep qualified personnel who are able to add to the effectiveness and success of the entire operation.

There are two categories of benefits provided by an employer, those that are optional (i.e., vacation days, sick leave, health insurance) and those that are required by legislation (i.e., social security, workmen's compensation, and unemployment insurance premiums). It is to the benefit of the practice manager to provide employees information on both types of benefits so the staff realizes there are real costs associated with employment that come directly from the employer.

Nonoptional or required benefits are usually the result of federal or state regulations. The employer can somewhat control expenses in those areas by improving documentation. In the case of unemployment insurance, it is important to document the actual reasons for termination (i.e., quit to take another job, discharged due to poor performance). The records maintained on employees can be used in an unemployment compensation claim by a former employee. The documentation of incidents can cut down on the premium paid by the practice as determined by the level of paid claims. Workmen's compensation claims for injuries on the job must also be documented immediately after their occurrence. It is important to have safety procedures in place and instruct new staff on preventing accidents and injuries.

Optional benefits the practice pays for or arranges are important components of the remuneration package of full- or part-time permanent staff. Not all practices can afford to or are large enough to be able to provide certain plans like group health, life, and disability insurance. There are associations that can provide group-type coverage through volume and special plans. Some employers can contract with health providers directly. It is wise for the employer to explore as many alternatives as possible: dealing directly with health care providers, life and health insurance companies, veterinary associations, and health maintenance organizations. Costs and coverage are so varied and complex that a review in this chapter would not be productive. Health and life insurance coverage is a benefit that employees desire and some view as a requisite. Chapter 10 covers the subject of practice and personal protection.

Another popular benefit is vacation, holiday, and sick leave. Leave programs are easy to administer and provide employees time off with pay. The employer can determine the holiday schedule when the practice actually closes. Typical holidays include New Year's Day, Memorial Day, Independence Day, Labor Day, Thanksgiving, and Christmas. Emergency clinics and some practices do not close. Employers can provide floating holidays (vacation leave in lieu of the actual holiday) to be taken at a time agreed upon by the employee and employer.

Vacation time is a benefit earned by employees in most businesses and organizations. The majority of vacation programs require that an employee work at least a year to earn 5 to 10 days of leave. After 5 to 10 years of service, employers typically increase the amount of vacation leave to 10 to 15 days per year. Again, leave programs vary tremendously. Another type of leave program can provide that sick leave be used for illness or medical treatment exclusively. Businesses that have sick leave policies normally provide the leave in addition to vacation time with a maximal accrual rate or specific rules for use. A new trend employers are trying is to combine vacation, sick, and personal leave, thereby providing "paid time off." The employee can then divide the time in any manner they wish. Employers who are using the plan indicate that abuse of sick leave is reduced. The majority of businesses and organizations view leave with pay as an important benefit that provides for security, renewal for the employee, incentives for longevity, and loyalty. It is a benefit most employees desire as much if not more than salary increases. Providing a leave program has a real cost in dollar terms; however, it is one of the most effective benefits that can be provided without any complexity outside of arranging for coverage for the absence of employees on leave.

Another benefit an employer can introduce without a great deal of effort is flextime. This is only possible when the coverage is deep enough to provide adequate staffing. Flextime provides employees the ability to work a schedule that meets their personal needs yet still provides coverage for the employer at times when the practice is open. An example of a flextime schedule for an employee who is pursuing a degree program part-time at a university could be working from 7:00 A.M. to 11:00 A.M. and then returning after classes at 2:00 P.M. and staying until 6:00 P.M. The advantage to the employee is the ability to continue his or her education and still have a full-time job. The employer could benefit by having increased coverage at times that are difficult to staff. Of course, this is just one example. The concept, however, can be a benefit to the employer and employee as long as both parties can agree and performance is not compromised. Other variations include 4-day, 10-hour shifts or 6-day, 6-hour shifts for employees with special needs and employers who want different coverage plans. Flextime can help a

working parent meet commitments for child care arrangements and provide employees the feeling that they are not just workers who have no control of their schedules.

In summary, benefit programs can be complex, hard to administer, and expensive or simple, inexpensive, easy to administer, or a combination of the two extremes. The practice manager needs to be creative, cost conscious, and understanding of employee needs and desires. The human resources of a practice are its most important assets. Good benefit programs can avoid turnover, which is expensive and time-consuming. Benefits must be viewed in relation to overall remuneration; salary should be blended with benefit plans that attract potential employees and keep loyal, productive workers.

New employee orientation, handbooks, and procedure manuals

Providing new employees with the right information at the right time is essential in the development of a good working relationship. Employees need to know the policies, procedures, and guidelines of the practice. New employee orientation meetings can help the practice manager in the orientation process. Having a formal meeting covering specific policies and general information is the most efficient way to ensure items are covered. It is suggested that an orientation checklist be used as the outline for the meeting. Figure 3-3 is an example of a checklist that can be adapted for any type of practice. The checklist covers policies and regulations including dress codes (if applicable), work hours, lunch and break policies, time clocks, and leave procedures. The system the practice relies on for increases in salary (merit, longevity, or other) should be communicated during the orientation period. If the practice has a probationary period, it should be detailed. Guidelines for promo-

ORIENTATION CHECKLIST

Name _____   Date _____

Position _____   Supervisor/Manager _____

Items to Be Covered During Orientation

General Information
_____ Hospital organization and structure
_____ Policy on breaks, lunch hours, smoking
_____ Parking regulations — staff, client, utility and maintenance areas
_____ Dress code as required (reception, laboratories, surgery, animal care, utility work)

Personnel Guidelines
_____ Salary and brief review of benefits
_____ Regulations on promotion
_____ Evaluation process
_____ Probation period for new employees
_____ Salary increases
_____ Disciplinary procedures

Policies and Regulations
_____ Working hours, workweek, weekends, or call policy
_____ Time clock (if applicable) or time sheets
_____ Requesting and reporting leave
_____ Accrual of leave — definition of sick, annual, LWOP, etc.
_____ Overtime requirements
_____ Punctuality, attendance
_____ Pay periods
_____ Holidays

Public Relations
_____ Importance of working effectively with clients
_____ Importance of working effectively with other staff members and veterinarians
_____ Working with referring veterinarians

Facilities/Safety
_____ Telephone system
_____ Building security
_____ Fire evacuation
_____ Workmen's compensation
_____ Reporting accidents
_____ Emergency assistance
_____ Restricted areas
_____ Tour of facilities, introduction of staff and coworkers

I acknowledge that the orientation meeting was held and the items above were discussed.

_____   _____
Employee's   Supervisor's
Signature and Date   Signature and Date

(Continued)

Figure 3-3. Orientation checklist

Administrative (Checklist for Office)

_____ Personnel folder
_____ Application form and/or resume
_____ Sick, annual, holiday leave record blanks
_____ Keys issued
_____ Mailbox, office space, or closet assigned
_____ Added to staff directory

_____
Signature of Manager

Termination (Checklist for Office)

_____ Personnel folder removed and filed, records completed
_____ Keys returned
_____ Deletion from staff directory

_____
Signature of Manager

Figure 3-3. Orientation checklist (Continued)

tions and job title changes should be outlined. It is also beneficial during the orientation meeting to review salary benefits, general organization of the practice, philosophy of management, and any other pertinent information. It is wise to have the employee ask questions and have two-way communication to ensure a common understanding of all issues. At the conclusion of the meeting the employee and the manager should sign a copy of the checklist, and the manager should date and then file it in the new employee's personnel folder. This action documents that the meeting occurred and the items were covered. The checklist can provide the manager backing in disputes over issues that might arise during the employee's tenure on the job.

After the orientation meeting it is good protocol to introduce the new employee to staff members who have not met the new individual. Tour the facilities and instruct the employee on safety and emergency procedures.

Handbooks and procedure manuals are useful tools for the practice manager. Handbooks can outline in detail the terms of employment and other items listed on the administrative checklist. The development of a handbook is time-consuming, but once completed, it needs to be updated only occasionally. It can provide a reference for both employee and employer by detailing the personnel program of the practice. Again, problems relating to employment issues can be resolved if detailed policies and procedures are provided in writing. Specific items that can be included are payroll periods, evaluation process, benefits, rights and responsibilities of employment, policies and procedures, and philosophy of the practice. The handbook's complexity and items covered should be only as involved as the personnel program of the practice.

Procedure manuals provide the employee detailed instructions on how to execute their responsibilities. They provide a cookbook approach to handling specific tasks and duties. Procedure manuals are also used as reference materials and actually document business practices. Developing a procedures manual can help the practice manager reorganize work methods.

The components of a good procedures manual include job descriptions for the work area, interrelationships between the position and sections in the practice, the actual steps in each procedure, and what to do in emergency situations. For example, a receptionist procedures manual could highlight the following topics:

1. Introduction
2. Opportunities for growth and development
3. Responsibilities of reception area and other sections
4. Job description
5. Procedures: admissions, information, data entry, medical records, discharge
6. Communication skills: standard responses, telephone etiquette, taking notes
7. Questions frequently asked with typical answers
8. Miscellaneous information: client management skills, emergency procedures, building evacuation plan in case of fire, and so forth.

The procedures manual should be given to the employee after the orientation session. Providing a manual to an individual can be the first step in the training process.

□
Training new employees

The amount of training necessary for a new employee to become effective on the job will vary tremendously from individual to individual and from one position to another. When an experienced individual is hired for a specific position, the training period can be shortened to learning the way the practice operates. On the other hand, if the practice has employed a person with little occupational knowledge, training will consume hours of time and will be extensive. Regardless of who is hired, it is important to have a plan in place to train the individual. A performance planning meeting (covered elsewhere in this chapter) should occur before the training begins. It is wise to have time set aside for specific training objectives, especially in areas of responsibility that are technical in nature and require special attention. In a complete training program safety issues and maintenances of equipment should also be incorporated along with the basic procedures. Outlining the training program in writing will assist the manager or supervisor in the process. If possible, dates and times should be scheduled into the outline. The goal of each training session should be clear and concise.

The direct supervisor or individual with the highest level of job knowledge should be responsible for training the new employee. The trainer should have the ability to notice problems in performance as well as praise good work and initiative. On-the-job training can be supplemented with reading pertinent information such as journal articles, textbooks, procedure manuals, and other professional publications. The qualities necessary to be a good trainer include strong communication skills, willingness to assume the responsibility, good organization, and perceptiveness. The trainer should build on success and emphasize the positive as well as point out problems to provide objective, constructive criticism.

Performance should be reviewed frequently during the training period. It is important for the trainer to be realistic about how much can be accomplished and not push the training period too fast. The trainer should allow the employee to do as much of the work as possible early in the training program. The trainer should be advising, watching, and instructing, not just teaching by example. Individuals learn quickly when they have to actually perform the tasks and duties for themselves. The trainer should always keep in mind the ultimate objectives for the position in relation to the final job description. The trainer should be sensitive to overtraining the new employee, which can be as big a problem as undertraining. The new employee should not be bombarded or overwhelmed to the point of questioning whether the job is going to work out satisfactorily.

There should be a conclusion to the training period (i.e., 3 months, 6 months, or a year when the employee is deemed to have completed the program). This should be coupled with the review of performance in the evaluation process. If, during the training period, the employee's performance is not satisfactory and progress toward reaching the goals for the position is limited, the employee may need to be discharged. It should be determined whether the employee has been given adequate time to master the assignment. The employee should have been given feedback along the way so that if discharge is necessary the personnel action will not be a surprise. This should be a rare occurrence, especially if the interview process was conducted well.

Training should not cease after the probationary period. In-service training programs should become a regular part of the personnel program. Technicians can become specialists in certain procedures and pass on new skills to other staff. The practice manager should encourage employees to join professional and technical associations. It is important to send staff to continuing education courses offered through veterinary associations. There are many seminars, conferences, and continuing education programs that can enhance the skills of professional, technical, and support personnel. Employees appreciate the opportunity of advanced training. The practice re-

ceives the advantage of improved or new skills, recognition for the employees, and a boost in morale.

Whatever methods a practice manager uses to encourage continuation of the learning process will keep the practice stimulated. Individuals that feel they can contribute to the effectiveness of an operation will tend to perform at a higher level.

□
Performance appraisal

The evaluation process provides the practice manager or supervisor the tools necessary for planning, measuring, and changing the performance of employees. The job performance evaluation form (Fig. 3-4) assists the manager in the process of providing structure and a mechanism to formalize the agreements during the planning process. Evaluation forms are only as good as the individuals who use them. If the process is not taken seriously or if it is treated as a piece of paperwork that has to be completed, its usefulness will be diminished.

In a basic performance appraisal process there are three requirements: (1) a performance plan with specific goals and objectives outlined in a planning session between the supervisor and employee, (2) feedback during the period between the planning session and review meeting, and (3) the evaluation or review meeting where performance is discussed and a rating is determined. The process should be viewed as a cycle, with the next planning session occurring at the end of the evaluation meeting.

The planning meeting requires two-way communications between the supervisor and employee with an underlying theme of improving performance and productivity and developing a common understanding of the goals and objectives of the position. The job description should be reviewed at each planning session and updated or modified if

JOB PERFORMANCE
EVALUATION FORM
VETERINARY HOSPITAL

NAME _____ JOB TITLE _____ Chief Technician _____

EVALUATION PERIOD <u>1-1-88</u> to <u>12-31-88</u>

REASON FOR REPORT: <u>Yearly Evaluation</u>

RATING SCALE

4	3	2	1	0
Outstanding	Very Good	Good	Poor	Unsatisfactory
Exceeds all expectations	Exceeds expectations	Meets expectations	Fails to achieve expectations	

PERFORMANCE FACTORS

	Proportion × Rating = Factor Assigned Rating
I. <u>Quality of technical work, patient care, technical preparation</u> <u>for procedures, emergency organization</u>	.30 × 3 = .9
II. <u>Maintenance of equipment and treatment areas, stock</u> <u>always available. Areas maintained between procedures.</u> <u>Equipment serviced.</u>	.20 × 2 = .4
III. <u>Relationships with people: Shows cooperation, respect,</u> <u>communications skills, courtesy and is a role model for others</u>	.15 × 3 = .45
IV. <u>Work habits: Shows punctuality, adherence to protocol, sup-</u> <u>port for staff, concern for safety</u>	.15 × 4 = .6
V. <u>Effectiveness of supervision: Leads, directs, evaluates one</u> <u>new technician and one part-time animal care attendant</u>	.20 × 3 = .6
VI. Other _____	.NA × NA = NA
Total	100% × Score = 2.95
	OVERALL SCORE: 2.95

Figure 3-4. Veterinary hospital job performance evaluation form

(Continued)

		SCORE TABLE
_____	Outstanding	3.5–4.0
___X___	Very Good	2.5–3.49
_____	Good	2.0–2.49
_____	Poor	1.0–1.99

Comments:

_____

_____

_____

_____

_____

_____

_____

_____

_____

_____

_____

_____   _____

Supervisor's Signature   Date

_____   _____

Employee's Signature   Date

Figure 3-4.   Veterinary hospital job performance evaluation form   (Continued)

changes are necessary. Performance factors should be identified on the evaluation form, with specific performance objectives outlined in writing. For example, a factor for a veterinary technician could be maintaining equipment and facilities and stocking supply cabinets. Specific performance objectives for this factor could include cleaning and storing equipment after each procedure, servicing the anesthesia equipment weekly, sterilizing surgical instruments each day by using the new protocol, stocking examination and treatment rooms each day, and ensuring adequate supplies of certain items. For the receptionist in a practice an example of a factor could be interpersonal relations. Specific performance objectives could include improving telephone skills, checking on clients in the reception area, showing interest and concern, keeping other staff informed of problems, and greeting clients in a particular manner. The examples given may or may not be pertinent to any particular practice. They are intended to illustrate how factors and performance objectives can be customized to an individual position.

Factors and objectives should be concise and provide direction. The number of factors used is totally dependent on how complex the position is and how detailed the supervisor wants each factor to be. Another consideration in the planning session is whether the supervisor wants to have the factors be equal or weigh them differently. For example, if you have had four factors, each should equal 25% of the overall evaluation, or if two were more important out of the four, you could weight them unevenly. Two factors could be 30% each; the remaining two could each be worth 20%.

The second phase in the evaluation is providing ongoing coaching and feedback. Telling employees they are meeting objectives or they need to improve their performance in a specific factor area is part of the evaluation process. It is also wise to have one formal midyear meeting to review the performance plan, change or revise it based on new responsibilities or priorities, and also provide feedback on how the individual is progressing toward goals and objectives. During the midyear meeting, it is important to ask employees how they perceive their progress.

The final phase in the appraisal process is the formal evaluation. Before the review meeting the manager or supervisor should fill out the evaluation form in pencil and, use a rating scale similar to the one found on the evaluation form (see Fig. 3-4). Each factor should be given a separate rating and, if appropriate, comments on performance detailed in the space provided or on an attached sheet. The rater should be careful when selecting a rating to avoid bias and preconceived notions. Observations, documentation of incidents, actual results, and examination of behavior should be the basis for the ratings. The evaluation session should be a balance of providing praise and constructive criticism. An honest appraisal will be respected by the employee. Overinflating or underinflating ratings can be counterproductive. Employees know their own strengths and weaknesses and in most cases will desire feedback that is based on reality and designed to improve performance.

The evaluation meeting should be held in private away from the distractions of the practice. Both parties should be prepared and know the meeting date several days in advance of the session. The supervisor should ask for a self-appraisal after discussing the ratings and should be prepared to change the rating if new, relevant information is provided. If the appraisal is fair and agreed upon, both parties should sign and date the form. The next order of business is to proceed to next year's plan by developing a new set of goals and objectives and updating the job description if necessary.

Special attention should be given to factors that need additional work in the upcoming year, and praise should be given in recognizing the outstanding work in a factor area the past year. Evaluation meetings with employees leave definite impressions on staff members. The meeting should be used as a motivational experience for all concerned. Showing a high level of concern, communication, professionalism, honesty, and willingness to respond to issues during appraisal meetings provides a renewal period and higher levels of interest and productivity. The evaluation process also aids the practice manager in long-term planning by assessing the strengths and weaknesses of the current staff, thereby providing possibilities for further delegation of responsibility and assisting in determination of salary increases based on merit. In summary, a solid appraisal system is essential in effectively performing all major personnel functions and is worth the investment in time and effort by the professional practice manager or supervisor.

□
Motivating employees

To realize the full potential of the staff, it is important to understand and use motivational theories and techniques. Each individual has his own personal goals and objectives and will respond differently to the varied approaches available. People work for many reasons including financial remuneration, achievement, recognition, and personal growth. Salary and benefits are important motivators that will influence an employee's performance. Increases in salary and other financial considerations like bonuses or employee benefit plans can increase productivity. The subject of salary and benefits has been covered in greater detail earlier in the chapter. This section will concentrate on less-concrete but extremely important motivational concepts and techniques.

There are many influences on whether an individual is satisfied with their job. If the salary and benefits are adequate and the individual is able to meet their financial requirements for housing, food, and the other needs, the individual's satisfaction on the job will then be related to the intangible rewards of the position. Typical considerations for the motivated employee will include the challenge of the position, recognition of work accomplishments, level of responsibility and authority attained, growth potential, and a sense of contribution. Not every position in a veterinary practice can provide employees an environment where they will be able to be motivated in terms of the aforementioned considerations. It is also important to recognize there are individual employees who cannot grow to assume higher levels of achievement or do not desire growth opportunities. A strong manager needs to develop a working environment that will maximize each employee's potential. In a world of changing values, individualizing your approach will assist the motivated employee who desires a high level of achievement as well as recognize the employee who wants to be a steady, hard worker and is happy in a more controlled, directed setting.

In general, the majority of professional and technical personnel want to work in an environment where they can be fairly autonomous. They want to know their responsibilities but also want to have a sense of control where they can exercise judgment and achieve high levels of performance on their own. The progressive manager will encourage this kind of activity and will recognize and support their efforts. The manager will respect employee input and acknowledge that their training and background can provide new ideas or improvements for the practice. If the veterinarian or technician wants to participate in local associations for development and advanced training, progressive practice managers will encourage it and will, if they can afford to, provide financial assistance for continuing education programs. The advantages to this approach are evident. Managers who tend to box up employees and limit growth can eventually be dealing with disenchanted individuals who are not challenged. Initiative should be rewarded to enhance an environment that should lead to improved service and operations. By broadening the horizons of the staff the practice can grow, and new services and procedures can be offered to clients. Today's practice needs to be prepared for tomorrow's world if it is to succeed and prosper.

Rotating assignments, cross-training, and adding new responsibilities can motivate employees who are in a job rut. By having the staff members train each other the practice will not only operate smoothly with reduced staff, it will also provide opportunities for growth, achievement, and recognition. Cross-training will cut through boredom and will create situations where the manager will be able to acknowledge the contributions of staff members who demonstrate diversified skills and abilities.

If this type of approach is new or foreign to the staff, changes in assignments could lead to stress and defensiveness. This should not dissuade the supervisor from cross-training. The practice manager needs to be a role model and can possibly rotate assignments with the rest of the staff. The manager or practitioner should sell their ideas and present a realistic view of the benefits and drawbacks of the changes. They should seek input in either group settings or individual meetings far in advance of the changes to address potential problems. The meetings should not lead to elimination of the proposed changes due to employee insecurity. The manager should always indicate that the situation will work out and adjustments can be made if necessary. Allow employees to become experts in certain areas. This will provide ownership in the change process and will provide recognition.

One of the most effective motivators can be a comment at the end of the day saying "you really did a great job today" or "thanks for the extra effort." Managers who have the right training and know when to provide direct verbal recognition usually have employees who respect them. Individuals who point out the positive when possible avoid employees who dwell on the negative issues. Building a spirit of pride and team effort can be the most important motivator an individual has without adding a penny of expense to the practice. This type of recognition is good for everyone from the animal care attendant to the co-owner of the practice. Thanking and praising people are contagious and will work through the entire organization. Showing interest in the employee's hobbies like baseball, skiing, and photography is a wise investment in time. Talking to them occasionally in the hall, reception area, barns, wards, or surgery suite will demonstrate interest. This strategy will help in the management role and will improve employee relations. Humor is also a good tool to use, especially in stressful situations. Telling a joke, sharing a funny thought, or even acknowledging a personality quirk leads to a comfortable working environment. Working relationships that develop in this manner tend to elicit loyalty and esprit de corps that will pay off when times are tough.

□
Communications and counseling employees

Effective managers realize communication between employees and management is essential to maintaining good working relationships. They also realize their methods in this area of responsibility rely on their own initiative. Employees desire two-way communications and should not be expected to start the communication process. The practice manager should open the door to invite communications, including setting up staff meetings and regular informal discussions on issues of importance. The manager or supervisor should encourage participation and keep meetings moving and productive. Sticky issues should not be avoided; honesty and objectivity on the part of the manager will be respected. It is important to maintain control of the sessions. Avoid getting into an argument with an employee. Provide explanations of procedures, changes, policies, and the rationale for decisions without becoming defensive.

During a meeting with a staff member or group of employees, it is critical to give the individual or group full attention. It is important to avoid working on other tasks or becoming distracted. If there is not enough time for the meeting, then reschedule it. Try to avoid dealing with personnel issues while working on a client's animal or in front of other staff. There is no quicker way to lose the respect of staff than airing problems in front of individuals who should not be involved in the discussion. Maintaining confidentiality is an important approach in dealing with personnel problems or sensitive communication.

There are times when managers must counsel staff members with personal concerns or problems. This is a natural role that many times is uncomfortable or difficult to handle. In a counseling situation the manager should maintain objectivity and avoid value judgments that could alienate the employee. One of the pitfalls to be avoided in counseling is getting directly involved in the problem by intervening or personally trying to handle the situation. A manager cannot make decisions for an employee. Managers should know their limitations in counseling the staff member. It is important to know when to back out and suggest professional support.

□
Conflict, resolution, and disciplinary action

There will be situations occurring where the manager disagrees with an employee's opinion. This type of interaction between a supervisor and a subordinate can be healthy. People can agree or disagree in a professional manner. When the disagreement turns into a conflict that is not resolved, the manager must then deal with the issue. There are common signs of unresolved problems including offhand comments, the staff member discussing the problem with clients or other staff not involved, and increased levels of gossip. The manager should take control of the situation by opening the lines of communication. If compromise will not jeopardize the manager's position or is in the best interest of the practice, negotiations can resolve the problem. If individual positions have hardened and there is no room for negotiations, then the employee must be warned to stop the inappropriate behavior so as to avoid disciplinary action. The manager should be sure the issue is worth creating a confrontation and should weigh the potential outcome of taking action. Gossip can be a destructive force on morale and employee performance and should be brought out into the open when out of control.

The wise manager knows not to listen too hard or to take everything too seriously. There is always an informal communication organization in a business, and it serves a useful function as long as it is understood and in control. There is no substitute for good judgment in knowing when to intervene and resolve conflict or letting an issue die due to lack of interest. By encouraging constructive criticism and having open lines of communication, gossip,

conflict, and related problems will seldom become important issues.

In dealing with disciplinary problems the number one rule to remember is that the practice manager or individual at the top is the role model and trendsetter in the practice. Managers live in a fishbowl. Their behavior is examined and evaluated. When an individual supervises others, a cardinal rule to follow is "Behave and conduct yourself as a professional on the job and expect no less from yourself than from any employee." The phrase "Do as I say, not as I do" will not work in the long run. Potential problems will be avoided by conducting business with integrity and honesty. Rank does have its privileges but should not be carried to extremes. Setting an example by coming to work on time, treating clients and staff with respect, handling money and receivables carefully, not breaking practice rules or policies, and maintaining good work habits will avoid inviting problems. Do not be seen out of control. It is fine to relax controls for special occasions; however, it should be clear to the staff that the change is an exception rather than the rule.

Discipline problems that are serious enough to warrant action affect businesses and organizations that are large or small. The small or large veterinary practice, however, should follow the same *basic* steps and procedures used by large businesses. The procedures may seem time-consuming, involved, or too much trouble to managers, but there are good reasons for having a formalized set of procedures. Having predetermined steps in a disciplinary action process protects the employer from claims of arbitrary decisions. It also provides employees a process that is fair and consistent from individual to individual, which protects against morale problems and claims of harassment or preferential treatment.

In setting up the disciplinary process for the practice, the manager should always have a complete set of employee records. Information that should be maintained includes the application form, orientation checklist, current address and phone number, dates of promotions, pay increases, and other personnel actions along with the notation and signature of the individual approving the action, leave accrued and taken, absences, evaluations, and other relevant records.

The word *discipline* has both negative and positive connotations. Viewing a well-disciplined drill team performing difficult routines in unison creates a positive feeling. On the negative side, discipline in the work setting suggests reprimands and punishment. The effective manager views disciplinary action as a tool to guide employees with performance or personal problems to full productivity.

Disciplinary action is one stage in a complete process. The usual steps consist of (1) informal warning, (2) formal warning with accompanying interview, (3) disciplinary action (sanctions), and finally (4) termination. The action taken to solve a problem is a judgment call in most cases. The general guideline to follow is to start with the lowest acceptable level that is appropriate for the offense. For example, if an employee strikes another employee or supervisor without provocation, termination would be in order. If an employee is an hour late for the first time in 1 year of employment, then an informal warning is probably appropriate.

The manager needs to review the cause of the problem and hear the employee's side of the situation before determining the course of action. An absence or tardiness could be the result of an unforeseen problem that has a justifiable reason. If the reason for the problem is poor, then the manager should document the problem by writing an incident report recording the nature of the problem, what behavior change is required, the time frame for improvement, and the consequences if inappropriate behavior occurs again. It is wise to provide the employee a copy of the documentation and file the practice's copy in the employee's personnel file.

Strategies to deal with problem employees

The practice manager, supervisor, or lead worker should never avoid dealing with the problem employee. The failure of managers to deal with small problems leads to larger problems. Managers need to be assertive and rely on the aforementioned approach. The manager cannot afford to be intimidated or avoid the problem because of a fear of hurting the feelings of an employee. The experienced manager will attempt to channel anger into changes in performance and attitude.

Absenteeism and tardiness directly effect productivity and can disrupt business if the behavior is not checked immediately. Having firm guidelines on requesting time off and calling in when unforeseen problems arise can curb problems. When an employee continues to come to work late and informal warnings have not helped, a formal warning and disciplinary meeting is in order. A written behavioral contract can be the outcome of a disciplinary meeting warning the employee that if the pattern of behavior continues the outcome may be discharge. In cases of continued absences due to illness, it is appropriate to ask for a physician's statement verifying that the employee is seeking treatment. In most cases requesting a release will eliminate inappropriate behavior unless the employee has a true medical problem. Falsification of physician verification procedures is cause for dismissal. Follow-up on your agreements and discussions protects your credibility. If the employee forgets to provide verification, the manager must insist on the documentation even if it is known the individual was sick.

Alcohol or drug abuse can affect the performance of an individual dramatically. It is rare that an employee will be caught at work partaking of drugs or alcohol. The signs that are apparent are the side-effects such as impaired performance, illness, deterioration of work habits, and other physical signs. Dealing with these types of problems depends on the severity of the abuse, willingness of the manager to deal with the problem, disruption to the practice, and legal issues in the case of drugs.

The strategy suggested to be used for the employee who is an asset to the practice is to confront the issue head on. The first step would be to meet with the employee and frankly discuss concerns. If the employee acknowledges the problem and is willing to correct his behavior and seek professional help, then a behavioral contract should be developed that outlines the problem including performance, work habits, and anything that applies to the situation. In the contract it should be a requirement that employees document and provide verification that they will seek professional help such as Alcoholics Anonymous meetings, rehabilitation program, or counseling from a physician or psychologist. The consequences of failure to meet the contract stipulations (sanctions or termination) should be written into the agreement. Using the counseling skills as described elsewhere in this chapter is important. The practice manager cannot accept responsibility for the staff member's life. If the individual refuses to acknowledge the problem and documentation on the individual's behavior problem is solid, the only available option would be termination of employment. Keeping alcoholics or drug abusers on your staff and hoping they will change their behavior on their own is a poor approach. The practice that avoids the issue will pay the price in loss of productivity, poor morale among the staff due to their carrying the individual's work load, and possible liability issues of the person working while impaired.

The employee who is caught stealing money or supplies should be dealt with swiftly. The individual has the right to provide an explanation before action is taken; however, if suspicions are proved or there is direct evidence, then immediate termination of employment is in order. Again, hoping the problem will remedy itself is unrealistic. Keeping an employee who cannot be trusted or is suspected by other staff members is a detriment rather than an asset, regardless of how good the employee's performance has been judged in the past. Preventive measures can discourage this type of problem. Make the opportunities to steal money or supplies difficult at best (also see Chapters 14 and 19). Avoid having petty cash available for personal use. Remember that the manager sets the example as the role model, especially in the area of ethics and honesty.

Another disciplinary issue that is difficult to deal with is behavior that results from attitude problems. Employees who at times become cynical or are negative should be warned that their behavior is unacceptable. The manager should try to discover the underlying reasons for the unacceptable behavior. Sometimes it is possible to remedy the situation without disciplinary action. If the behavior continues, then the manager or supervisor should document the problem and meet with such individuals to explain that their attitude must improve or termination of employment will be necessary if the pattern continues. During the meeting, a copy of the written documentation of incidents should be provided to the employee. If the employee's attitude does not improve, then the manager should discharge the employee.

Insubordinate behavior or refusal to do certain types of work should be dealt with immediately. If the request is legitimate and the response is out of order, then the practice manager should confront the employee directly. The dispute should be discussed and the alternatives provided to the employee.

The individual then needs to make a decision whether he will comply or face the consequences outlined in the conversation. If the employee complies, then the manager should followup the problem by documenting the situation in a letter of corrective action that indicates that insubordinate behavior is inappropriate and if the behavior is repeated the employee will be terminated.

These strategies are intended to depict typical incidents. Each manager has to handle situations his own way. The employer should, however, be consistent, willing to confront problems head on, objective, and predictable. The personnel actions in a disciplinary process should be related to the severity of the problem. Managers should keep in mind that employees should be treated the way they would want to be treated in a comparable situation.

Termination procedures

The final step in a disciplinary process involves discharging the employee. If the practice's disciplinary program has been followed and the decision has been made to terminate the employee, it is important to complete the records properly. A memorandum should be written and attached to the documentation in the personnel record which indicates the reason for termination, a review of the history of the problem(s), last working day, and a brief statement summarizing the overall view of the individual's performance to the termination date. The memorandum provides a permanent record should there ever be a reason for review of the case, as in unemployment compensation claim, request for reference material from another potential employer, or some type of legal action.

It is important to notify the employee immediately of the decision in a private meeting. Honesty is the best policy, and the individual should be told frankly the reasons for the deci-

sion. The manager should be prepared for the meeting by having the final paycheck available, asking for appropriate signatures, and requesting keys to the building. If the individual has any equipment off the premises, the individual should be asked to bring it to the meeting. The meeting should be conducted in a professional manner and should be brief and concise. If the individual is concerned about a future reference or employment verification and asks your willingness to provide one, it is important to tell the individual what will be stated. End the meeting quickly, and then escort the individual out of the practice.

□
Exit interviews

It is a good personnel management practice to interview employees who plan to terminate employment. Employees who are discharged typically are not interested in an exit interview. The employee in most cases will not be motivated to extend contact. The exit interview is recommended for all employees who leave the practice of their own accord. Not every exit interview will be a productive session. The meeting is intended to provide information in an open, honest exchange. Some employees who intend to leave may not be willing to share information, may have hurt feelings, or may feel uncomfortable discussing their concerns.

The topics for an employee exit interview include the good and bad points of the job, remuneration for the position, reasons for leaving, the employee's ideas for change to improve the practice, attitude toward management, and the employee's overall assessment of the experience. There are risks involved in an exit interview. The employer must be willing to hear the individual's thoughts objectively without judging the response during the session. Employers may not like what they hear, even if it is an honest appraisal. The individual leaving the practice may feel uncomfortable or guilty for leaving and may not be in the frame of mind to have an open discussion. It is important for the manager to be sensitive to these issues and maintain control of the meeting by using good judgment and changing topics when necessary. The meeting should be upbeat, positive, friendly, and professional. The meeting should be held in private. The positive aspects of the working relationship should be stressed. The manager should thank such employees for their willingness to share the information provided. After the meeting concludes the manager should record the information exchanged. The ideas provided, concerns addressed, and feelings expressed can assist the open manager in improving the management of the practice by implementing good ideas from departing staff members. If the reasons for departure are valid, it is wise to take advantage of the suggestions by changing procedures. Effective managers are able to accept constructive criticism and want to improve the performance of the practice as well as their own individual attributes.

□
Summary

The personnel program in a veterinary practice is a necessary component in effective management. It should only be as involved or complex as it has to be — related to the size of the practice. The functions of planning, organizing, and controlling and the use of a problem-solving approach should be the basis for all procedures instituted in a personnel program. There should be a reason for every policy, or methodology; otherwise it is not necessary.

The practice manager should decide that it is better to be respected rather than just being one who has to be liked. The effective manager will be willing to be consistent; lay out goals and objectives; delegate responsibility with authority; direct activities; be honest, communicative, and accessible; be willing to listen; and have the ability to make fair decisions. The effective practice manager will motivate employees by giving them credit for their ideas and initiative and know when it is wise or fair to accept the blame for a problem. Regardless of the practice size, the importance of having a personnel program is essential. The success of a practice relies on the effectiveness of the human resources employed. There is no procedure that can replace good judgment. Personnel management is as important in a practice that employs 2 staff members as it is in one that employs over 25 individuals. The personnel program that a practice uses is a tool that is only as effective as the individuals that use it. The accomplished manager will view personnel management as a top priority.

Chapter 4
□
Real estate selection – management

Walter R. Gillespie

Practice location

There is an old cliche pertinent to selection of real estate for any business venture that says the three most important factors are location, location, and location. This dictum is no less true today in selection of a site for an animal hospital, providing the term *location* is used in its broadest definition. An excellent *geographic* location within a community or rural area could be very undesirable without other vital attributes. For example, one of the first considerations would be the need for veterinary service in the area being surveyed. If a given area is already saturated with animal hospitals in proportion to the animal-owning population, it would probably be a poor choice for a new facility. There may be some exceptions to this concept in very large metropolitan areas where strips of commercially zoned areas are embedded in high-density residential areas, but as a general rule it would be valid in most localities.

Another important consideration should be the ease of ingress and egress for clientele. In the case of small-animal hospitals this may make the difference as to which veterinarian some clients patronize, especially older clients (who now constitute a large percentage of the volume of many small-animal practices). Many clients are reluctant to fight traffic and congested areas to visit one veterinarian when another has a location providing much easier access. In the case of large-animal hospitals, ease of entering and leaving as well as providing space for maneuvering, loading, unloading, and parking stock trucks or trailers that will transport animals to and from the facility is an important consideration. An adequate lot size to provide space for buildings, parking lots, kennels, stock pens, landscaping, and future expansion is essential in picking a location. The type of neighborhood and neighboring businesses can be a very important consideration in choosing a building site. Selecting a location situated next to a potential nuisance-type business such as a tavern, adult movie theater, noisy auto body repair shop, and so forth may create a less than favorable atmosphere for future clientele. Conversely, selecting a location surrounded by attractive, well-kept homes and business properties can only enhance the overall appearance of the area to your potential clients.

Another aspect of veterinary facility location is the importance location plays in advertising the presence of a veterinarian in the area. Locating on or within visual distance of a well-traveled thoroughfare or in close proximity to a heavily frequented business (such as a convenience market or other shopping area) can be very instrumental in informing the public of the presence of veterinary services. This type of exposure will have decided effect on the rapidity of increasing the volume of client calls. This can be very important when a practitioner is starting a new practice in any area. It is becoming increasingly difficult to locate desirable areas where there is a real need for veterinary services due to the increasing number of new veterinarians entering the profession and all of them looking for ideal practice sites. This factor accentuates the need to make an exhaustive search for as close to an ideal spot as possible to start a practice. To do less than this may severely limit the future growth of the business.

Zoning

The very first thing to consider when seeking the ideal location to establish a veterinary facility is zoning law requirements of that mu-nicipality. Real estate must either be already properly zoned or subject to being rezoned (which may be a very lengthy and expensive endeavor). The unfortunate part of any rezoning attempt is that veterinary hospitals still have the stigma of being a noisy, odorous, nuisance-type operation. Many zoning ordinances concerning animal hospitals are predicated on this basis and often do not make any real distinction between small-animal clinics, full-service small-animal hospitals, and large-animal hospitals. There is a real need to educate planning and zoning departments of many cities regarding modern veterinary facilities that are designed, in most cases, to operate in a clean, odor-controlled, noise-abated atmosphere.

Type of neighborhood

The neighborhood in which a veterinarian is considering a substantial investment in real estate should be viewed with an eye to the future. In many cases this real estate will be one of the largest investment vehicles the practitioner will have to provide retirement income at the end of a practice career. A neighborhood in a transition phase from residential to commerical or industrial may not be worthy of prime consideration. That type of change could spell trouble for building the practice and possibly also result in decreasing real estate values. Of these two investment considerations, the danger to the future value of the practice may be the more critical long-term financial problem. In most cases, the eventual value of a given veterinary practice will far exceed the value of the real estate upon which it is located, though both values should certainly increase, assuming the continuing effect of inflation.

In considering the future sale of a practice it is necessary to realize it can be difficult to divorce the practice itself from the real estate. Very often, a large part of the value of a veterinary practice may be closely associated with the *location* of the real estate. All too often, by the time a practice has matured and a sale is being contemplated there is no other viable, properly zoned, available land in the proximate area to which the practice could be moved. Attempting to move a practice out of the immediate neighborhood could risk the possibility of losing a substantial number of clients. The net result of this type of situation, in many cases, is that it becomes almost impossible to sell the real estate separately. To do so would jeopardize the value of the practice unless it *could* be moved to a new location a very short distance away. The time and money expended to make a thorough investigation of the future trend of both the demographic changes and the property utilization changes in the area will certainly help in making a more logical decision.

Room to expand

One of the common problems that occurs, due to a lack of foresight by many young veterinarians starting a practice, is failure to provide for eventual expansion of their physical plant. It is often difficult to visualize the future need for more space in a new practice, especially in a rather sparsely settled, developing area. It would certainly not be wise to overbuild in a new practice situation. The important thing is to provide room for future expansion and to locate the building on the property in such a manner that it could be more easily expanded if and when demand for more room occurs. Not only should you consider eventual expansion of the building area but also give some thought to the probable need for increased parking areas and additional livestock pens as well. Time spent in planning utilization of space with this thought in mind can save a lot of frustration when the time comes to expand the facility.

Property maintenance

Selection of a location for new construction or remodeling of a veterinary facility is of prime importance in establishing a practice. Once a physical plant is in operation, the next major consideration regarding this expensive investment is proper maintenance of the property, both building and grounds. Well-established day-to-day maintenance procedures will pay handsome dividends to owners of the practice and real estate. The practice will benefit from the appearance of a well-kept building and nicely groomed landscaping and grounds. Owners of the real estate will benefit from reduced expense if repair and maintenance schedules are properly followed. People notice when attention is given to proper housekeeping, decorating, and gardening details. Clients are people, and these impressions play a big part in what they think of the practice and personnel associated with the facility. Impressions they form along these lines correlate closely with their impressions of how their animals are being treated at the facility. Establishment of good maintenance procedures should receive high priority in the management of any veterinary operation. The last part of this chapter will deal with the subject of real estate management.

This chapter deals with the selection of a site for the establishment of a *new* veterinary facility and management. Purchase of an existing facility and practice is covered in Chapter 7.

☐
Real estate selection

Purchase vs. lease

The decision between purchasing or leasing property to build a veterinary hospital is often decided by availability of funds. Building a new facility, whether it be new construction or remodeling an existing structure, to serve as a veterinary hospital requires a large outlay of capital that must be available before starting the venture. Sources of this capital are often limited due to reluctance of many lending institutions to lend money to a person for a business with no established track record. Money is more easily obtained in the case of a young veterinarian borrowing to buy an established practice with a good track record of high earnings. Lending institutions may require collateral or a qualified cosigner to guarantee the note when buying real estate for the purpose of establishing a new practice.

Purchasing

Many people feel that the outright purchase of property (rather than leasing) is most desirable because of the potential for long-term property value escalation and resultant accumulation of equity as a favorable investment vehicle. As equity grows, it becomes a ready source of collateral for borrowing funds for emergencies or for remodeling or expansion projects. Ownership of a piece of property can allow more freedom in utilization of the property for such things as subdividing or erecting other buildings for rental purposes.

Leasing

On the other side of the fence are those who feel leasing will enable the owner of the practice to conserve capital that may be used for other purposes. If available funds are limited, leasing could provide more funds for erecting a larger facility or remodeling an existing building to a greater extent as well as allowing for more and better equipment, furniture, and fixtures. With the high cost of land and construction or remodeling as well as equipping and furnishing a hospital today, leasing can be a valid approach to getting a new practice started. If a lease *is* being contemplated, it would be prudent to secure a long-term, re-

newable lease with an option to buy after a given number of years. Regardless of which method is used to acquire the property, it is imperative to have legal counsel in preparing the contract and to thoroughly understand the purchase or lease agreement before signing the document.

The age of the veterinarian and estimated length of practice life that he or she is contemplating could have a bearing on the decision whether to buy or lease the hospital site. In the case of a young person with a long practice life ahead, it may well be better to strive to purchase. The older doctor might want to lease a facility to keep expenses to a minimum in order to conserve capital in anticipation of approaching retirement.

Shopping centers

The location of the proposed facility may dictate whether the site may be purchased or leased. In a shopping center location a lease would normally be mandatory. Many of the larger shopping centers will lease for a certain annual sum plus a percentage of gross income the business generates. Cost per square foot of space can be rather high and will vary with the size and prestige of the center. The lessee normally must bear the expense of construction of or remodeling leasehold improvements to create the veterinary facility. A shopping center may have much stricter requirements regarding design and operation of the veterinary facility than would be encountered in a freestanding building located on a separate piece of property. The main advantages of a shopping center location for a veterinary clinic would be nearly unlimited parking and high visibility. These two factors can be very helpful in getting a practice started. Shopping center locations are becoming more commonplace for a variety of reasons.

One of the more common uses of a shopping center clinic is for a satellite facility operating in conjunction with a large animal hospital. The shopping mall is an ideal location for a satellite that does not require a lot of square footage due to the nature of its operation. A shopping center facility requires only a minimal number of rooms. It should function as a simple examination/diagnostic/vaccination and minor surgical facility. Satellite clinics refer most of their cases to the central hospital for more sophisticated diagnostic/surgical/treatment services.

Another rather common use of a shopping center site for a veterinary clinic is by an older practitioner who has left his original busy practice and wants to continue to practice at a slower pace. The older veterinarian can then do as much or as little as desired and refer the rest to surrounding colleagues. Probably the most common type of shopping center practice is that of the young veterinarian who wants to get out alone but does not have the finances to buy a piece of property and finds leasing a viable way to start a practice. An example of a veterinary clinic in a shopping center location is shown in Figure 4-1.

It may be possible to locate developers who have recently purchased a large parcel of land

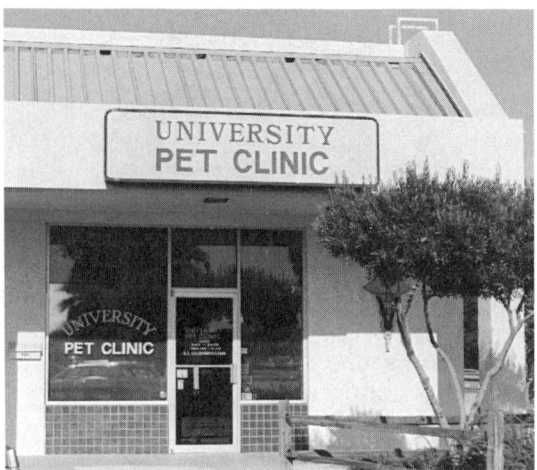

Figure 4-1. *Veterinary clinic in a shopping center location*

in a desirable area. If a shopping center – type development is being planned by the developers, it may be possible to interest them in either selling or leasing a small portion of the parcel. An illustration of such a site may be seen in Figure 4-2. Needless to say, the availability of a shopping center site would apply to a small-animal clinic.

Purchase of a site with excess land

In some cases veterinarians may locate a piece of property having all the attributes that they are looking for to establish a practice, but it may be a much larger parcel than is needed for the veterinary facility (including any reserve area for future expansion). With some ingenuity it may be possible to arrange financing in a manner that would allow construction of the veterinary facility along with some commercial space on the same property. The commercial space could then be leased or sold to help finance the cost of the land and the veterinary building. Development of the excess portion of the property may not occur until a number of years later, depending upon the financial situation of the people involved and demand for such space in the area. Not infrequently a real estate investment opportunity will present itself in the immediate vicinity of or on occasion right next door to an established animal hospital. If it is possible to acquire the property at an advantageous price, the veterinarian may be able to develop the site into an added source of income. An illustration of the result of this type of approach may be seen in Figure 4-3.

The veterinarian constructed the animal hospital shown in Figure 4-3 many years ago and built a successful practice. At the time the veterinary facility was first established, this area of the city was just beginning to develop. The area has now become well developed, and the owner recently elected to remodel and enlarge the original hospital and at the same time

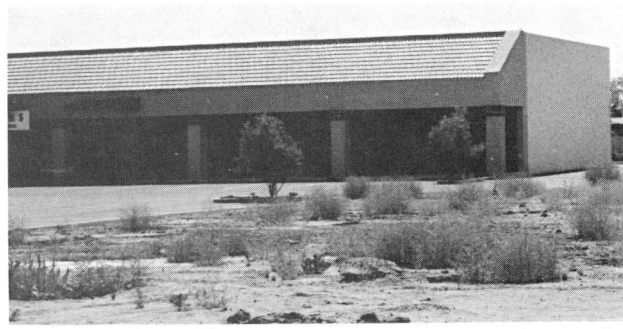

Figure 4-2. Potential location for a veterinary clinic in a developing shopping center

develop the adjacent piece of the property. The two-story commercial building was built next to the hospital and is presently being leased as a retail bridal shop. Income from this lease is paying for the cost of the new building as well as the cost of the hospital remodeling. This is a good example of prudent utilization of an oversized piece of property that was originally purchased for use primarily as an animal hospital but with eventual further development in mind. In a situation such as this as well as with any new construction, it is of the utmost importance to locate buildings in such a manner as to provide the most versatility for any future development. One consideration in this respect is that of maintaining separate access and parking for the animal hospital and also for the commercial development. Should an opportunity arise in the future that would make it beneficial to sell off the commerical

portion, it would be very important to be able to separate the two parcels into two intact entities with the least inconvenience to either one.

Large-animal sites

Locating a desirable piece of property on which to build a large-animal facility is a very different problem than that encountered by the small-animal doctor. The very nature of the large-animal practice dictates it be located in an area proximate and accessible to livestock owners. Zoning regulations in most parts of the country are quite strict regarding the location of large-animal hospitals. They are commonly prohibited from locating near residential areas or even near certain types of commercial operations such as hotels, motels, or restaurants. They must provide adequate controls to prevent offensive odors and noise. These restrictions tend to force them to locate in agricultural areas near livestock farms or close to horse racing tracks. Modern large-animal hospitals are, for the most part, well-designed, architecturally attractive, and functional facilities that are a credit to the areas in which they are built. Figure 4-4 shows an example of this type of modern large-animal hospital.

Very often large-animal facilities will offer varying degrees of small-animal service to their clients. Some large-animal facilities have very complete small-animal hospitals incorporated into their buildings. This arrangement is

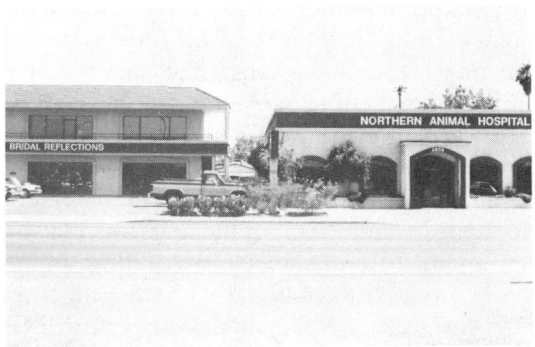

Figure 4-3. Example of commercial development on veterinary hospital real estate

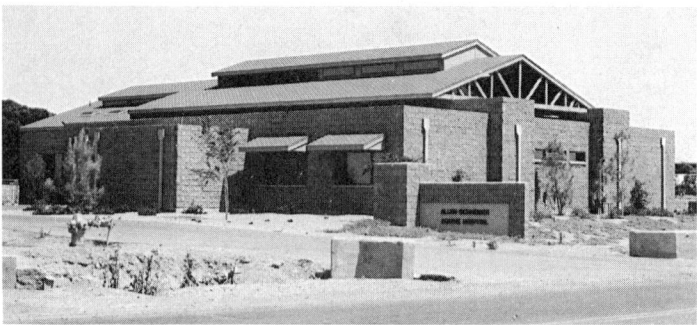

Figure 4-4. *Modern large-animal hospital*

found more frequently in outlying rural communities rather than in metropolitan areas where an abundant supply of pet hospitals exist.

Whether leasing or purchasing a piece of property, it will be necessary to research existing city or county zoning regulations and applicable building codes to be certain the site will conform. Property should be checked for any deed restrictions or easements that may have a detrimental effect on the proposed use. It would be wise to find out in advance if the subject property exists within a flood plain. In the event of a proposed purchase it would also be prudent to get a survey of the property.

☐
Building size requirements

New construction

Before beginning the search for a hospital site there are some important decisions to make regarding the proposed facility. One of the first items of consideration will be the approximate size of the building being contemplated. Assuming new construction is being considered, a decision will have to be made regarding whether to build the entire, complete hospital initially or to build only the essential portion first and provide for later expansion to complete the project. If the area being considered is a relatively undeveloped one in a growth stage, it may be well to consider building a minimal portion of the hospital to begin with and include plans for later expansion in the original design. On the other hand, if the area is well established and the need for veterinary services appears sufficient, it may be better to build the complete hospital initially if finances permit. In either case the total size of the completed building will need to be known in order to plan for adequate site size. Parking lots, landscaping requirements, and building code setbacks must be taken into consideration. As a rule of thumb, the building should take up no more than 25% of available land. It is most beneficial to employ a design consultant or an architect who has experience in animal hospital design to plan the facility.

Design will vary a great deal depending on the type of practice being planned. Practice type can range from that of a solo practitioner in a shopping center pet clinic to a multi-veterinarian group practice in a full-service animal hospital. Design may range from an exclusive small-animal clinic or even from an exclusive feline practice to a mixed general practice for large and small animals combined. Available finances often dictate the type and size of facility being planned. All of these factors play an important role in the size of building being contemplated and will influence the selection of a site on which the animal hospital will be built.

Many factors will dictate the size and number of individual rooms in any animal hospital. The type of practice, amount of financing available, size of lot the building will be located on (which in turn will dictate the total building space available), and individual preference of the veterinarian building the facility all play a part in hospital design. Long-term plans will also be instrumental in deciding the initial planning of a building in which to start a practice. If the area is new and the owners of the practice anticipate a large growth in the practice over the years, then they should plan accordingly in making decisions of building size and eventual expansion.

For the purpose of estimating the minimal lot size needed on which to locate a small-animal hospital, the approximate size of the building must be known. In order to plan the building size, one must make some estimate of dimensions of the individual rooms. In a small-animal hospital the *minimal* size of various rooms may be as follows:

Reception room	12′ × 16′	192 sq. ft.
Receptionist office	9′ × 10′	90 ″ ″
Examination rooms (each)	(2) 8′ × 9′	144 ″ ″
Laboratory/pharmacy room	8′ × 10′	48 ″ ″
Treatment/x-ray room	10′ × 20′	200 ″ ″
Surgery room	12′ × 15′	180 ″ ″
Rest room	4′ × 5′	20 ″ ″
Kennel room	10 × 20′	200 ″ ″
Storage room	10′ × 12′	120 ″ ″
Private office	10′ × 10′	100 ″ ″
Mechanical room	8′ × 10′	80 ″ ″
	Total =	1374 sq. ft.

These figures could represent the *minimal* square footage needed to build a small facility, either freestanding or in a shopping center environment. Design of the floor plan can easily change any of these figures. Many times room usage can be combined, and often certain areas such as the laboratory and pharmacy can be incorporated into a large hall area behind the examination rooms. The possibilities are numerous and will vary with each designer or veterinarian.

At the other end of the building size spectrum is the multiple-veterinarian, small-animal, group practice hospital. An example of this type of hospital is shown in Figure 4-5. This recently constructed hospital has 6440 total square feet of floor space. The new hospital is the result of expansion of this group practice that had outgrown its previous facility. The owners were very fortunate in locating this property just around the corner from their old practice site. This is, of course, the ideal way to move a practice location and be ensured of keeping your clientele.

The building includes a semiseparate boarding and grooming facility consisting of 1500 square feet. The veterinary facility has a full-time staff of four veterinarians and a part-time veterinary specialist who spends time at several area hospitals. In contrast to the minimal-sized rooms listed before, this hospital has spacious rooms throughout the building. For example, the reception area is a very sizable 32 feet by 38 feet and has a large free-standing receptionist's office in the center.

There are four examination rooms that are 10 feet by 12 feet and a surgical suite that is 15 feet by 20 feet. Adjacent to surgery is a scrub room and pack sterilization area that is 9 feet by 12 feet. The pharmacy, treatment, surgical preparation, and workroom areas are all combined in one large multipurpose room that is 22 feet by 23 feet. There is a separate x-ray room, 9 feet by 12 feet, and a grooming room for hospital patients that is located within the kennel area, which is 24 feet by 44 feet.

The building has an apartment/lounge/lunchroom area that is 12 feet by 32 feet and a spacious private physician's office, 14 feet by 18 feet. Small storage closets and cabinets are

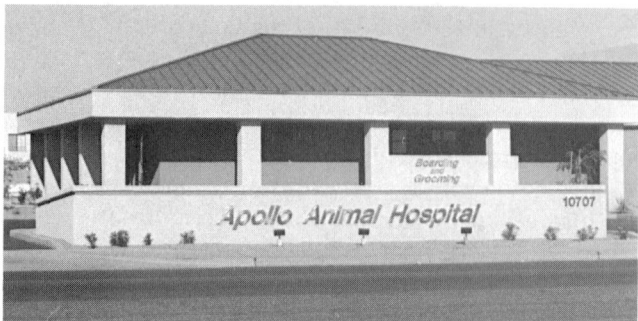

Figure 4-5. Multiperson, group veterinary practice

located in convenient areas throughout the hospital. Numerous other rooms such as the mechanical room, a large central storage room, and rest rooms are also included. This building is situated on a 29,000-square foot lot and, as mentioned earlier, uses less than 25% of the available lot space. This leaves adequate room for parking lots and attractive landscaping and gives an attractive appearance to the entire veterinary hospital facility.

Remodeling

If you locate a piece of property that fits most of the criteria for a desirable hospital site and has an existing structure on it, consider the possibility of remodeling the building to fit your needs. Again, it would be very important to consult with a good architect to determine the feasibility of conversion. A remodeled building will never be the same as a building that is designed specifically for a veterinary hospital, but the cost of remodeling is usually much less than new construction, and it is possible to end up with a very workable facility at a much reduced price. See Figure 4-6 for an example of a home remodeled into a successful animal hospital.

This older house was located on a piece of property properly zoned for an animal hospital. The veterinarian purchased and remodeled it by closing in the carport, adding some additional plumbing, and making some changes in the interior walls and doors. Parking lots and a street sign were put in. The owner and his family lived in the building for 2 years after the practice was started. Additional remodeling was done periodically as the practice grew, and eventually the hospital was expanded to include the whole house, part of which had been used as an apartment. The new kennel addition was added 5 years after the practice opened. The remodeled facility continues to serve a busy practice very adequately as it has for over 25 years.

Remodeling can be a viable consideration. It may, however, be nearly as expensive to make major alterations to an older building and bring electrical and plumbing systems up to code requirements as it would be to erect a new building. Cost will be dependent on the

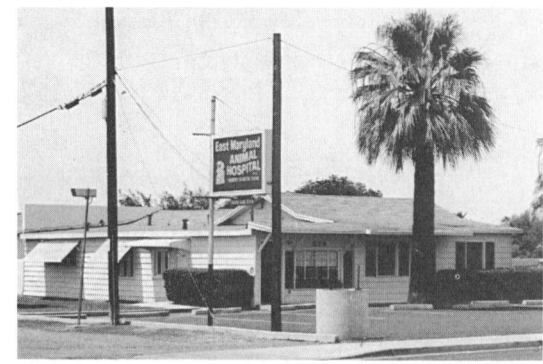

Figure 4-6. Veterinary hospital remodeled from an existing home

degree of alteration required. If operating on a low budget this could be one avenue to explore.

□
Hospital site selection (established or developing areas)

The search for an ideal site on which to place an animal hospital entails many considerations by the potential builder. The financial situation is one of the prime factors in determining what areas may be suitable. Real estate values normally vary according to degree and type of existing development that has occurred in a particular area.

Established areas

Well-established areas normally have a much higher cost per square foot. A substantial part of this higher cost may be attributed to the fact that many amenities of urban development are already in place and have previously been assessed. These amenities may include paved streets with flood control drains, sidewalks, electric power, street lighting, water and sewer systems, police and postal substations, parks and recreation areas, and other features and services that undeveloped areas have not yet acquired or paid for. Developed areas will provide a much greater potential client density and offer greater visibility for the new hospital, both of which should provide for more rapid growth of a new practice. They would not normally be a viable area of consideration for a large-animal hospital due to their higher population density, which could conflict with zoning requirements.

Developing areas

The fringe areas of a city that are in the path of future development will yield very desirable and less expensive sites for locating a veterinary hospital (large or small animal). If the area being considered has not yet been annexed into the city, there is a good possibility zoning may be more favorable for a veterinary facility. Very often county zoning requirements are less strict than those in cities. Land values will be lower at the time of purchase or lease, though there will likely be periodic ongoing capital expenses to provide the amenities of development described earlier. These expenses will manifest themselves in such things as street and sewer development districts that assess property owner taxes to fund the programs. A practice started in this type of area will undoubtedly grow at a slower pace initially. Client numbers and visibility will be low until development occurs around the hospital. Site selection will be much easier in undeveloped areas simply because of more numerous available locations.

Some criteria to consider in looking for an ideal location might be the direction of growth of the city, which often can be determined by location of proposed major thoroughfares and intersections, planned sites of shopping areas, proposed flood control projects (if any), planned industrial areas, and so forth. This type of information can be obtained by visiting the planning and zoning department of the municipality. Try to determine where the center of the city will be in the next 10 years. Find out whether any large-scale land use such as new airport construction, proposed city parks, and so forth is being planned in the area under consideration. The more information available about the area, the better judgment will be in selecting a location. Another source of information is the real estate department of various lending institutions (banks, savings and loan associations, and mortgage bankers). In some cases utility companies may be of help because they need long-range plans to stay ahead of growth in the area. Additional information can be found by contacting planning and development departments of the telephone, gas, and electric companies.

Plan for ease of accessibility

The benefits of the hospital being visible in order to let animal owners in the area know veterinary services are available have been previously discussed. A word of caution is in order about locating on a street that may become a major thoroughfare. If the street is *too* busy, ingress and egress become very difficult and can actually dissuade clients from patronizing that facility. Use careful planning to provide for easy access and easy exit for future clientele.

Determining property value

After a location has been selected, the next step is to determine a fair price for the property. The ideal but more expensive method would be to get an appraisal (which a lending institution will probably require at the time of loan application). There are several advantages of a formal appraisal. The appraisal firm will do a very thorough job of researching recent sales of like parcels of land in the area. They will compare similiar (and dissimilar) features of respective sales compared with the subject property. They can provide an estimated value based on various methods such as cost, income, and market approaches. They also will be able to give a reasonable assessment of the nature of the general area regarding its stability and any trends in real estate values, upward or downward. The cost for this type of professional help will be several hundred dollars, depending on the firm and the time expended in making the appraisal.

If funds to purchase the property are available from sources other than a lending institution, such as savings or from a family member,

for example, it may be possible to forego the formal appraisal. A personal informal property appraisal could be made by using some recent sale comparisons of similar properties in the area. A real estate person would be very helpful in getting the necessary information and assisting with the informal appraisal.

Title insurance

Title insurance must be obtained before closing the sale. This insurance will ensure a clear title to the property being sold. The title company examines the deed and guarantees that no liens or other encumbrances have been placed against the property. If for any reason a question regarding the validity of a clear title should arise in the future, the title company would then be responsible to protect the buyer.

The cost of obtaining an appraisal of the property, cost of title insurance, and cost of the plans of the proposed building are all expenses of the borrower.

□
Obtaining real estate financing

Once the value has been established and the price agreed upon, the next step is to arrange financing (assuming the property will be purchased rather than leased).

If there is an existing mortgage on the property with favorable interest rates, it may be possible to assume the mortgage and simply continue to make the payments. The balance of the purchase price must then be negotiated. The seller may require the balance in cash, and the buyer may then have to secure a loan to make the payment. If the seller is willing to carry a portion of the sale amount, at mutually acceptable conditions, then the immediate need will be arranging for the down payment.

Cost of borrowing money

It is always wise to shop around for the best interest rates available for a commercial loan because they vary considerably from one source to another. The lender may put a "stop" on the loan at the end of 5 years and require that terms be negotiated again at that time. Another commonly used method of making loans is to tie the interest rate to the prime rate (1 to 3 percentage points above prime is commonly used). These two methods are the result of volatile fluctuations in interest rates that have occurred over the past few years.

Lending institutions are reluctant to lend money for the purpose of a down payment and will likely require collateral or some qualified person to cosign such a note. If the seller wants cash for the sale, then most lending institutions will normally require the buyer provide the down payment. They will lend the buyer the balance needed, up to about 75% of the cost or appraised value of the land and the proposed building, whichever is *lower* (actual cost or appraised value). Some lenders will lend up to 75% to 80% of the cost or appraised value, whichever is *higher*. If the latter type of loan can be arranged, then it can often pay for furnishing and equipping the hospital as well as construction. Most lending institutions will require a "first position" or "first mortgage" on property before lending money. This would enable them to take over the property in case of default by the buyer and sell the property to satisfy their interest. They would, in essence, be paid first to the extent of their monetary interest in the property.

Another cost of borrowing money, in addition to interest charged for the loan, is the "points" the lender will charge to make the loan. A point is equal to 1% of the total amount of the loan and is paid at the time the money is given to the borrower. The number of points charged will vary from time to time based on the economy, current interest rates, degree of risk involved in the loan, and so forth. Presently, banks are charging about 1% up front for the interim financing and 1% when the total funds are committed. It is not uncommon, however, for lenders to charge 3 or more points on some loans.

Preparation for the loan interview

Before beginning a search for financing the purchase of property, a complete package of pertinent information should be prepared regarding the proposed business venture and the borrower's qualifications, integrity, and probable ability to repay the loan. This package of information should contain, but is not limited to, the following:

1. Building plans and brief explanation of type of business
2. Personal history, including scholastic achievements and degrees, honors and awards, employment history or experience (especially in the veterinary field), marital status, number of children, civic club memberships, and so forth
3. Personal financial statement
4. Past 3 years' tax returns (most lenders will require this)
5. Personal credit references
6. Cash flow projections: estimates of income and expense the new business will be expected to maintain
7. Capitalization (beginning balance) amount of money available to the business upon commencement of operation
8. Additional pertinent information that would substantiate the need for a veterinary facility in that particular location. This could be animal census figures for the area, lack of other veterinarians servicing the area, traffic counts, and so forth.

Information presented to lenders should be concise and limited to pertinent facts that can be used to make a decision regarding the loan. Do not overwhelm them with excess paperwork.

Once the pertinent information has been gathered, it should be well organized in a folder. The next step is to make appointments with commercial real estate loan officers of as many different lending institutions as possible. Shop as thoroughly as possible, and do not commit until information has been gathered from all potential institutions. Be prepared to leave a copy of the information folder with each person contacted. Also, be prepared to wait because most lenders will take some time to come to any decision regarding larger loans.

There are some clauses a borrower should strive to have included in the loan contract. One is that there be *no prepayment penalty,* and another is that the loan *be assumable by another party.* These items may not seem to have much importance at the time the loan is obtained. They can, however, be very helpful at the time of a future sale. This would be espe-cially true if interest rates have risen substan-tially and the borrower should desire to refi-nance or pay off the debt prematurely. It can also be of great benefit in the sale of the prop-erty if the buyer can assume a low-interest loan during a high-interest rate period. The lender may not wish to make these concessions, but they are negotiable.

Loan repayment terms

Selecting the term of repayment of a loan can be a very important decision. It is true that the longer the term of repayment, the smaller the monthly payments. Close examination, how-ever, of relevant differences between a 30-year payoff and a 15-year payoff reveals some very interesting facts. A borrower should consider the cost of longer-term payoffs before com-mitting to any specific payment period. If it is at all possible to make the relatively small in-crease in monthly payments, the rewards for a shorter term can be substantial. The examples shown in Table 4-1 use 15- and 30-year periods

Table 4-1
Comparison of 30-year vs. 15-year amortization of a loan
assuming repayment of $200,000 at 12% interest

	30-Year Payoff	15-Year Payoff
Monthly payment	$2,057.23	$2,400.34
(annual payment)	$24,686.76	$28,804.08
Buyer's equity Accumulation		
End of 5 years	$4,673.56	$32,695.32
End of 10 years	$13,164.01	$92,092.80
End of 15 years	$28,588.57	$200,000.00
Total interest paid over term	$540,601.07	$232,060.50

For an increase in the monthly payment of $343.11 (17%) which would amount to $4,117.32 annually, the loan could be amortized in half the term, and the equity would increase much faster. The total cost of the loan (interest paid) would de-crease by more than half.

for illustration, but the results are relative to any two payoff periods.

□
Real estate property management

Proper maintenance of a veterinary facility is essential for many reasons. Visual perception to clientele is probably one of the most important. The first impression of a veterinary practice clients will form will be the appearance of the building and grounds as they approach the parking lot. The appearance of the inside of the building will be noted as the client waits in the reception area and examination rooms. Cleanliness and orderliness of the inside and outside of the hospital will have a profound effect on most people. Building and grounds' appearance can be a major factor in the decision to return for future services at that facility.

Other reasons for proper maintenance procedures are to ensure the comfort and safety of the people and animals located within the building. Poor waste management procedures and general clutter in kennel and barn areas can result in noxious odors as well as potential fire hazards. Improper handling and disposal of hospital waste materials can cause other types of accidents as well as possibly lead to infectious disease problems. Failure to maintain electrical and plumbing equipment can cause serious consequences for occupants of the building as well as financial problems for the property owner. Slippery floors due to improper waxing or standing water can cause serious injury from a fall and could result in a liability action against the hospital owner. Failure of heating or cooling systems in extreme conditions of heat or cold can disrupt normal business functions and potentially cause serious health problems in very ill animals. Inadequate performance of air-conditioning systems can create personnel problems that can result in poor performance or in some cases even the resignation of good employees.

Use of maintenance schedules

One of the first procedures the manager of a veterinary hospital should institute is a maintenance plan. This plan should provide schedules that go into as much detail as possible regarding proper maintenance of all the various systems in the hospital as well as the building and grounds. An example of a general maintenance schedule is shown in Figure 4-7. This type of schedule can be modified to serve any type of veterinary facility and is merely one of many ways to set up a maintenance chart or schedule.

Responsibility for maintenance procedures

Once a schedule has been devised, it is of utmost importance that someone be responsible to see that it is properly completed. There are various ways to use maintenance schedules to ensure they will be followed. The size of the practice and hence the number of employees will often dictate the specific type of maintenance program that will be used. Figure 4-8 illustrates another example of a periodic maintenance schedule that includes items that need to be done on a weekly or less-frequent basis. The schedule is designed so that the person responsible for the procedure has a place to initial it and put down the date of completion. If the schedule is followed regularly, it provides a record of maintenance that will help ensure proper care of the facility and equipment.

Employee training (maintenance procedures)

It is essential that all new employees receive proper and thorough training in their maintenance duties. Employees who have previously

	Daily	Weekly	Bi-weekly	Monthly	Semi-annually	Annually	As/Date needed
Janitorial (building)							
Exam table pedestals — clean	✓						/
Bathrooms/toilets — clean	✓						/
Floor lamps — clean	✓						/
Floors — vacuum/sweep/mop/buff	✓						/
Laundry (surg. drapes, gowns, towels) — wash	✓						/
Washer/dryer — clean and empty lint trap	✓						/
Porches — sweep/hose off	✓						/
Sinks/countertops — clean	✓						/
Soap/alcohol bottles — fill	✓						/
Stock exam rm refrig's — (vaccines, drugs)	✓						/
Towel dispensers — ck/refill	✓						/
Trash — empty containers/put in new liners	✓						/
Waste baskets/trash cans — clean/sanitize		✓					/
Windows — wash			✓				/
Walls & woodwork — wash			✓				/
Wall hangings — clean/dust			✓				/
A/C air filters — replace				✓			/
A/C vents — clean/dust				✓			/
Hot water heaters — drain				✓			/
Light fixtures — clean/dust				✓			/
Refrigerators — defrost/clean				✓			/
A/C & furnace blowers — clean/oil					✓		/
Cabinets & Doors — wax/polish					✓		/
Drapes, curtains — wash/clean					✓		/
Floors — strip/wax					✓		/
Fire extinguishers — have tested						✓	/
Grounds maintenance							
Lawns/planters — pick up trash	✓						
Parking lots — pick up trash	✓						
Lawns/plants — trim/mow		✓					
Lawn irrig. system/bubblers — check					✓		
Lawns/plants/trees — water							✓ /
Lawns/plants/trees — fertilize							✓ /.

(Continued)

Figure 4-7. *Veterinary hospital general maintenance schedule*

Parking lots — resurface/restripe							✓ /
Sign(s) — replace light bulbs, paint							✓ /
Building exterior — repair/paint							✓ /
Roof covering — repair/replace							✓ /
Special equipment							
(Follow manufacturer's recommendations)							
Film developing tanks — clean/change solutions							✓ /
Automatic film processors							✓ /
Anesthetic machines							✓ /
bellows and tubing — wash/rinse							✓ /
gas vaporizers — service as needed							✓ /
Microscopes — clean and service as needed							✓ /

Figure 4-7. *Veterinary hospital general maintenance schedule* *(Continued)*

worked in other animal hospitals need to be properly instructed in how to do things the way the new hospital owner or manager requires. Failure to properly train maintenance personnel can result in slipshod work and poorly maintained premises and can lead to employer–employee problems. Employees cannot be expected to do a job properly unless they have been properly instructed. This same premise applies to outside contractors who are doing scheduled maintenance work for the hospital. They need to be instructed in what work is to be done and the way in which the hospital manager or owner expects it completed. Additional information concerning employee training may be found in Chapter 3.

Veterinary technicians (certified or registered) should not be asked to do menial janitorial or kennel duties. This underutilization of skilled personnel is a waste of payroll dollars and can result in friction and ill feelings among lay staff. Technicians should be responsible for maintaining special equipment, supervising the preparation of sterile packs,

and so forth. An exception to this rule may be the new practice that does not have a staff large enough to avoid duplication of duties. Utilization of the veterinary technician is discussed in Chapter 12.

In the larger practice, one method of maintenance scheduling is to create various maintenance zones in the hospital. The zones might be arranged as follows:

Zone A: Public areas of the building that clients frequent (waiting area, receptionist's office, business office, exam rooms, and public restrooms)

Zone B: Hospital work areas (surgery, treatment, x-ray, pharmacy, laboratory, and doctors' offices)

Zone C: Kennel area (ward rooms, dog runs, bathing, and grooming areas)

Zone D: Exterior building and grounds (including porches)

Each zone may be assigned to specific employees on a permanent or rotating basis. Rotating zones has the advantage of having all

	Frequency	By/Date	By/Date	By/Date	By/Date	By/Date	By/Date
Janitorial (building)							
Waste baskets/trash cans — clean and sanitize	Weekly	/	/	/	/	/	/
Windows — wash	Biweekly	/	/	/	/	/	/
Walls & woodwork — wash	Biweekly	/	/	/	/	/	/
Wall hangings — clean/dust	Biweekly	/	/	/	/	/	/
A/C air filters — check & replace	Monthly	/	/	/	/	/	/
A/C vents — clean/dust	Monthly	/	/	/	/	/	/
Hot water tanks — drain	Monthly	/	/	/	/	/	/
Light fixtures — clean/dust	Monthly	/	/	/	/	/	/
Refrigerators — defrost/clean	Monthly	/	/	/	/	/	/
A/C blowers — clean/oil	Semiannually	/	/	/	/	/	/
Cabinets and doors — wax/polish	Semiannually	/	/	/	/	/	/
Drapes/curtains — clean/wash	Semiannually	/	/	/	/	/	/
Floors — strip/wax	Semiannually	/	/	/	/	/	/
Pest control — insecticide fog kennels/wards	As needed	/	/	/	/	/	/
Grounds maintenance							
Lawns/plants — trim/mow	Weekly	/	/	/	/	/	/
Lawn irrigation system/bubblers — check	Semiannually	/	/	/	/	/	/
Lawn/plants/trees — water	As needed	/	/	/	/	/	/
Lawn/plants/trees — fertilize	As needed	/	/	/	/	/	/

Item	Frequency						
Parking lots — resurface/restripe	As needed	/	/	/	/	/	/
Sign(s) — replace light bulbs, paint	As needed	/	/	/	/	/	/
Building exterior — repair/paint	As needed	/	/	/	/	/	/
Roof covering — repair/replace	As needed	/	/	/	/	/	/
Pest control — insecticide spray premises	As needed	/	/	/	/	/	/
Special equipment							
(Follow manufacturer's recommendations)							
Film developing tanks — clean and change solutions	As needed	/	/	/	/	/	/
Automatic film processors	As needed	/	/	/	/	/	/
Anesthetic machines	As needed	/	/	/	/	/	/
bellows/tubing — wash/rinse	As needed	/	/	/	/	/	/
gas vaporizers — service as required	As needed	/	/	/	/	/	/
Microscopes — clean/service as needed	As needed	/	/	/	/	/	/
Fire extinguishers — have tested	Annually	/	/	/	/	/	/

Figure 4-8. *Veterinary hospital periodic maintenance schedule*

employees cross-trained in maintaining various parts of the hospital and grounds. This can be beneficial during vacation periods and in times of employee illness. Cross-training will also make the job of training new employees easier.

Another method of job delegation is to assign specific duties throughout the hospital to individual employees who may be more adept or suited to specific types of maintenance work. These duties include floor maintenance, general cleaning, kennel work, yard work, and so forth. Regardless of how scheduled work is assigned, it is very important to have someone of authority in the practice (veterinarian or hospital manager) who will be responsible for seeing that assigned tasks are properly done and at scheduled times.

Use of outside contractors for maintenance

An alternative to using in-house personnel for janitorial and yard work duties is to utilize an outside janitorial service or a yard service. In the event outside contractors *are* used, they should be furnished a copy of the appropriate maintenance schedules, and someone in the practice must be responsible to see that the schedules are being completed. If the janitorial service will be working in the building after regular hours without supervision, its personnel should be bonded.

Electrical, plumbing, and air-conditioning systems should all be included in schedules for routine maintenance. Specialized equipment will require regular maintenance to keep it working trouble free.

Pest control procedures

Pest control can be a very important routine maintenance item, both inside and outside the animal hospital, and should be included on the schedule. Any establishment that houses animals, even for short periods of time, is providing a natural habitat for infestations of animal parasites. Control of fleas and ticks on the premises should be a high-priority item. One of the quickest ways to alienate a small-animal client is to allow an animal to be released from the hospital with any type of parasite on its body. Regardless of how well the surgery or treatment of that animal went, it can all be negated the moment the client finds the animal infested with even one parasite that it picked up at the veterinary facility. In some parts of the country external parasite control can be an ongoing, frustrating problem for all hospital owners. There are many approaches for controlling this problem, and it is important to find methods that work best in a specific area and make sure they are rigidly followed.

One control method is that of fogging the kennel areas with an insecticide. Attaching a timer to a fogging machine and letting it fog the empty kennel rooms one at a time has proved effective in both tick and flea control. Extreme care must be taken to keep animals and people out of the area until the fumes have been completely aired out. This same method can also be used to fumigate the same areas with disinfectant fogs to aid in controlling viral outbreaks of respiratory disease. In some hospitals that board animals this procedure is often used before and after heavy boarding seasons. It may also be necessary to use an insecticide dip on every animal on the premises if a number of animals in the hospital are discovered with ectoparasites and the problem appears to be getting out of hand.

In the large-animal hospital care must be taken to control rodents and flies. Fly control can be maintained through regular cleaning schedules, hand-applied insecticides, electric insect killing devices, or automated timed-release spray systems. Rodents can be effectively controlled through employee-applied bait systems, professional exterminators, or resident feline patrol.

Importance of using schedules

The schedules in Figures 4-7 and 4-8 are merely examples of one way to set up an ongoing control of maintenance procedures. There are many ways to design a chart that will accomplish the necessary result. The importance of using schedules is that maintenance items are not neglected as often as when left to hit-and-miss methods. Things left until employees "get around to it" are rarely "gotten around to."

Some items need to be examined, cleaned, or restocked on a daily basis, whereas others only require attention weekly, monthly, semiannually, or less frequently. Unless a schedule is established and followed, many maintenance jobs will not be done, and problems will erupt, usually at inopportune times. The items that require more *infrequent* attention are most often the ones that do not get *any* attention. Some examples of this include changing of filters in air-conditioning return air ducts, semiannual oiling of electrical motors in air-conditioning equipment, checking of fluorescent light bulbs for signs of deterioration that can lead to damage of older-type electrical ballasts (and possible fire), draining of hot water heaters on a monthly basis, checking fire extinguishers on an annual basis, cleaning and servicing furnaces before winter use, defrosting freezers, and so forth. Failure to properly maintain these items in the animal hospital can lead to equipment failure with resultant undue expense. Occasionally, severe problems such as flooding from plumbing failure or fires from electrical malfunctions may develop from a lack of routine maintenance. Diligent use of well-designed maintenance schedules can be of great help to ensure proper and timely care of equipment, buildings, and grounds.

Conserving energy and utility costs

Some routine procedures such as maintaining clean filters in air-conditioning systems and the timely repair of leaking faucets can result in substantially lower utility costs. This is accomplished by allowing more energy-efficient operation of the air-conditioning equipment and better conservation of water.

Energy conservation can also be aided appreciably by maintaining good control of any air loss (hot or cold) through cracks around door and window openings. Weather stripping, caulking, and seals around these and other openings through walls should be inspected on a regular basis and repaired or replaced as needed. Refrigeration pipes and ducts that are exposed to outside or attic air should be kept well insulated. Automatic door-closing devices on all outside doors help to prevent unnecessary hot or cold air loss. These door closers serve a dual function because they can help prevent the escape of loose animals from within the hospital.

Careful attention to the placement of trees and large shrubs for efficient shading of the east and west sides of the building in hot climates can be a very energy efficient procedure. The use of deciduous trees and shrubs can be very beneficial in providing shade in summer and allowing sunlight to help warm the building in winter.

Sun-protective awnings and reflective films on windows will also provide good reduction in energy expense during summer months. Many new devices have become available in the past few years to aid in reducing high-energy costs. Air-conditioning (refrigeration) "precoolers" are a good example. They use an evaporative cooling effect on the air that enters the refrigeration unit and thereby decrease demand on the refrigeration unit in cooling air to the required temperature. Solar water heaters are another example of energy-saving devices being used in many parts of the country. Solar energy is being used, to a much smaller extent, to air-condition entire buildings. Use of this form of energy is still in its infancy but should increase steadily as new technology is developed.

The use of electronic light sensors (electric eyes) to control security lighting will ensure timely illumination of the premises each evening and will shut off the system at dawn to conserve electricity. Installation of lawn sprinkling and planter bubbling systems connected to a timer clock will enable proper watering of outside vegetation with a minimal amount of wasted water. Periods of watering can be changed with the seasons, thereby eliminating careless over- and underwatering.

Maintaining a good appearance

Maintenance of various components of the building itself should be of prime importance to the owner of the practice. This is one of the best methods of advertising the quality of the practice to the clientele. People will judge the quality of a business by the appearance of the building and grounds. A building with a neatly painted exterior, well-maintained roof, and clean windows, floors, walls, and ceilings that is tastefully decorated inside and out and situated on well-maintained, nicely landscaped grounds will convey a message to clients that this is a high-quality business establishment.

Periodic redecorating of interior rooms, especially "client contact" rooms, can be very rewarding. A change in wall colors or floor coverings and changes in some or all the wall decorations and occasionally even the furniture will relieve the boredom and give the hospital a new look. Aside from the primary pur-

pose of improving the look for clientele, these changes have a beneficial effect on the staff as well. Providing a pleasant atmosphere for employees to work can result in increased levels of performance and less tension.

Importance of prompt repairs

Prompt attention to making repairs of damage to any part of the building is very important. Failure to do so will soon result in a run-down or worn-out appearance of the facility. Even very minor damage such as a broken floor tile or a cracked window pane, if allowed to go unrepaired, will convey a message of lack of concern by management. Major repairs such as replacement of damaged or aged roof covering and repainting of the building are important from the standpoint of preservation of the capital investment in the facility. Damage to the roof or exterior of the building should be covered by insurance, but routine wear-and-tear maintenance costs are not and can amount to considerable expense. Roof repairs are usually made rather quickly due to potential damage to ceilings and other internal contents of the building. Routine painting of the external part of the building too often is delayed because of procrastination on the part of the owner who sees the building daily and doesn't realize the extent of its deterioration in appearance.

□
Summary

In this chapter methods have been discussed to aid in selection of a site for construction of a veterinary facility. Various ways have been suggested to establish the value of a given piece of property and to approach the problem of obtaining finances with which to build the facility. The importance of proper maintenance of the facility once it is in operation has been reviewed. It has been pointed out that there are many considerations and many decisions to make in selecting a location, acquiring financing, and building and properly maintaining an animal hospital. Each veterinarian, or group of veterinarians, will approach the problem in their own particular way.

Chapter 5
□
Computer utilization in veterinary practice

George M. Angleton

The principal purpose of this text is to identify and discuss criteria for the development of a successful, modern, quality veterinary practice. One criterion involves the use of a process termed *integrated information utilization* (IIU). In the most direct sense IIU is a process that involves extracting individual packets of information from multiple sources, weighting these packets according to needs, integrating these weighted packets into a single packet of information, and then condensing the information in the single packet into a useful format or procedure.

In the modern veterinary practice attempts to effectively use the IIU process may at times appear unproductive. When one concludes such an effort is unproductive, then a determination of causes must be made. In general, these causes may be classified in one of two ways: either adequate tools for using the process are not available or available tools are used ineffectively. In either case, the costs in terms of time and other resource commitments associated with attempts to use the process may become excessively high. Attempts are then made to contain these costs. Containment of costs under these conditions results in a decrease in the efficiency of the processing of pertinent information. The consequence is that practice management decisions are then made with only a fraction of the available information.

The effective practice manager does not need to be reminded to optimize the use of information in making decisions. The practice manager has the inherent responsibility to continually seek ways for optimizing the utilization of available information and to do so in a cost-effective manner. The practice manager must also implement new procedures to increase the productivity of personnel and improve the effectiveness of management and clinical decisions. This means the effective practice manager will need to understand the process of IIU and seek ways to increase the efficiency of its use.

The most economical route to follow for achieving the goal of increased efficiency for IIU is to incorporate the use of automated information processing. In general, this means incorporating the use of computers and related technologies into the day-to-day activities of a veterinary practice. In this chapter some of the concerns related to the usage of computers in veterinary practice management are discussed. These discussions will emphasize the use of computers in processing information used for making managerial decisions, maintaining accurate fiscal records, and supporting routine office and clinic operations. In discussing IIU from a practice manager's point of view, it needs to be recognized that the IIU process could also be used to process information as it pertains to clinical procedures for purposes of optimizing patient care.

Finally, this chapter will not become involved with specific hardware configurations, software packages, or vendors marketing hardware and software. The reason is that any reference book dealing with the merits of specific hardware configurations or a specific software package tends to be quickly outdated. In many cases, material discussed in such a book may be out of date before publication. Hence, for the material presented in this chapter to have any long-term application it will be necessary to develop a perspective for the role of computer technology in a program designed to progressively upgrade the process of IIU with the realization that both hardware and software are undergoing a rapid, but nonetheless continuous evolution.

In this chapter, space does not allow for extensive speculation as to futuristic computer support. Historically, such projections have been meaningless. It is worth noting that the residual market value of most computer equipment marketed 3 years ago is now worth about 10% of its original value. The primary use of such equipment is for spare parts. When a veterinary practice is to be computerized from scratch, essentially no used equipment is purchased. This means that the costs of computerization need to be amortized over a 3-year period. At the end of 3 years, it is likely the equipment will be replaced and the old equipment will be disposed of as junk, even though it may still be functional. It may be well to remember that when a computer system is purchased, big or small, the newly acquired system needs to be treated as a "disposable computer system."

The buyer should be skeptical of computer support systems development based on promises of vendors. Existing systems seldom perform as flashy demonstrations lead one to believe. A high percentage of vendors' promises never make their appearance on the market. Hence, in designing a system, it is well to remember "What you see is what you get." Be prepared to make the system work, knowing that a completely new system will be available in 3 years. The new system may materialize either through total replacement of the existing system or a continual upgrading of components of the existing system.

□
The role of computerization in a veterinary practice

There is only one reason for computerizing a veterinary practice. Computerization will increase the efficiency with which information is processed and will provide the mechanism whereby progress can be made toward achieving the goal of IIU. It should be noted that the term *IIU* has a significantly different meaning than the perhaps more familiar term of *Inte-*

grated *Information Processing* (IIP). The term *IIP* places an emphasis on the mechanics of processing information. The term *IIU* places emphasis on the utilization of information. IIP may be considered an integral part of IIU, or a subset of IIU.

The veterinarian or practice manager is primarily interested in information utilization. In regard to information utilization, the sources from which information can be gathered are clients, product bulletins, veterinary literature, and observational data. Observation data can be stored in client medical records, procedure files, or in product files. Needed data are then retrieved from data files and used to support necessary or desirable practice management activities such as generation of appointment schedules, maintenance of inventory records, or updating accounts receivable and accounts payable files.

Computerization of a veterinary practice will lead to enhancements for one or more of the following processes: (1) collection of observational data, (2) maintenance of data files, (3) retrieval of information, and (4) utilization of information. The goal of computerization should be the establishment of a program that will perspectively and progressively allow for simultaneous enhancements of all four processes. The simultaneous enhancement of all processes represents IIU. In regard to the last of these four factors, it needs to be kept in mind that utilization of information eventually involves decision making. One needs frequent reminding that the computer is only used to obtain summaries of information that in turn are used along with other sources of information in the process of making decisions.

Historically, computerization of a professional office has meant implementing an automated billing system using computer technology. Originally this meant that billing information was manually transported to a distal central computer site for remote entry of data and subsequent processing. An enhance-

ment to this procedure was realized when it became possible to transmit the same data to the distal central site over telephone lines by using electronic data transmission procedures originating in the office. Today, the same information can be sent electronically to computer systems located in the same office in which the information is generated, that is, to computers located within the offices of the veterinary practice.

A natural consequence of developing the use of computers primarily in support of billing activities has been that the concepts for the use of computers in practice management have developed along the same lines. Namely, many office managers continue to think of computerization within the restrictive framework of developing an automated billing system. It is important that these office managers broaden their perspectives and realize that computerized billing procedures represent only one segment of IIU.

Before making a casual commitment to computerization, it is very important the office manager consider responsibilities. In taking a brief look at these responsibilities, terminology associated with computerization need not be used. The reason for this is that computerization is an activity to be used in reaching a goal, namely, IIU. This goal has always existed.

Practice managers must realize that they have the responsibility for organizing the flow of all information in the practice. This has always been the case and will always continue to be so. This responsibility is not affected as a result of changes in the tools that become available to expedite the flow of information. For practice managers to meet these responsibilities effectively they must naturally keep informed about the tools available for managing this flow of information. As new tools become available, the cost-effectiveness of their use must be continually evaluated. Acquisition of tools and incorporation of their use must be done in a timely manner.

Caution must be exerted though. At times, some practice managers tend to become overly enthralled with a tool simply because it is the latest item to appear on the market. Frequently, inadequate attention is given to how such items will benefit the overall flow of information in the practice. Such managers become better known for their collection of "white elephants" than for their effectiveness in information processing and utilization. In this case white elephants are defined as mementos of expensive items that did not perform as promised.

Caution must also be exerted in the other direction. A more conservative approach to the acquisition of new tools is to delay their acquisition until the effectiveness of their use has been demonstrated with complete certainty. The person who follows this strategy is probably worse off than the person who always wants to acquire the latest device on the market. This person will probably wait for 5 years after the introduction of a new product before purchasing the product. With the continuing rapid technological evolution of business management products, such a practice manager will become better known for their collections of "antiques" than for his progressive management.

The perceptive manager will be well organized relative to the flow of information within the practice and, for that matter, between practices. Many aspects of the flow of this information can be computerized; however, care will need to be exerted not to computerize one aspect without considering the interrelationships of information flow. It is no longer appropriate to deal with billing activities in a manner separate from management of medical records, scheduling of appointments, inventory management, practice management analyses, office automation, and other activities that involve information processing.

Once the decision has been made to move forward with computerization, one needs to pause and ask the question "Do I really know the role of computerization in practice management?" To answer this question the practice manager must be aware that computerization does not mean that all practice personnel are expected to become programmers. In fact, it does not mean they have to become very knowledgeable in the relative merits of operating systems or other special programs that control computer operations. In addition, computerization does not mean that users have to become very knowledgeable in the repair and maintenance of computer equipment. In the long run, one needs to realize that only a very limited amount of knowledge concerning the electronic and mechanical aspects of computers needs to be acquired before initiating a meaningful program for computerizing a veterinary practice.

The purpose of computerization in a practice is to generate efficient and effective processing of information. This means that the practice manager will need to become aware of all aspects of the procedures involved in processing practice information before computerizing the procedures. The practice manager will have to acknowledge that the goal being sought is IIU. Once the manager understands the tasks to be done, he or she will then have to acquire knowledge relative to the specific functions that can be performed by computers. The eventual approach to be used in the computerization effort will need to be one with which the combined inventories of white elephants and antiques are kept to a minimum.

□
Analysis of needs for computerization

An analysis of the needs for computerization in a practice must be performed very carefully. Such an analysis requires knowledgeable input from everyone who will be involved in the use of the system. Equivalently, this means everyone on the staff. It is also important to recognize that computerization will affect the complete staff. The practice manager must become knowledgeable about the potential for use of computers in the practice and then will have to share this knowledge with the entire staff. The learning process can proceed in a variety of ways.

The first step should be to read and distribute articles on veterinary computing. A meaningful second step involves visiting sites where computers are used in support of management activities similar to those of a veterinary practice. It is important to note that these sites need not be restricted to veterinary practices. There are many medical and dental offices that have been computerized. Very few have used identical approaches to computerization. Hence, by making visits to several sites, one can tap an extensive source of pertinent information.

A third step would be to invite hardware vendors, software vendors, system consultants, and other available knowledgeable individuals to present miniseminars in their specialty areas. These seminars should be conducted at the site being computerized to ensure that all staff members have access to the same information.

A fourth step involves the practice manager developing a generalized flowchart for auto-

mated processing of practice management information. Such a flowchart needs to be reviewed by the staff. The flowchart should be constructed in modules. This will ensure that the system can be implemented in stages and later enhanced in a modular fashion.

The initial flowchart for computerization of a practice should reflect only the needs of processing information. At this stage, specific hardware components need not be referenced. An illustrative flowchart is given in Figure 5-1. This flowchart addresses client management activities only. The flowchart would become more comprehensive as needs to computerize other activities materialize.

The upper box of the flowchart refers to client information that needs to be stored online to be interactively accessible in support of functions listed in the lower boxes. Detailed supporting documentation must be generated for each of these boxes. This activity needs to be completed before proceeding to the next step.

The fifth step would then involve having a consultant systems analyst perform an analysis of the proposed system. The systems analyst would identify the type of software package modules needed, options for acquiring hard-

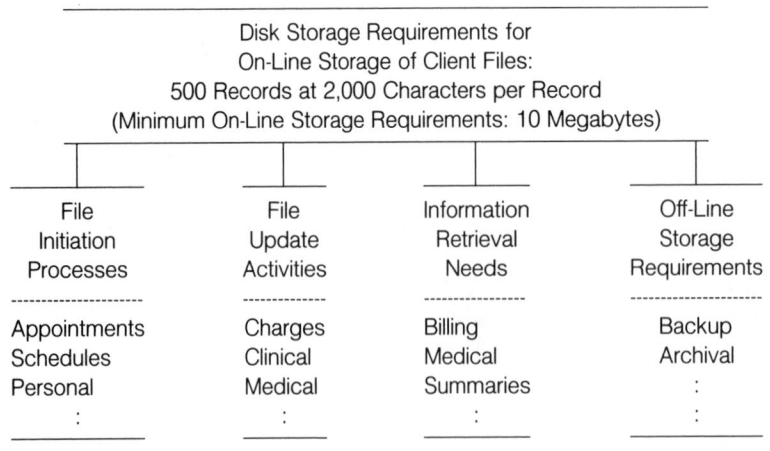

Figure 5-1. *Illustrative flowchart for computerizing client files*

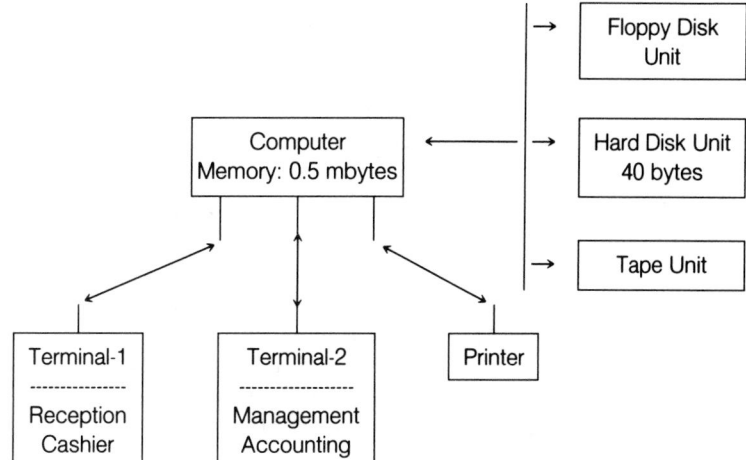

Figure 5-2. Schematic diagram for computer hardware to be used in managing client files

ware components and how they should be interfaced, and priorities for obtaining items and finally make recommendations relative to training and outlining procedures for implementing the system.

Figure 5-2 is a schematic for computer hardware that could be used in support of the information processing flowcharted in Figure 5-1. The computer is interfaced with two types of peripherals. The first type includes the disk units and the tape unit. These units are used to store information processed by the computer. The second type of peripherals are the input/output (I/O) devices of the users. In this illustration the I/O devices consist of two terminals and a printer. Undoubtedly, a systems analyst would design a system such that it could be expanded to support additional I/O devices.

If the costs of computerization are to be kept within reasonable limits, procedural steps equivalent to those just given must be followed anytime a new system is acquired or an existing system is significantly upgraded. This is true whether a manual system is being upgraded to a new or revised manual system or to a newly designed computer-based system. It is also true when an existing computer-based system is being upgraded to another computer-based system. Unfortunately, because computer systems tend to become obsolete within a period of 3 years, the practice manager needs to be prepared to repeat this analysis process about once every 3 years, especially if the practice is experiencing growth.

A major reason for adhering to this protocol for upgrading is that the costs for implementing a conversion tend to be very high. As will be noted later, all office procedures will be affected, and extensive retraining will have to be performed. Many managers are not aware of the complexities associated with a conversion at the time a commitment is made to computerization. As a consequence, it is not unusual for a business to acquire an expensive computer system and then not be able to use it. Once a significant monetary loss is experienced as a result of a non-successful computerization effort, it becomes difficult to maintain a continuing positive attitude toward computerization.

Another excellent reason for adhering to this protocol involves the risks incurred during a conversion process as far as maintaining the integrity of client and management data files is concerned. Records can easily be lost, resulting in loss of revenue or loss of client information. For example, a conversion representing many hours of effort will appear to be essentially complete when one of two problems can occur. Either human error occurs, or an equipment malfunction takes place that results in a complete loss of converted material. There are many ways for this to happen, especially when the conversion is not implemented according to acceptable guidelines.

Another undesirable event that occasionally takes place is that some of the converted information becomes unusable. Such problems generally manifest themselves when special data base update programs or retrieval programs are used for the first time. This type of problem can become difficult to resolve. In many cases the problem may not be resolvable without making additional purchases of hardware and software or seeking the services of a computer specialist. This after-the-fact treatment of such a problem is usually quite costly in both time and money.

There are still other significant snafus that can arise when the needs for IIU are not carefully assessed. For example, all too often the new system is designed to meet the needs of the previous system. The conversion then may only lead to increased efficiency of performing existing tasks. When this happens, very little forward movement toward IIU will be achieved. Consequently, the benefits associated with computerization may at best be marginal.

It will be impossible to avoid all pitfalls and roadblocks along the path of computerization. To minimize the risks of such hazards, however, it is extremely important that the practice manager realize that successful computerization of a veterinary practice involves making a commitment to IIU and developing an overview of information utilization.

☐
Software alternatives

The manager who lacks perspective might look upon the management operations as a set of independent operations with no relationship existing between any two operations. Alternately, another manager might identify subsets of operations that are interrelated and then manage as if there were no relationships among the subsets. On the other hand, a manager might realize that relationships exist among all operations and consequently manage by taking advantage of all interrelations. There are alternatives for selecting computer software that correspond to such alternatives for management. If the goal for computerization is IIU, then the manager will need to adhere to the interrelational style of management.

Regardless of the style of management, computerization will require the manager to construct flow diagrams outlining the flow, or lack of flow, of information within the practice. Flow diagrams are basically charts consisting of boxes and lines connecting the boxes. A given box contains a description of how information is processed when it is passed into that box and also the criteria for determining which box or boxes shall receive the processed information. Flowcharts should be constructed in such a manner that each box represents a module of activity. This means, regardless of the scheme developed to process the information in one box, that decisions should not affect the scheme for processing the information in another box. Until these flowcharts are generated, the practice manager runs the risk of making conflicting decisions. If the conflict is not resolved before the acquisition and implementation of computer hardware and software, the result may be unused equipment. Such has been the case for many small businesses.

Computer programs represent the translation into computer code of flow diagrams of logical processes describing, for example, practice management operations. Computer code represents collections of strings of binary (0, 1) numbers used to control the electronic operations of a rather sophisticated calculator in performing numerous calculations very quickly. The results of the calculations are then translated into code that can be translated into electronic signals used to control the operations of a variety of output devices. These devices include video display monitors, printers, plotters, tapes, disks, and automated control of equipment.

A computer program selected by a practice manager represents the translation of a detailed flow diagram created by a systems analyst or programmer into a computer language. This flowchart is generally not made available to the user. So to speak, it contains trade secrets. Such programs need to meet the specifications for information processing as given in the generalized flow diagrams developed under the direction of the practice manager. These computer programs will function at best according to the limitations of the programmer's flow diagram. Most likely, not all of the options detailed in the flow diagram will be incorporated into the actual computer program. The programmer will probably indicate that they may be added at a latter time.

For a variety of other reasons, including programming errors, the logic that is actually included in a computer program may not represent a one-to-one translation of the logic in the flow diagram. Accordingly, the program may have logic errors or "bugs." Detection of bugs is sometimes difficult. Frequently, the user discovers a bug after using a program for several months. Once a bug is discovered, the party responsible for generating the program must make the correction. This process is referred to as "debugging" a program. Some-

times the debugging process can be very complicated, time-consuming, and consequently expensive and hence not done in a timely manner. This may mean the user will have to learn to use a program that is correct most of the time.

Using a computer program that represents an incomplete translation of a logical process or under certain circumstances generates output containing errors will lead to frustration on the part of the user. This, in turn, will have a significant negative impact upon the attitudes of the staff members who are trying to accept computerization of the practice management. Hence, it is very important that quality software be selected. The selection of quality software should be done in collaboration with a knowledgeable person. This may mean that the practice manager will have to use a paid consultant.

Software selection

There are two major tasks in selecting computer programs. The first is to evaluate the *functionality* of the program, that is, the flow sheet or logic for the program. The second task is to evaluate the *reliability* of the program and the integrity of the organization responsible for maintenance of the program. Cost should not be considered a major factor in software selection. The reason cost is not a major factor is that a well-written program will lead to the generation of revenue; a poorly written program will lead to a loss of revenue.

In evaluating the functionality of programs, the practice manager needs to continually evaluate goals for IIU. If monthly billings, maintenance of medical records, inventory control, processing of accounts payable, correspondence (word processing), budget control, and other activities controlled by the practice manager are treated as separate unrelated areas of management, then individual programs for each of these areas will probably be acquired and used. In fact, many practice managers may perceive some of these areas of activities as not being interrelated. This is indeed unfortunate because effective modern practice management demands that these interrelationships be identified and that efficient management procedures be developed with respect to these interrelationships. That is, the principles of IIU will need to be used.

During the past decade, most programs written in support of management operations provided support of only one activity at a time. That is, billing programs, inventory control programs, accounts payable programs, and others were written without regard to mutual utilization of common information. There are numerous reasons for this. In the early 1980s, the use of computers was not perceived as a key element in practice management. About that time, though, a few practice managers realized computers could be used in support of billing services. Accordingly, programs with the scope of application restricted to billing operations were written in response to market demands.

At that time there was also another major reason for writing programs with a restricted scope of application. This was related to the limitations and costs of computer hardware available in the early 1980s. As will be discussed later, these restrictions have now disappeared. As a result, programs incorporating some of the principles in IIU are now on the market. More comprehensive programs can be expected to be available almost on a daily basis. Hence, the practice manager, who a few years ago had to forego IIU to computerize, needs today to gain a firm understanding of the principles of IIU. Programs will shortly become available that will support IIU to a level beyond conceptions established before computers existed or when computers were used to support isolated segments of practice management activities.

Word processing

Astounding progress in the development of software has taken place within the last 5 years. For example, consider the changes in word processing and spreadsheet analysis programs. Five years ago word processing programs were very limited in scope and performed rather poorly. At that time word processing was highly oriented toward magcard electric typewriters, a few stand-alone word processing systems, and a rather limited number of systems that supported centralized word processing.

Today, the whole perspective of word processing has changed. Both the software and hardware options needed to support word processing have been developed to the point that they support a wide range of user needs. Word processing is being used increasingly by almost all professionals. Thus, it probably goes without saying that almost everyone involved in supporting practice management will need to become proficient in word processing. Word processing should no longer be considered solely a secretary's tool. Those so inclined to think this is the case really need to take time to reappraise their concepts of the role of word processing in the more comprehensive picture of information processing.

Word processing programs have become comprehensive relative to the generation of all types of documents. These programs are able to be used with almost any type of printer on the market. As a result, they can be used to generate numerous office forms that formerly had to be generated by professionals. These programs can also be used to generate multiple copies of documents that formerly required the use of multipart paper. Hence, proper use of word processing to support these functions can lead to an appreciable reduction in the costs of office forms.

In reference to the generation of standard text material, word processing capabilities are again quite comprehensive. For example, most worthwhile word processing programs feature a spelling check dictionary. Such programs allow users to access a standard list of words to be compared with text words generated by the user. If a text word is not found in the dictionary, the program displays words having spellings similar to the text word. The user is then able to select a displayed word to automatically replace the text word, manually change the spelling of the text word, or if appropriate, enter the text word into the dictionary. As word processing programs become more comprehensive, the options for computer-assisted editing of text material can be expected to become almost unbelievable.

Spreadsheets

The growth in the development of spreadsheet programs has paralleled the growth of word processing programs. Five years ago, spreadsheet programs tended to be used in a rather restricted sense, primarily in support of basic accounting activity. For the most part, spreadsheet programs were conceived to be an accountant's tool, in the same sense word processing was conceived to be a secretary's tool. The amount of data that could be processed at any one time and the options for processing the data were severely limited.

Spreadsheet programs now support a very large number of office functions. They are becoming an important tool for routine use by both management and accountants. In fact, spreadsheet programs are now becoming routinely used by any staff member involved in the mathematical manipulation of numbers. Spreadsheet programs can be designed to support accounts payable and receivable activities. Likewise they can be used in generating budget reviews and budget projections. They can be used in the construction of tables including both text and numeric data. Almost all spreadsheet programs today allow for sophis-

ticated generating of summary reports that incorporate the use of business graphics. The term *business graphics* until recently referred to bar charts, histograms, pie charts, line charts, and other basic graphic modes for displaying business information. Today the term is being defined in a much broader sense. Graphic displays can easily incorporate the use of an almost unlimited number of symbolic notations or figures. In other words, as with word processing, spreadsheet analysis programs are becoming increasingly comprehensive.

Comprehensive practice management software

These dicussions on the evolving comprehensive nature of word processing and spreadsheet programs illustrate trends taking place in all computer programs of interest to the practice manager. It should be noted, though, that the discussions were presented in such a manner that might lead one to think that word processing and spreadsheet analyses represented unrelated activities. A few years ago, operationally this was the case. Today, this is not true. Word processing programs increasingly include spreadsheet capabilities as part of the word processing capability. Or perhaps it is the other way around. At any rate the two types of programs are beginning to merge. In fact, the integration of word processing and spreadsheet analysis programs is becoming sufficiently common for a new generic name to be applied to the programs. For veterinary practices, the generic name *comprehensive practice management software* (CPMS) could be given to programs representing such integration. This acronym, CPMS, will be used for discussion in this part of the text.

Rapid strides are being made in the development of CPMS. There is an ongoing trend to integrate all facets of practice management programs. New perspectives are being given to the development of programs formerly used in isolation to support specific management operations. The list of operations for which isolated computer programs have been written include billing, accounts payable, accounts receivable, payroll, inventory, medical records, laboratory data processing, and others. The current trend for development of software is to integrate these programs into a single package. That is, software is now being developed from a broader perspective in recognition of the need of CPMS.

With these points in mind, it should not be surprising to note that tremendous strides are being made in data base management packages. These data base management packages are being developed in a way that may change how all practice management programs are written. In general these new data base management packages are referred to as *fourth-generation languages,* or 4-GLs. There are essentially no 4-GLs of outstanding quality on the market today. However, there are several 4-GLs available that may be characterized as having average or reasonable quality.

Once 4-GLs of outstanding quality become available, the practice manager will find even greater opportunities for achieving the goal of IIU. For example, within about 3 years, the practice manager who has developed a skill for flowcharting information and who possesses the self-discipline to ensure that the flowcharts remain current (both with respect to current operations and desired operations) will be in for some very pleasant surprises when dealing with software vendors who develop computer programs using quality 4-GLs. These surprises will include (1) the ease and options for creating data input screens, (2) the options for distributing data to different files, (3) the options for retrieving data from multiple files, and (4) the options for generating reports containing text, data, and graphics.

The pace of development for CPMS can be expected to accelerate over the next few years.

The practice manager is going to be challenged in attempts to keep abreast of these developments. It is a challenge that is going to have to be successfully met if available tools are to be used effectively in support of IIU. The practice manager is going to need help if the challenge is to be met. For the established practice manager this may mean attendance at workshops. Unfortunately, at this time many workshops are rather poor at presenting pertinent, practical information. On the other hand, progress is being made in the improvement of the quality of these workshops, but this progress is slow because of a lack of interested and competent people needed to develop such workshops. Moreover, progress is directly related to market demand, that is, demand for practice managers to move forward, with automated information processing to be used in support of IIU.

☐
Hardware alternatives

The practice manager has the responsibility for developing a complete overview of administrative information processing as it applies to the practice. Once this is accomplished, the manager may begin to compile an information base that outlines alternatives for computerizing information processing in a manner commensurate with stated goals. This information base needs to include the results of costs analyses, benefit analyses, and performance analyses relative to the use of computer hardware. Only after this is accomplished will it be possible to generate an ordered list of alternatives for moving forward with computerization. This list will then be used to establish priorities for phasing in the acquisition of computer hardware.

Once this information base is in place, surprising as it may seem, it will probably become apparent that there are rather limited sets of alternatives for selecting computer hardware to meet the defined needs. The reason for this is that the prioritized list of steps to be followed in the computerization effort will likely contain specifications for the use of certain software packages. These specifications may be rather restrictive, especially if the long-range goal for the computerization effort is IIU. Unfortunately, the number of acceptable software packages available today to support this effort is quite limited. In fact, it is highly unlikely that software adequate to the needs of IIU will exist before 1988, or possibly later.

There is no need to procrastinate, however. In order to even partially meet current needs, a set of unified software programs appropriate for use in a veterinary practice needs to be identified. This means that the manager, in conjunction with a consultant, will probably need to identify software packages that can use common data files. The reason for this is that a data file generated by one program might not be able to be used by a second program without modification of the data file. Furthermore, as might be expected, not all software packages will run on all computer systems. Hence, the identification of sets of software packages needs to be made with respect to also identifying the hardware configurations on which the programs can operate. Thus, the software specifications will tend to dictate the choice of hardware alternatives, that is, the type of computer components to be acquired.

For any given component of a specified hardware configuration, the products of any of several vendors might be selected. In general, the hardware offerings of the various vendors will tend to be quite similar. Likewise, there will not be a lot of difference in the costs of equivalent pieces of equipment. With this in mind, the best route to follow in the selection of hardware is to select hardware that will meet all of the known requirements and at the same time contains additional performance features that will allow for implementing some desirable options. In addition, the hard-

ware should be obtained from a vendor of established reliability and accessibility, even if there is a slight additional cost. For the most part, price differences in computer hardware should not be the basis for selection of equipment or vendor.

One reason for ignoring price differences in the acquisition of hardware is that once a component is purchased there is little opportunity for exchanging it for a more appropriate piece of equipment. If a component of hardware is not acceptable for any reason, then the most likely alternative will be the outright purchase of a new component. A second reason for ignoring price differences is that hardware investment is really only a small fraction of the total investment being made. The initial and ongoing costs of the software, software updates, training, hardware maintenance, and operations management will each represent larger investments of time and money than the costs of hardware. It is the investment in these other factors that needs protecting. Acquisition of quality hardware from an accessible vendor or dealer almost always translates into an appreciable reduction in the costs to the practice of these other cost factors.

In establishing the needs for computer hardware, it is important not to loose sight of the goals for computerization. Computerization involves acquiring information processing capabilities to meet defined requirements. This means computer software or programs designed to perform specific computer operations will have to be obtained. The assumption is made that the appropriate software will be purchased. It is quite unlikely that the manager, or anyone else in the practice, will become directly involved in generating the core programs to be used to control information processing. Core programs include those used for billing, inventory, word processing, accounting, and other management activities. To one degree or another, the computerization effort will involve assembling pieces of compatible equipment. Thus the information processing equipment has to be compatible relative to the use of core software as well as able to become connected electronically. It also has to be compatible with respect to the expected growth of computerization within the practice.

Growth of computerization within a practice can take place on several levels. The lowest level of development can be characterized in terms of a computer system consisting of a small personal computer, a matrix printer, and a dual-component floppy disk drive. During the time span 1981 to 1984, such a system would have been exciting to have but somewhat frustrating to use. A small practice involving a single clinician and an administrative clerk probably would have found that using such a system was of real value relative to managing some of the fiscal matters of the practice. Today, using such a system would not generate much excitement, but the level of frustration would probably be much higher.

These frustrations result from restrictions placed upon the effectiveness and the efficiency with which information is processed. Evolution in the development of computer hardware is a result of the continual attempts to favorably modify these restrictions. There will always be restrictions. Hence, there will always be the frustrated user. There are some identifiable factors that influence these restrictions and at the same time tend to identify categories of frustrations. The practice manager needs to be aware of them at the time the hardware configuration is being designed and purchases are being made. Several of the more important of these factors will be discussed.

Single-user vs. multiuser systems

The three-component system referred to earlier is a single-user system. This means that only one person can use the system at a time

and only one person at a time can have access to the information stored on the computer. This is equivalent to having a file cabinet containing hundreds of files subjected to the use restriction that only one file at a time can be examined by a single designated person.

Today, it would be a mistake for a practice manager to acquire a single-user system. The options for acquiring a multiuser system are becoming more numerous every day; however, a lot of software and related hardware are still being marketed for single-user systems. A practice manager who moves in this direction will most likely be purchasing an antique.

There are good reasons why vendors try to sell single-user systems. All computers operate under the control of a category of software referred to as the *operating system.* The operating system controls the access to disk units, printer, and video display terminals. The operating system along with system software is also used to interpret programs written in languages such as FORTRAN, Pascal, COBOL, or PL-1. In other words, the operating system constitutes the interface between the computer hardware and the user programs. As might be expected, the operating systems for single-user systems are much easier to develop than are those for multiuser systems.

An insight into the complexity of a multiuser system can be gained by noting that a typical mulituser system contains a single *central processing unit* (CPU). The CPU performs all of the computations. In a single-user system, the CPU usually supports only one activity at a time. In a multiuser system, the CPU will support several activities, still one at a time, but in a sequential manner whereby millisecond or shorter time slices are allocated to each activity. Developing an operating system that will support multiuser functions in an efficient manner is very costly. In addition, modifying programs for use in a multiuser environment is also costly and time-consuming. Hence, it is not unrealistic for a vendor to market an existing product, even when other vendors have a more desirable product. So it is with single-user systems vs. multiuser systems.

Today, the operating systems for multiuser systems are sufficiently advanced and of such a high quality that it is unlikely a practice manager would even consider a single-user system. If the practice resources are such that it is not realistic to acquire a multiuser system, then a single-user system capable of being upgraded to a multiuser system through the addition of hardware components could be acquired. That is, a multiuser system should be acquired that is configured around a CPU having expandable memory options and having one terminal, one quality printer, and an adequate disk drive system.

Disk systems and tape systems

The principal components of a disk system are (1) rapidly revolving disks upon which large volumes of data may be stored, (2) an arm that may be quickly positioned over any sector of a disk, (3) a read–write head located on the end of the arm that is used to transfer information between the computer and the disk, and (4) a controller board installed in the computer that is used to control the movement of the arm and the transfer of information between the disk and computer.

The principal components of a tape system are (1) several hundred feet of computer tape upon which large volumes of data may be stored, with the tape being wound on a tape reel; (2) a cabinet containing two spindles upon which tape reels may be mounted and are then used to rapidly move magnetic tape between the two reels in such a manner as to pass specified segments of the tape in front of a read–write head; (3) a read–write head that is used to transfer information between the computer and the disk; and (4) a controller board installed in the computer that is used to con-

trol the movement of the tape and the transfer of information between the tape and computer.

In some aspects there is not much difference between a tape system and disk system. They are both used to store large volumes of information to be processed by the computer. The principal difference between the two systems is the manner in which the information is accessed. This difference results in information being much more rapidly accessible on a disk system than a tape system; however, the costs of storage are much cheaper for the tape system. For these reasons disk systems are used for on-line storage of information when a computer is being used to process information. Tape systems are generally used for off-line storage of information to be processed at a later time or to create a backup for information stored on a disk. There are exceptions to this statement, but they really do not apply to the computerization efforts of a veterinary practice.

The exceptions relate to the fact that floppy disks and other removable disks may also be used to provide off-line storage of information. Off-line storage of information on removable disks is somewhat expensive and should be reserved for use with relatively small volumes of information. A veterinary practice needs to be prepared to store large volumes of information, both on-line and off-line.

The continual technological advances for both disk systems and tape systems for use with office systems of interest to the practice manager are impressive. Both the volume of information stored and the speed with which the information can be processed continue to increase rapidly. At the same time the costs per unit of information stored are decreasing. Hence, the net costs to the practice manager for storing increasingly large volumes of data on tapes and disks are remaining somewhat constant. The practice manager needs to be prepared to take advantage of this opportunity of having ever-increasing amounts of data available to support the process of IIU.

The rapid increase in disk storage capabilities can be illustrated by comparing typical disk applications in 1980 with those for 1986. The floppy disk units in use in 1980 were typically used to store about 0.25 megabytes (mbytes) of information. One byte equates to one character of information. By 1984 disk units capable of storing 10 mbytes of information were in common use. By 1986 disk units capable of storing well over 100 mbytes of information were available for use on office computer systems.

Whenever large volumes of data are stored on disks, they need to be backed up on tape. Fortunately, developments for tape storage have kept abreast of those for disk storage. As the capabilities to store increasingly large quantities of information on disk have materialized, tape systems have also been developed to handle comparably large quantities of information. In conjunction with the increase in storage capabilities, there has been an increase in the speed with which information can be accessed. This is true for both disk and tape systems. Of interest to the practice manager is the fact that compact tape systems for use with large disk systems are readily available. In addition, they are rather easy to use.

Quite obviously, computerization of a veterinary practice will involve acquiring a disk unit. There may be some debate over determining the size of the disk unit. Because office managers have tended to be slow in grasping the concepts of IIU, disk systems seem to be selected on the basis of meeting only the perceived existing needs. This means many offices are acquiring 10-mbyte and 20-mbyte systems. In a multiuser environment, the practice manager will quickly realize that the minimum disk that should be acquired is a 100-mbyte system. Since the initial investment and the corresponding ongoing costs for a 100-mbyte system are only slightly greater than

those for smaller systems, there is little justification for going with a small system.

One reason for the continuing increase in the volumes of information being stored on-line is related in part to the need to store more text data on-line. Both word processing and the processing of uncoded text data for medical records contribute to this need. In addition, more and more accounting information is being stored on-line that includes descriptive information. Another reason for this continuing increase is that data files are becoming both increasingly large and numerous. Data files are also frequently stored in multiple formats. This results in redundant storage of information at times. The redundancy is justified on the basis that it facilitates user access to information.

Another factor that leads to increased disk size requirements is the need to reserve approximately 25% of the disk space for manipulation of data files. Whenever sort routines or word-processing programs access data files, ancillary data files are created. Some of these files may be large. In working with these files, large blocks of contiguous disk space will be needed. Finally, disk space must be allocated to the on-line storage of operating system programs and user programs. The disk space needed to support such program storage can easily exceed several megabytes.

Equally obvious to the need for the acquisition of a large disk unit should be the need for the acquisition of a tape storage unit capable of rapidly backing up the information stored on disk. Unfortunately, this means someone is going to have to perform these tape operations. That is, someone on the staff is going to have to develop tape backup procedures and then become a computer operator. This requirement will have to be managed for both the very small as well as the moderately large computer systems. The systems analysis or hardware consultant working with the practice manager needs to be perceptive relative to these developing needs. If dealt with in an informed manner, managing a so-called large disk system will not be a difficult task.

Printers

Printers of interest to the practice manager may be given the broad classifications of (1) impact, (2) matrix, and (3) laser. It is important to note that the technological developments for printer systems are also keeping pace with the technological developments for the other components of computer systems. Accordingly, it should not be surprising to find out that a 3-year-old printer has little if any market value.

Impact printers are most frequently used in support of activities where fully formed characters were desired, in contrast to the dot matrix characters produced by matrix printers. Thus, impact printers have traditionally been used to support word-processing activities. Impact printers operate at speeds of 30 to 50 characters per second. In use, the maximum output rate of these printers is about one page every 2 minutes when producing documents containing standard text. The output rate decreases dramatically when special features of word processing programs are used, features such as boldface, underline, super- and subscripts, and overstrikes. For the most part, the technological advances and the pricings for matrix and laser printers are such that there is little justification for the acquisition of an impact printer, especially for a veterinary practice. A good impact printer with an automatic sheet feeder and a silencer will require an investment of about $2500. Even with a silencer it will be noisy and will require 10 to 12 square feet of floor space.

Matrix printers became popular because they could print at much faster rates than impact printers. Print speeds for matrix printers of interest to the practice manager range from 50 to 300 characters per second. Most matrix printers operate in at least two modes: draft

copy mode and document mode. In the draft mode, most matrix printers produce characters at the rate of about 150 characters per second, with spacing between the matrix dots of the characters being quite noticeable. In the draft mode, documents can be generated at the maximum rate of about two pages per minute.

When a matrix printer operates in document mode, the spacing between matrix dots is reduced, generally by having the printer reprint characters coupled with a slight shift in the position of the matrix. Some printers allow this process to be repeated three times. The output then closely resembles that produced by impact printers. Reprinting of characters reduces the maximum speed for the production of documents to less than one page per minute. Matrix printers, along with impact printers, can be used to complete multipart forms. The processing of multipart forms represents standard operational procedures for many business offices; however, a veterinary practice might not need to generate significant numbers of multipart forms, especially if the production of duplicate forms would be an acceptable alternative to the processing of multipart forms. A significant cost reduction can be achieved by printing second and third copies of documents as opposed to obtaining duplicate copies through the use of multipart forms.

Matrix printers are noisy and need to be enclosed in silencers. In general they will require the same floor space allocation as an impact printer. A wide-carriage matrix printer designed for moderate use with a silencer will represent an investment of more than $1200. If the primary justification for the acquisition of a matrix printer for a veterinary practice relates to its occasional use in the production of multipart forms, then a matrix printer costing less than $400 might be sufficient for purposes of processing multipart forms. If this is the case, then the practice manager needs to give consideration to acquiring a laser printer.

Laser printers are a very attractive alternative to impact and matrix printers. Most of the common laser printers produce characters in the same mode as a copy machine. In fact, some devices are available that can function as both a copy machine and a printer. Documents can be generated at the rate of more than six pages per minute, which is equivalent to about 300 characters per second, with all characters having the appearance of being fully formed. Hence the through-put speed for quality documents is several times faster than for matrix or impact printers. A laser printer represents an investment of between $2000 and $3000. This is about twice the investment required for a matrix printer. However, the difference in initial costs will be quickly recovered in a heavy-use environment. Laser printers are quiet. They can be placed on a counter; hence, they do not require the same allocation of floor space as do other printers. A wide variety of character fonts are available for use with these printers. This means the printers can be used not only for routine printing but also for generating special forms used for reporting client information.

The practice manager needs to carefully evaluate the relative merits of the three types of printers. Again, cost differentials between the various types of printers should not be a major factor in the selection. The laser printer represents at most an incremental cost of $1000 over that for a matrix printer. There is essentially no cost differential between an impact printer and a laser printer. In regard to other factors favoring the acquisition of a laser printer, office productivity can be expected to be significantly greater with a laser printer than with any other type of printer. For example, the total time commitment required to print a letter on a laser printer is less than a minute. The total time commitment required to obtain a quality printout of a letter on a matrix printer is more than 3 minutes. The time differential can be attributed to the difference in the print speeds of the two printers and also to the fact that stationery has to be inserted into a matrix printer whereas the laser printer feeds stationery automatically.

Display terminals

Display terminals are frequently referred to as CRTs (cathode ray tubes) or VDTs (video display terminals). VDTs consist of a visual display device usually referred to as a monitor and a keyboard. Again the technological advances in VDTs are such that their useful marketable life expectancy is about 3 years.

They are used for interactive entry of information into data files stored on disks. Interactive in this case means that the information in the data file is modified as soon as data is entered from a terminal. VDTs are also used for interactive display of information previously entered onto disks. They serve these functions for both single-user systems and mulituser systems.

There are a wide variety of VDTs on the market. Again the practice manager should seek the input of a knowledgeable person before selecting VDTs. VDTs may be classified in two categories. The most common category of VDTs is that where a *cathode ray tube* is used for display purposes. The second category of VDTs, one that is gaining in popularity, is where a variation of *electroluminescence* is used to display information on a flat screen. The footprint, that is the desk space requirement, for the flat-screen VDTs is much less than for cathode ray tube VDTs. However, the resolution and other common features of interest to most users favor the use of the latter in an office or practice environment. Flat-screen VDTs are used extensively with portable computer systems. Not only are the space requirements less for a flat screen but the weight of a portable computer is considerably reduced when a flat screen is used.

In selecting a VDT, particular care should be

given to the resolution characteristics of the monitor. Because users of the terminals can be expected to spend many hours looking at the screen, it is important to obtain a high-resolution screen. Economizing on the cost of a monitor is the incorrect thing to do. Productivity in the use of a VDT can be directly related to the quality of the VDT. In this regard, it is also important to evaluate the usability of the keyboard of the various terminals. Again, a VDT characterized by a keyboard with low usability will contribute to a decrease in productivity.

In addition to specifying the resolution characteristics of a terminal, several other options need to be considered. One of these is referred to as the *compressed print option.* The standard terminal can display up to 80 characters of information on one line. A terminal with the compressed option can display up to 132 characters or more of information on one line. This option is used extensively in processing spreadsheet and accounting information and also in the preparation of tables for documents.

VDTs should also have *graphics* capabilities. Modern business practices are making increasing use of graphics displays. Likewise, word processing programs are now incorporating graphics capabilities. Again, the incremental costs of obtaining a VDT with this option is small. It should be noted that as the routine use of graphics displays increases it will be necessary to acquire printers that can generate copies of the graphics.

There are other options to be considered. One of these is the color of the characters displayed on the screen. Originally, VDTs displayed characters in white on a black background. Today, there are many options relative to the selection of colors for display of information. Again, these options need to be carefully evaluated. In fact, one might give consideration to going to a color monitor, one that will allow information to be displayed in a variety of colors and shades. In general, though, color monitors can cause severe eye fatigue if used for extended periods. They probably should not be used in an office environment.

Considerable attention also needs to be given to positioning or locating the VDTs in an office. Reflections from improper lighting can cause a variety of problems, the biggest problem being that of making errors during the input of information. It is also important that functional furniture be acquired. Time needs to be allocated for evaluating furniture. Again selection of furniture needs to be made with the intent of optimizing the production of the user, not with regard to minimizing the initial costs.

Computers

The computer is the device that performs all of the data processing. It contains a CPU and *memory.* Computer programs and data are stored on disk and are retrieved by the computer to be temporarily stored in memory of the computer. The operating system then directs the processing of data according to instructions given in the programs, with all of the actual processing being performed by the CPU. All devices such as disk systems, tape systems, VDTs, and printers are peripheral devices. The computer needs to be recognized as being a separate item. This statement applies to both single-user systems where only a personal computer is being used as well as multiuser systems.

CPUs are characterized by the speed with which they perform computations. For the most part, the speed of the CPU is not an important factor. The reason for this is that all vendors attempt to maximize the speed of their CPU. The result is that there are not appreciable differences in the processing speeds of CPUs for products introduced within any 12-month period. Again a systems consultant can advise the practice manager on the merits of a particular CPU at the time equipment is being evaluated.

The size of the memory is probably a more important factor than the speed of the CPU. Many programs of interest will require the computer to have a large memory. For this reason, memory size should never be less than 0.5 mbytes for single-user systems and small multiuser systems. The memory requirements for multiuser systems can be considerably greater than 0.5 mbytes. In the case of a multiuser system, care should be taken to acquire one that allows for the addition of memory boards. If the processing speed of a small multiuser system becomes slow, which it eventually does as the use of the system increases, usually the first enhancement needed to speed up the system is the addition of memory.

□
Personnel support

It is a well-accepted fact that personnel are the most important resource of any organization. This means, for example, if a veterinary practice is going to move forward with IIU then the people involved in the process will be the movers. Furthermore, to optimize the contributions of personnel to an organization's goal, they must be given quality tools with which to do their jobs. In addition, they must be given training relative to their job responsibilities and recognition for jobs well done; they must be informed of the consequences for a job not well done; and above all they must be given freedom to set priorities and procedures for achieving job responsibilities.

There is, however, one other factor in personnel support that spells success or failure when implementing a computerization program. This factor involves the attitude and convictions of the practice manager. The practice manager needs to be aware that implementing and sustaining a meaningful computerization effort can be a formidable task, at least initially for an inexperienced person. As experience is gained, the unpleasant aspects

of the task tend to disappear. Once this occurs, everyone involved with the use of the system will tend to experience a sense of pride and ownership. This sense of pride and ownership can only come about, however, if the practice manager gives solid direction and support for the development and implementation of an IIU system. The practice manager cannot enter into such an activity with a passive attitude toward computerization. If this happens, the result will be a passive system used in a passive manner.

If achieving some reasonable degree of IIU is an organizational goal, then appropriate quality tools must be provided to the personnel responsible for implementing and using the system. Two of these tools have already been discussed. They are appropriate quality hardware and appropriate quality software. Although these are indeed important tools, they are not the most important tools. The most important tool is knowledge. Everyone on the staff, including the practice manager, must have knowledge relative to the use of the system. Not everyone needs to have the same knowledge base. But everyone does need to obtain a knowledge base relative to their expected interactions with a system.

It is the responsibility of the practice manager to identify and support training programs in applied computer technology. These training programs should be presented to personnel as learning opportunities. Those people who indeed consider such training an opportunity to achieve self-improvement and at the same time provide support to organizational goals will usually acquire a meaningful knowledge base for performing computer-related tasks. People who do not look upon such training programs as an opportunity of any kind will most likely not acquire the knowledge base needed to meet their developing job responsibilities. These people will have to be assigned to tasks where interaction with computer equipment is minimal. Unfortunately for these people, during the next decade the number of tasks that do not require interaction with computer support equipment will all but disappear, especially in the area of practice management.

Support of training activities will be a continuing responsibility. As new people are hired to fill new positions or positions are vacated by experienced people, it will be necessary to cycle these new people through established training programs. In addition to the required training of new people, it will also be necessary to provide ongoing training to permanent staff. The practice manager always needs to be cognizant that computer technology is continuing to change rapidly. Accordingly, updated hardware and software are being used in support of IIU and, as a consequence, the opportunity to provide more and more extensive IIU. Hence, training of all personnel is an ongoing requirement.

The practice manager needs to select training programs very carefully. In some cases, an adequate training program may involve a staff member becoming thoroughly familiar with procedures outlined in a syllabus generated by other office personnel. In other cases, it may require staff being sent to workshops. Workshops can be expensive. Not counting personnel time, workshops can cost from $200 to $2000. Nonetheless, if the knowledge base of an individual as used to meet specific job responsibilities can be appreciably enhanced, then the cost of the workshop is an investment that has almost immediate dividends. This is especially true where practice management procedures are being implemented in support of IIU.

□
Feasibility analysis for computerization

One of the principal components of performing a feasibility analysis for computerization involves identifying cost factors. The nature of cost factors can be expected to vary over time. They can also be expected to vary according to the size and management style of the practice.

As indicated before, computerization of a practice was originally perceived as a billing activity. Initially practices used computers located off site for computerized processing of billings. The personnel requirements for managing a computer center were supplied by people located at the remote site. Under these conditions, the operational management costs to the practice on a per client basis were much lower than would be the expected management costs on a per client basis for computer systems maintained and supported within a practice. Formerly, all the practice had to do was forward billing information to the billing center where the information was processed along with information from other businesses. Although the actual processing costs were low, the costs of compiling and transmitting information became high because there was a need for multiple recording of billing information. Computerization of the practice should result in a significant reduction in the costs related to duplicate processing of information. Thus, the data input costs can be expected to decrease for a system maintained within a practice. These and many other cost factors need to be identified and evaluated in performing a feasibility analysis for computerizing a veterinary practice. For some of these factors, computerization will result in increases in costs to the veterinary practice; for other factors there will be decreases in costs. The practice manager will be responsible for implementing the use of a computer system that will result in a positive balance for the combined costs of all factors.

Cost factors can be categorized as follows: (1) hardware, (2) software, (3) personnel, (4) personnel training, (5) space allocation for hardware and personnel, and (5) management orientation. Generalized comments pertaining to these various categories of cost factors are made throughout this chapter. The most important of these comments is the one stating that a systems analysis needs to be performed by a competent systems analyst. A well-performed systems analysis will identify the costs for each of these factors along with alternatives or options that will allow for modification of these costs, both initially and over time.

In looking at cost factors over time, the practice manager needs to remember that computerization is a dynamic and evolving process. As already indicated, computer hardware tends to become obsolete within 3 years; thus it is important that a systems analysis take this into account and define a path for upward migration of computerization. Most vendors are not concerned with the user's needs 3 years in the future. Consequently, when the practice manager allows a de facto systems analysis to be performed by a vendor, the practice manager runs the risk of having to start anew the computerization process within 3 years.

A second principal component for performing a feasibility analysis for computerization of a veterinary practice involves defining a new and additional role for the practice manager. The new role is related to supporting the process of IIU. Once this is done, then a decision has to be made as to whether the practice manager will accept and effectively manage the responsibilities associated with this new role.

Achieving the goal of IIU will most likely require the installation and support of a computer system in the offices of the veterinary practice. Once this is done, the practice manager needs to realize that a computer center has been established and that the practice manager now also assumes the title of director of a computer center. The director of a computer center has many responsibilities. The practice manager will have to recognize and effectively manage each of these responsibilities.

If the practice manager is going to become a director of a computer center, then a definition of a computer center needs to be formulated, or at least a concept needs to be established. Conceptually a computer center may be envisioned as being located in a limited-access room having a controlled temperature and humidity. The focal point of a computer center is the computer. A computer might be envisioned as being a large machine capable of processing large volumes of information very quickly. Information to be processed by the computer is stored on disk systems and tape systems generally considered to be part of the computer system. VDTs are used to enter information into the system and to display information retrieved from the system. Printers are used to obtain hard copies, that is, permanent copies, of retrieved information.

The computer center operations are supported by staff members who perform a variety of functions such as

1. Managing the computer system through a console. In large systems, a dedicated VDT is used for this purpose. In small systems, the user's VDT would be used for this purpose.
2. Coordinating the hardware maintenance of all components of the computer system.
3. Maintaining documentation for all phases of operations involving the use of the computer system
4. Maintaining a tape or removable disk library to be used for storing information off-line and to support routine backup procedures for information stored in the computer system
5. Performing data base management functions including establishing verification procedures to ensure the integrity of the stored data
6. Consulting with users relative to use of the system.
7. Integrating all aspects of computer oper-

ations. This task is usually performed by an operations manager using guidelines established by the director of the computer center.

If these concepts are used to define a computer center, then it appears that a single-user computer system sitting in a veterinary practice also constitutes a computer center. That is, all of the functions and activities just mentioned need to be performed in support of a single-user system as well as for a large multiuser system. It is important that the practice manager recognize this need. The probable consequence of not doing so will eventually be disaster.

In the single-user system, a single person becomes the director of the computer center, the operations manager, the computer operator, the user consultant, the data base manager, as well as the user. For such a user, these combined responsibilities will eventually become difficult to manage, and hence all or part of these responsibilities will have to be delegated to appropriate personnel. These personnel must have the knowledge base to meet the responsibilities. As a system evolves from a single-user system to various degrees of multiuser systems, these same factors have to be taken into account.

In addition to coordinating the operations of a computer center, the practice manager in fulfilling the role of director of the computer system will have to assume other responsibilities such as the following:

1. Identifying and training a computer operator or operators
2. Identifying and training data entry personnel
3. Identifying, acquiring, and updating software packages
4. Identifying, acquiring, and upgrading computer hardware
5. Directing and coordinating system analysis procedures

6. Budgeting for the ongoing operational maintenance costs of a computer system
7. Maintaining a realistic knowledge base relative to the use of computer technology in the office management environment
8. Developing a broad perspective relative to IIU

In reality, the role of being the director of a computer center is not a new role for the practice manager, nor need it be an overwhelming role. Possibly, without realizing it, the practice manager has already been the director of a computer center in that he or she has been the director of information processing. Unfortunately, the tools available for processing information have severely restricted the ability to collect and process information. Incorporating computers into the information-processing system merely allows more information to be processed, and as a consequence, the practice manager assumes a responsibility for managing additional resources. Hence, the position of director of information processing now has the additional identifiable components of responsibilities that collectively can be used to define the subposition of director of a computer center.

Identifying the cost factors and the management responsibilities are the two most important activities involved in performing a feasibility analysis for computerization of a veterinary clinic.

One other factor that also applies to designating any system is common sense coupled with a comprehensive viewpoint. Once a decision is made to move forward with computerization, the practice manager needs to allocate time for thinking, planning, and reviewing. There is really no need to rush into an activity, especially one that is as dynamic as computerization. A carefully formulated and implemented plan for computerization will right from the start result in increased efficiency of operations, better management of fiscal matters, and improvement in the use of the process IIU.

☐
Summary

The discussions on computer utilization in a veterinary practice presented in this chapter focused on the need for the practice manager to understand the process of IIU before delving into the computerization process itself. It was pointed out that the practice manager is indeed the director of information processing for a clinic, a responsibility that exists independent of how the information is processed. It was also pointed out that resources usually available to the practice manager for the processing of information are generally not adequate for supporting a high level of IIU. Computerization of a veterinary practice provides the resources to support an appreciable upgrade in information processing, and as a result, computerization of the practice provides the opportunity to process practice information in an integrated manner and, hence, to use it in an integrated manner (i.e., to pursue a goal of IIU).

A major consequence of computerization of a veterinary clinic is that the practice manager also becomes the director of a computer center. This means that the practice manager will need to commit time for obtaining an understanding of the role of computerization of the practice and then commit resources for performing an analysis of the needs for computerization. At the same time the practice manager will need to become aware of the alternatives for acquiring and using both software and hardware. The manager will then need to assimilate all information and use it to evaluate the feasibility for computerizing the practice. Finally, once the decision is made to computerize, the practice manager needs to make sure adequate support will be provided to personnel relative to training and defining job responsibilities.

The primary responsibility for success or failure of a computerization effort rests with management. In the case of computerization of a veterinary clinic, this means the practice manager needs to keep abreast of the continuing rapid changes and enhancements of the use of computers in veterinary medicine. Keeping abreast on the broad front of computerization can be very time-consuming and probably not very beneficial to meeting the primary goals of practice management. Perhaps the best first step to be made toward keeping informed is to interact with other veterinarians who have common goals toward the use of computers. This can be achieved through participation in the activities of the American Veterinary Computer Society (AVCS) and reading the monthly AVCS newsletters that appear in the publication *Modern Veterinary Practice*. The AVCS is an unbiased organization committed to promoting the understanding and utilization of computers in the veterinary profession.

Chapter 6
□
Marketing your practice and the profession

Dennis M. McCurnin

Most professionals, including veterinarians, feel uncomfortable with the idea of marketing because the scope of activity has been poorly understood. Oftentimes, *marketing* connotes *advertising*. However, advertising is only a portion of the total marketing picture.

Professional marketing has numerous definitions, but the one that will be used here is "the communication of professional services and goods." Veterinarians who graduated before 1970 were taught in veterinary school that it was unethical to advertise. Those graduating between 1970 and 1980 were advised about limited advertising (marketing) through the use of practice handout materials, business cards, service reminder letters, and so forth. Graduates after 1980 were exposed to a variety of professional marketing tools that included institutional advertising.

During the 1980s veterinary practice became a more competitive environment as the economic conditions of the United States changed. Also, during the 1970s government-supported veterinary school expansions increased the number of new veterinarians entering practice careers in the 1980s. The increase in practicing veterinarians along with the static population growth and slow growth economy increased the competition for the traditional practice market.

Individual practices felt the increasing market pressure, as evidenced by stable or declining caseloads and level or slow-growth gross incomes. By the early 1980s the American Veterinary Medical Association (AVMA) addressed the perceived shrinking veterinary practice market by hiring a marketing management consultant firm, Charles, Charles and Associates, Overland Park, Kansas. In July 1983, a report on the veterinary services market was published for the AVMA.[1]

The information contained in the Charles, Charles and Associates report was not used extensively until about 1985. The use of market information became of intense interest after the Veterinary Medical Manpower Study was published in 1985.[2] After the manpower information, which confirmed most practitioners' feelings, a renewed interest in professional marketing became evident.

During the mid-1980s many practitioners became increasingly concerned about maintaining their market share in the face of increasing economic pressures. Some veterinarians panicked and attempted unsound marketing methods. The era of low-cost vaccination clinics, low-cost elective surgeries, and merchandising began.

The panic strategy of a few practitioners began to affect the attitudes of many veterinarians. The effect oftentimes was to oppose *all* marketing activities. A few very successful practitioners, however, were able to establish continued practice growth during this same period by using sound marketing methods.

After the initial panic of the early and mid-1980s, state veterinary medical associations and the AVMA began to organize marketing seminars and long-range planning. More and more veterinarians began to discover professional marketing as another practice management tool to be used along with good personnel management and sound accounting practices.

This chapter will attempt to discuss the role of professional marketing in veterinary practice. The marketing field is changing so rapidly that it is difficult to summarize the subject of marketing in one chapter; nevertheless, the importance of proper marketing application to veterinary practice cannot be overemphasized.

□ Professional marketing

Numerous publications have been written about commercial marketing. Departments of marketing exist in most business colleges that are devoted to the research, study, and dissemination of business marketing information. All successful businesses have marketing departments for the promotion of company products and services.

Professional marketing has been practiced for years, just as business marketing, but designated by a different name. Most professionals referred to marketing techniques as *public relations* programs. Physicians, dentists, attorneys, and veterinarians, all referred to their specific practice- or association-level marketing programs as public relations activities.

Practice vs. institutional marketing

Marketing programs can be carried out at both the practice level and the association (institutional) level. Most veterinary practitioners were conducting practice marketing techniques long before the institutions. Specific examples of practice marketing would be using client reminder service cards, distributing handout materials to clients, and so forth. An example of an institutional marketing program would be the promotion of National Pet Week by the AVMA or state VMA.

Internal vs. external marketing

In addition to practice vs. institutional marketing programs another division can be made for marketing: *internal marketing* vs. *external marketing*. Internal marketing programs are those activities that promote a specific practice to current clientele. External marketing programs are activities directed outside the practice to both client and nonclient.

□
What is professional marketing?

Professional marketing consists of all activities supporting the communications of professional services and goods. Marketing includes client relations; appearance of the hospital, clinic, or ambulatory vehicle; listening to the owner's opinions; convenient practice location; polite support staff; offering full-service care; sending client service reminders; being neat and clean; using business cards; sending newsletters; providing nutritional and dietary management; providing emergency service; offering pet and livestock supplies; giving career talks at the high school; having producer or client educational nights; being involved in a community service club; using the yellow pages of the telephone book; providing handout material to clients; having an attractive and well-located building sign; sending thank-you and sympathy cards to the appropriate clients; appearing as a guest on radio or television shows; writing a newspaper animal column; using attractive letterhead stationary; becoming active in professional veterinary associations; joining the AVMA Political Action Committee; group advertising in the newspaper about the annual rabies vaccination clinic; and so forth. The examples of marketing are so numerous that this chapter could become a continuous listing. A grouping of various methods along with the utilization technique would, however, be more useful for the practitioner. It becomes obvious that not all subjects can be addressed, but the aforementioned list will start the brainstorming process.

Professional marketing has now become a part of practice and should be used with the same skill and progressive techniques as medical, diagnostic, or surgical procedures. Continuing education in the areas of marketing and practice management are as necessary as any other veterinary medical discipline. The question is no longer "*Should* we market" but "*How* should we market."

The profession needs to continue to be acutely aware of professional ethics and maintain the highest degree of professionalism. Professional marketing is not opposed to that position and philosophy when properly applied. The first step must be to accept marketing as a useful practice tool. The next step is to gain an understanding of the techniques available and then apply those techniques to the practice and the profession.

Marketing education

The educational process for professional veterinary marketing must be targeted at (1) the veterinarian and veterinary technician, (2) the veterinary student, and (3) the general public. The process of educating the veterinarian has begun. Most national, state, and local VMAs have offered courses in marketing. These courses have been well attended, and those in attendance have been given a clearer definition of the marketing process. Acceptance and utilization of the material presented have been successful in pet practice (small-animal and equine) but more difficult in food animal practice. Economic concerns are more of a factor in food animal practice than in pet practice. Therefore, many of the techniques used in pet practice are not as applicable to food animal practice. Specific new programs are being developed for the food animal practitioner such as the Integrated Reproductive Management (IRM) program, which was developed by the Idaho Veterinary Medical Association.

Veterinary educators have somewhat ignored the needs of veterinary students in the practice management and marketing areas. Most veterinary schools find it difficult to obtain professors skilled in practice management and marketing. If professors had such skill, most would be in private practice. Veterinarians skilled in management techniques, however, are now being developed in both institutional and practice settings.

The veterinary technician plays a vital role in the overall marketing of professional services. In most practices the technician or receptionist probably spends more time with the client than does the veterinarian. The client must gain confidence in the practice before he or she will allow a full range of services to be performed on their animal or return to the practice at a later date for additional or follow-up services. The client gains confidence first through the receptionist; it is reinforced by the technician, and then is established by the veterinarian.

The need to introduce management techniques and marketing philosophy into the educational process of both veterinarians and veterinary technicians is well founded. Most institutions have recognized our historical shortcomings in these subjects. All members of the veterinary practice team must be skilled in management and marketing.

Students in most colleges of veterinary medicine are now exposed to practice management, client management, and professional marketing courses. These courses should be team taught by both knowledgeable professors and practitioners. The importance of this material should be stressed during the freshman year in veterinary school and followed by practical courses during the junior and senior years.

Once the veterinarian, veterinary technician, and veterinary student have been exposed to marketing concepts, a practice philosophy must be developed that will allow clients to become educated about veterinary services. This same supportive veterinary marketing philosophy must also be developed in national, state, and local veterinary medical associations. For the entire professional marketing concept to be effective, the profession as a whole and each veterinarian within the profession must be clear about the type of service offered in veterinary medicine.

The business of veterinary medicine

One of the most critical questions a practitioner should ask is "What business am I in?" To be able to conduct a successful business one must be clear about specific business objectives. Some practitioners believe they are in the animal medical business. Furthermore, they believe that as long as a high-quality medical and surgical skill is delivered, the client will continue to use their service on the basis of the quality of service alone. Fortunately, clients today are well-informed consumers and are looking for both quality and value. The average client lacks the professional background to accurately judge the quality of medical or surgical services performed; however, they do have the ability to judge the quality of care *they* received personally and the value of the service received.

Veterinary medicine is in the *people service business.* The profession cares for animals but provides professional services to their owners. If the veterinarian understands that he or she is in the people service business, a completely different orientation will take place. When clients call on the phone, for example, they are not interrupting the veterinarian's time in the examination room or surgery room; they are the reason for the examination room and surgery room being there. Veterinarians do provide high-quality professional service to animals, but only after the agreement and support of the owner–client.

The professional success of most veterinarians is the result of *interpersonal skills* rather than strictly clinical skills. The ability to relate to people and their problems will allow one the opportunity to practice high-quality veterinary medicine.

When practice is viewed as a people service

business, then marketing of those services becomes possible. The product to be marketed is *high-quality, people-oriented, professional veterinary medical service.*

□
Professional marketing techniques

The profession must be guided into a long-term productive marketing program that will benefit both practitioners and nonpractitioners. Marketing techniques must benefit the profession as a whole to enable maximum success. The overall program must promote the *benefits* of veterinary services rather than the specific service.

If one were to compare a program of the benefits of immunization to one that sold a vaccination, the long-term effects are evident. The program that details the benefits of immunization can build in a physical examination, dental care, nutritional management, and so forth on an annual basis. The approach of selling a vaccination is just that—promoting a vaccine.

The program of promoting the benefits of a high-quality, people-oriented, professional veterinary medical service must be the goal. Nonpractice positions will also profit from professional marketing because the public is becoming informed about what veterinarians know and do. When the general public becomes better informed about veterinary medicine, additional career opportunities will develop.

Nonpractice marketing

In the United States each year approximately 75% of our veterinary school graduates enter private practice and 25% enter nonpractice positions, whereas in Japan 75% of the graduates enter nonpractice positions and 25% enter private practice. The Japanese have found veterinarians to be highly skilled and trained in nontraditional employment areas.

Some of these nontraditional areas are milk processing, public health epidemiology, zoological administration, agricultural toxicology, fish production, and so forth. The responsibility for identifying new nonpractice positions lies with both organized veterinary medicine and the colleges of veterinary medicine. A portion of the perceived glut of veterinarians must be directed into productive and rewarding nonpractice positions. The colleges and schools of veterinary medicine must start an *academic marketing program* that will identify and train graduates for these new careers. Veterinary career exploration must take place during the freshman year in veterinary school to allow proper plans for career diversification.

While some specialization could occur during the senior year in veterinary school, many positions may require postgraduate education. Emphasis should be placed on identifying new positions that do not require additional postgraduate training. During the past 10 years the financial remuneration as reported by the AVMA has been greater on the average for nonpractice positions than for practice positions.

As a part of the academic marketing program, colleges of veterinary medicine must also recruit students into veterinary medicine who have nontraditional backgrounds. Students who have a background in nutrition, toxicology, sales, research, fish production, and wildlife are much more likely to continue in these areas after veterinary school if challenging jobs are available to them upon graduation.

In addition, all veterinary schools must actively support the marketing efforts of organized veterinary medicine. University professors must become more involved in actively supporting veterinary association marketing efforts to allow the profession as a whole to become more effective in the marketplace.

Knowledgeable and dedicated veterinary professors can become a valuable resource to marketing efforts in the areas of promoting new research techniques and acting as authoritative sources of information for newspapers, radio, and television. The nonpractice areas of veterinary medicine can become a valuable resource to the practice areas while benefiting from the practice marketing programs.

It is hoped that new careers can be identified in the nonpractice areas by having a more informed public concerning the practicing veterinarian. An uneducated marketplace is a nonexistent market.

Practice marketing

Practice marketing cannot become a "bag of tricks" to be pulled out as a last resort when all else fails. Marketing must become a practice and professional philosophy that is driven by client needs. The profession must understand the needs of the client both in pet practice and food animal practice. A compromise must be reached between what we think the client needs and what the client feels they need.

A marketing plan

The first step is to determine client needs. One must listen closely to services being asked for by each client. Determine what service trends are going on within the practice in response to economic growth of the community. As an example, both spouses usually work today. As a result some people are unable to seek veterinary care during the traditional 8:00 A.M. to 5:00 P.M. time period. The typical client also has less free time to devote to shopping around at several stores for items when all items could be purchased at one convenient location. By listening to clients and observing service needs, the practitioner may opt to extend the practice hours two evenings per week and open later in the mornings on those days. The practice may also expand services to in-

clude boarding to offer more service at one location.

The practice owner must determine the direction of the marketing plan by listening to client needs and gathering additional facts about community trends. The marketing process will then be guided by current facts and information. Once the client needs are assessed, the *marketing mix* must be established.

Marketing mix

The marketing mix consists of four major areas: (1) product, (2) place, (3) promotion, and (4) price. Each component affects the other, and all four affect the client (Fig. 6-1).

Product. As was discussed in The Business of Veterinary Medicine section of this chapter, the product that veterinary medicine has to market is "high-quality, people-oriented, professional veterinary service." What the client really wants is a healthy animal. The relationship of the owner with the animal drives the need for care. Some clients are driven by economics (food animals, performance horses), whereas other clients are driven by emotion (small animals and pleasure horses). In addition, some clients do not seek care at all because they have no strong relationship with the animal. The animal can become a *disposable* item when no relation exists.

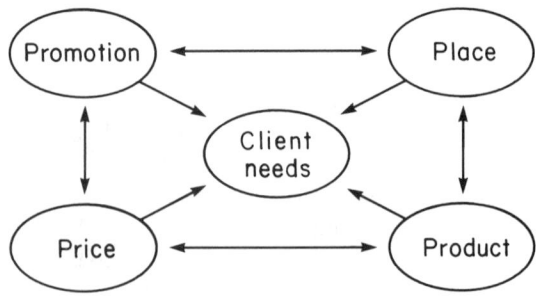

Figure 6-1. Marketing mix controlled by the practice

The product must be designed to meet the needs of the client. Our product must rely on state-of-the-art information delivered in a personal manner that treats the current problem yet stresses a prevention program. We must be in both the treatment and prevention mode. In addition, the product (service) must always be delivered at the same level of quality. It is more difficult to establish consistent levels of quality control for a service than for a product. Product quality is also affected by the price and place where the product is sold. Clients do not have the ability to judge professional service quality but do make judgments about the facility, price, and result.

Place. The location of the practice and the nature of the facility affect the market mix. In a competitive market clients will be looking for convenience and value. The location of a practice is a key factor in practice growth. Clients want high street visibility and easy access to parking from the main street. Building maintenance and care of the grounds, plantings, and parking areas are clear signals to clients about the quality of service to be found inside the facility.

Ambulatory veterinarians must be acutely aware of the cleanliness of the outside of their vehicles as well as the inside of the box. Clients make judgments on the cleanliness and organization of the instruments, equipment, and drugs found inside a mobile facility.

Also included in the place area of the market mix is personal attire and hygiene of each staff member and veterinarian. Clients can easily judge the level of cleanliness and will resist returning to a facility that contains filth and odors.

The place is also affected by the product and promotion areas of the marketing mix. A facility that delivers a high-quality product (service) will take on a different appearance and mood than a facility that promotes a poor-quality service. The promotion of the place will become much easier and more effective when the facility is maintained in the highest of standards.

Promotion. The promotion of a practice is the ability of the staff to understand the product and express that information to the client. Each person in the practice needs to know exactly what business the practice is in. The promotion of the service needs to be in the form of the benefits of the service rather than promotion of the service itself. Through promotion, the sale should be made at the program level rather than at an individual service level, thereby promoting a total health program rather than a single service.

Promotion is also the attitude of the veterinarians and staff within the practice. Even if everyone in the practice understands the product and takes pride in the place, the promotion of the practice will fail without a positive, helpful, concerned, caring attitude. Everyone in the practice must be a "people person" who enjoys problem solving while working with animals.

The ability to promote the practice is affected by the place and the price. Promotion of the practice and its services is much more effective when the facility is first rate. The facility will sell itself. Price is an important element that affects promotion. Most people understand the adage "You get what you pay for." Most clients, however, are willing to pay a little more for quality service when the service is promoted properly.

Price. The consumer is price sensitive to most purchases. As consumers become more educated about the product, their sensitivity to price increases (Fig. 6-2). If consumers are poorly informed about the product, however, the evaluation is reduced to price. Consumers of veterinary service do not usually have the knowledge and ability to judge the quality and benefit of professional service. Consumers of

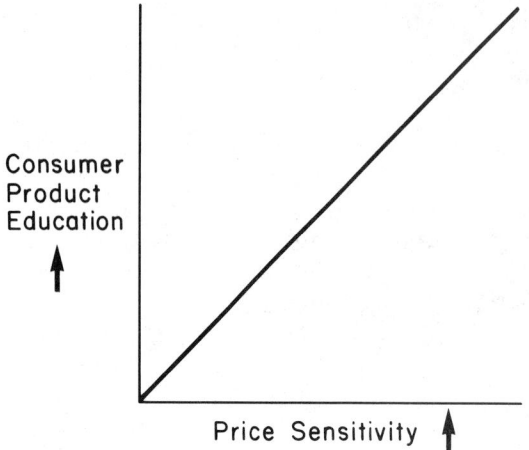

Figure 6-2. *Relationship between consumer education and price sensitivity*

veterinary service are, however, able to judge the price of the service by calling several veterinarians.

If the consumer only knows enough to ask the price and the response from each practice is only the price, then the decision will be based on price. The response from the practice when asked about the cost of spaying should be based on information first and fee second.

A typical response to the consumer question about the cost of spaying might be: "When we perform an ovariohysterectomy, an inhalant anesthesia is used because this is the safest on the animal during major surgery. We also recommend a screening blood test to evaluate kidney and liver function before anesthesia. The surgery is done using sterile techniques, and the animal is continuously monitored for heart and respiratory function. We hospitalize the animal for one night after surgery and perform a final physical examination before release. Our fee for the surgery, laboratory work, anesthesia, monitoring, and hospitalization is X dollars."

Providing such information allows the caller to be informed about the service, which permits them to base their decision on more information than just price. Unfortunately, many practices respond to the price question with a negative fee answer. When the consumer calls, the practice has an opportunity to educate another person rather than just provide a fee quotation.

Both promotion and product affect price. Consumers are constantly weighing the price against the value and benefit of the product. When the consumer is provided with more information about the product (promotion), the price can become a secondary issue. The quality of the product (service) must be the highest possible and must be provided with personalized attention (client relations) to allow a value to be placed by the consumer. If both promotion and product are working together, the consumer will understand both the value and benefit of the service, thus providing an educated evaluation of the price. It becomes difficult to refuse, on price alone, a high-quality service that has great personal value.

Controlling and understanding the marketing mix (product, price, promotion, place) will allow the veterinarian to become more competitive in the marketplace. Professional marketing techniques are the tools necessary to accomplish the task. Skillfully applying marketing techniques at both the practice and institutional (association) levels will allow the profession to expand the market share rather than continuing to compete for the same traditional share.

□
Specific marketing techniques

Marketing techniques will not overcome the effects of poor client relations within a practice. Unless client communication and client orientation are practiced on a client-by-client basis, marketing will be unsuccessful.

Professional marketing can be divided into

internal marketing and *external* marketing. Internal marketing techniques are the day-to-day activities that occur within each practice, whereas external marketing includes techniques used outside the practice. The purpose of both internal and external techniques is to enlarge the potential market.

Internal marketing

Internal marketing is aimed primarily at the existing client base. These techniques are intended to educate and inform current clients about various veterinary services and service programs. The following methods are meant to serve as an idea base and not as a complete listing of techniques.

Client relations

The *most* important technique to use in any marketing program is personalized, sincere client care. Most clients require as much attention and care as the patient. Clients today want both high technology and high touch. Personalized service that places emphasis on each individual client will allow the opportunity for excellent communication to be established. Both veterinarian and technician must be skilled communicators as well as technically skilled professionals. A very detailed discussion of client management is found in Chapter 2.

Practice appearance

The visual appearance of the clinic, hospital, or ambulatory vehicle is the first outward signal to the client of the potential quality of service. Everyone is an expert at spotting a run-down building or property. Looks can be deceiving, but how often are outside appearances used when first selecting a restaurant, motel, or grocery store? Without additional information oftentimes the outward appearance becomes a critical issue.

In making an overall marketing plan, one must consider the appearance of the building (repair, paint, cleanliness) and the grounds. Plantings and grass must be neat and trimmed and the parking lot clean and well signed for parking. The interior of the building must also be clean, well cared for, and odor free. Silent messages are sent to clients through the appearance of the facility.

The large-animal practitioner has the same image to maintain in the practice vehicle as in the clinic. The vehicle should be clean, dent and rust free, and in excellent repair. The interior of the vehicle must also be clean in both the driver's compartment and equipment and drug storage areas. Dirty and disorganized bottles of medication send signals of poor-quality medicine to the layperson.

A practice facility does not have to be new or have the latest equipment to project a positive image. The older facility that has been given proper care and maintenance will exhibit a strong marketing message of "we care" to people passing by each day.

Practice location

In the overall marketing plan, practice location is not an item that can change without moving the practice; however, the current location might be able to be enhanced by improving the building signs and parking areas. The building sign should be professional in appearance and very visible from both directions as people approach the property from the street (Fig. 6-3). The outside of the building may be improved visually by adding additional landscaping items such as trees, shrubs, and flowers (Fig. 6-4).

Practice location is very important to building a practice. Location on a main street near a shopping area is ideal (see Chapter 4). As people do their regular shopping, they pass by the veterinary location and take in the aesthetics of the property and the sign. These forms of marketing (advertising) are continuously and silently working to promote the practice. To be

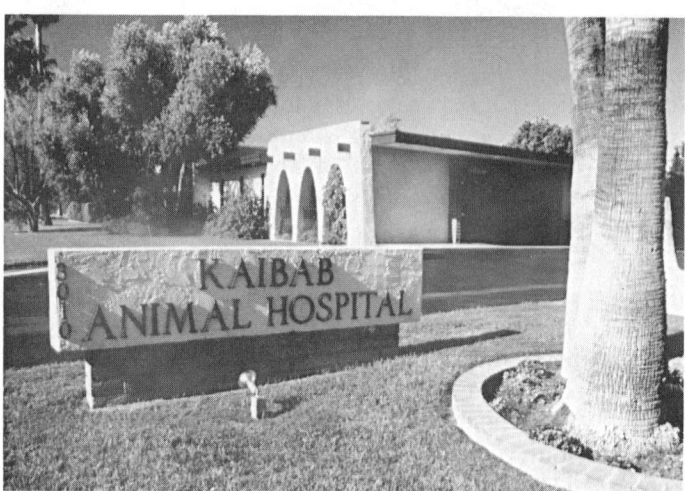

Figure 6-3.   Professional sign with high visibility from street

able to continue to do their job, they must be in excellent repair.

Support staff utilization

Most of the internal marketing carried on within a practice will be through the support staff. The support staff activities will augment the efforts of the veterinarian in client relations and personal appearance. It is primarily the staff who will be responsible for recommending services or goods and following up on hospital programs that require appointments or individual client contact. The staff will be regarded as an extension of the veteri-

narian and must have a professional approach to client management. Additional information on utilization and management of the support staff can be found in Chapters 3 and 12.

The support staff can deliver the majority of client education. Handout materials, visual aids, and a slide–tape presentation will help the staff in their educational efforts. The staff will need detailed information about the various health care programs from the veterinarian. To be able to promote the product, everyone needs to be clear about the product.

Professional sales point displays can add another level of service for clients. These dis-

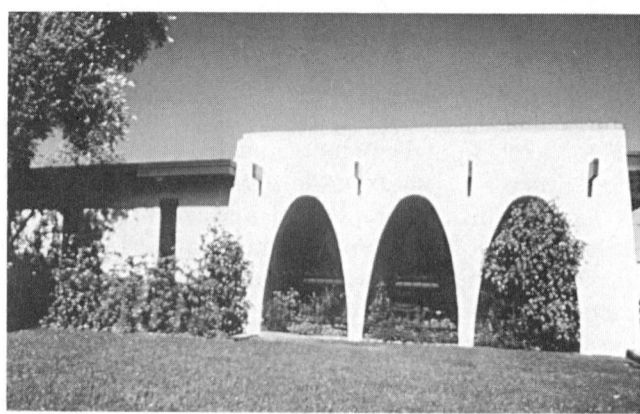

Figure 6-4.   Neat, attractive landscape greatly enhances hospital exterior

plays need continuous monitoring by the support staff to allow "on-the-spot" professional information. Areas in which the support staff should have in-depth knowledge include nutrition, parasite control (internal and external), grooming aids, dental care, immunization programs, rearing orphan animals, and so forth. In addition, the support staff must be on constant lookout for new clients and additional services. Staff members who are active in dog or horse clubs have continual access to potential new clients. New clients may not be aware of services offered, so all staff members must be willing to provide program information at any time. If certain key support staff members are given a small percentage of income from all new services and new clients they provide the practice, a new wave of enthusiasm may develop in everyone.

Personal appearance

The personal appearance and hygiene of each staff member are reflections of the quality of the practice (Fig. 6-5). Clients quickly relate personal appearance to the sanitation level and quality of the practice. If staff members do not care enough to change a dirty smock, why should they care enough to provide the highest quality service? Personal appearance marketing works just as building appearance: an outward signal of internal activity.

Listening to the client

Listening is a communication art that must be developed to the fullest extent. When practice personnel listen to the needs of the client, they will have the opportunity to build the type of services clients really want. Listening is a very difficult skill to develop because our own biases come into play. Oftentimes the real concerns of the client are lost or dismissed without complete consideration.

Clients ask for full-service practices so they will not have to spend their own time looking for various needs. In a large-animal practice this may mean computerized record management or computerized nutritional evaluations provided by the practice. The small-animal practice might expand into boarding of animals or offering more convenient evening hours.

Senior citizens are watching their expenditures more closely than ever before, so providing a 10% seniors' discount might meet their

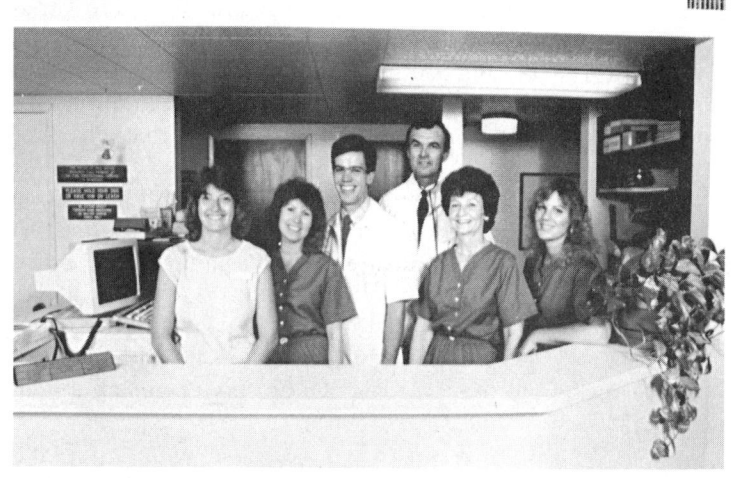

Figure 6-5. Personal appearance of the professional team is extremely important

needs. Listening to the client and offering the type of service needed will allow practice marketing to be more effective.

Product delivery service

In the past, food production veterinarians have concerned themselves with 8% of the animal population (the diseased animals) and have overlooked 92% of the potential market. Dr. Byford Wood of Breese, Illinois, reviewed his practice area and listened to client needs.[3] The veterinarians in the practice realized their income had been derived primarily from food-producing animals in an ever-changing agricultural economic scene.

During the past 25 years, Dr. Wood's practice had remained at a 1½-veterinarian work load. In 1982 the practice philosophy was changed to meet some of the agricultural changes; there was more activity in management areas focusing on nutrition, herd health, and production record keeping. This change required market-packaged information and product programs and was enhanced by a regular delivery service.

Clients are contacted by letter and telephone immediately before the scheduled delivery date. Client needs are received, and an order is taken. This type of service provides the opportunity to meet the client other than over a sick animal. A significant amount of veterinary service has been requested as a result. The practice has evolved from a two-person sick call general practice to a business group centered around six veterinarians and nine lay employees.[3]

Full-service care

Listening to client needs will verify that clients want full-service care when possible. People are exposed to 1-hour photo processing, 1-hour eye glasses, 7-Eleven, fast-food restaurants, K-Mart, Target, drive-through banking, and so forth. Convenient, fast, economical,

one-stop shopping is the rule for families in which both husband and wife work. People are now asking for this same type of convenient service in their veterinary care. In a small-animal practice full-service care would include prepurchase counseling about pets, human–animal bond counseling, pediatric care, preventive medicine, nutritional counseling, boarding, geriatric care, dentistry, bereavement counseling, cremation service, plus full routine veterinary care. The service would extend from womb to tomb.

In a large-animal practice full-service care might include prepurchase evaluations, housing management, computerized record service, nutritional consultation, product delivery service, herd health management, integrated reproductive management, plus full routine veterinary care.

In a full-service practice various programs can be packaged for marketing. The goal of marketing is to sell a *program,* not an individual service. A small-animal practice might have a complete health maintenance program for new puppies. This program carries into adulthood and on into the geriatric period. The health maintenance program could include an annual physical, nutritional counseling, dental care, immunizations, and so forth. Nutritional counseling would include pediatric care, obesity control, and adult and geriatric care as the patient's life cycle matures. As clients continue their regular contact with the practice to purchase diet foods, the practice has a regular opportunity to market other health care services.

In the full-service food animal or equine practice the program should include evaluations of housing, pasture management, nutritional management, reproductive management, herd health, and so forth from prepurchase evaluation to sale. Clients want more than a vaccination service or sick animal service.

Direct mail contact

Client reminders

One of the more successful early attempts at practice marketing was through the use of a vaccination reminder system for small animals. During the early discussions on the use of a recall system, many practitioners felt it was unprofessional to send a reminder card to clients because it was advertising. No one was considering the service provided to the client and the animal. Most veterinarians thought only of how it would appear to other veterinarians.

Charles, Charles and Associates discovered that sending vaccination reminders was more important to clients than having boarding facilities or an attractive building.[1] Clients want to be reminded when specific services are to be done; however, clients prefer reminders be by mail rather than phone.

A reminder system is a major marketing feature of most practice management computer software packages. A system that only has the capacity to generate one reminder is not nearly as valuable as a system that will produce a second and third level of accountability. Using a system that will allow a second or third notice to be sent will greatly increase the service return rate.

Most veterinarians now accept the use of a reminder system as a valuable marketing tool for routine immunizations. The reminder system must now be expanded to include other routine services for the client. Additional usage in small-animal practice could be in the areas of dentistry (routine cleaning), annual physicals, geriatric care, hip dysplasia evaluations, heartworm evaluation, and so forth. The suggestion of an annual physical examination may appear on the surface to be a poor recommendation in light of physicians now recommending fewer annual physicals; however, considering that dogs and cats age seven to

nine times as rapidly as humans and that in most instances the diligent veterinarian is able to find a potential problem on almost every physical examination, many clients will take advantage of the service when offered. When performing the examination the veterinarian must explain and demonstrate the findings to the client (i.e., potential problem with ears, eyes, teeth, anal sacs, hair coat, obesity, and so forth).

Small-animal geriatric care is another relatively untapped marketing area. When patients reach a specific age (i.e., 7 to 8 years of age), a reminder letter could be sent to the client to provide information on specific conditions to be monitored. The letter could approach the client by "Congratulations, Blacky has just become a senior canine citizen. When dogs reach about 8 years of age, the care necessary to prevent and monitor disease changes. We would like to provide the following information to allow Blacky to enjoy his new senior status: . . . ." This letter could be developed on the word processor and recalled by the computer at a specific age.

Another area in which a reminder system could be used is to recall young animals that have been previously vaccinated but not yet neutered. The recall of unneutered animals is an opportunity to market ovariohysterectomy and castration services. This reminder may attract some clients who would otherwise go to a low-cost spay-and-neuter clinic. A personalized word processor letter could detail specific features on the service not possible from spay-and-neuter clinics.

In food animal and equine practices, recall systems could be developed to follow up on seasonal problems (i.e., vaccinations, deworming, pregnancy checks, dehorning, teeth floating, and so forth). Special seasonal services could also be featured such as ration evaluation and preconditioning programs. Too often clients do not fully understand the need for potential services. A reminder for a specific service may initiate a call from the client, which allows additional information to be provided by the veterinarian.

The use of a recall system allows the market to be segmented (targeted). An example of market segmentation would be to send all feline owners a reminder about leukemia vaccination.

Sympathy and thank-you communications

A very personal marketing approach is to use sympathy and thank-you types of communication appropriately. One may choose to use commercially prepared cards or develop a letter format on the word processor that can be personalized. Regardless of the format, the use of personal messages to specific clients for specific purposes has an everlasting positive effect.

In the case of a new client referred by a current client, a note or card to both the referring client (thanking them for the referral) and the new client (welcoming them to the practice) is very appropriate. The sympathy card or note is helpful to demonstrate open concern for the feelings of the client during their emotional loss. The expression helps the client deal with the loss and also allows the client to understand the "I care" attitude of the practice.

Letters, notes, or cards can be prepared by computer-generated lists or by the technical staff. Only the professional staff need to sign the prepared material.

Newsletters

In a recent newsletter service evaluation of 253 veterinarians the following information was obtained.[4] Nearly three out of four veterinarians (73%) had never used a client newsletter. Only 16% of the veterinarians in the study were currently using newsletters. The interest in a client newsletter was highest among veterinarians and practices with the following characteristics: (1) in practice 20 years or less, (2) two or more veterinarians in the practice, (3) larger practices (at least 2300 clients per veterinarian), and (4) computerized client lists. These characteristics indicate that newsletters have the most appeal among progressive veterinarians with larger practices.

Among the veterinarians interested in newsletters, the top priority for the newsletter was to educate the client. The most important newsletter topics in order of preference were (1) preventive medicine, (2) geriatric care, (3) dentistry, (4) disease conditions, (5) training, and (6) human–animal bond. Respondents also preferred to sent out a client newsletter on a quarterly basis.

Charles, Charles and Associates have reported that the use of newsletters is related to an increased number of clinic visits by dog owners.[1] The utilization of newsletters will increase client activity through improved understanding and education about veterinary services. Educational goals for newsletters should be to inform animal owners of signs of illness, make seasonal animal health care recommendations (i.e., heat stroke in summer), and review health care programs. Many clients do not understand how to tell whether an animal is ill or in serious condition. This lack of knowledge is especially true for cat and horse owners.

When experiencing abdominal pain from colic, the horse is difficult for the average client to evaluate. Unless the owner is familiar with the specific signs of abdominal pain, the horse's condition may become critical before attention is sought. It is also difficult to tell when cats are ill. Normally cats sleep a lot, cover their feces and urine, and tend to be loners. It becomes difficult to really know when they are ill unless you have a little knowledge.

Newsletters will allow the client to be exposed to specific pieces of information that will help the owner to know when to call a veterinarian for help. Total health care plans can also be explained to allow the owner to be aware of full-service health care that extends beyond vaccinations. The newsletter should help market the benefits of healthy animals.

Newsletters can be sent to specific segments of clients in the practice computer base; however, they can also be provided through a hand-generated list. Most veterinarians do not have the experience or time to compose a compete newsletter three or four times per year. Careful thought should be given to purchasing a professionally edited newsletter ser-

vice. Several services are available from which to choose, with direct mailing from the publisher to the client as an option (Fig. 6-6*A* and *B*).

Each newsletter should be personalized by the practice to allow the reader easy access to the practice's location and phone number. Another advantage newsletters have in overall marketing is the ability to reach the nonuser. This is actually a form of external marketing. If the client receiving the newsletter passes it on to a nonclient friend, the nonclient has an opportunity to be exposed to various veterinary services.

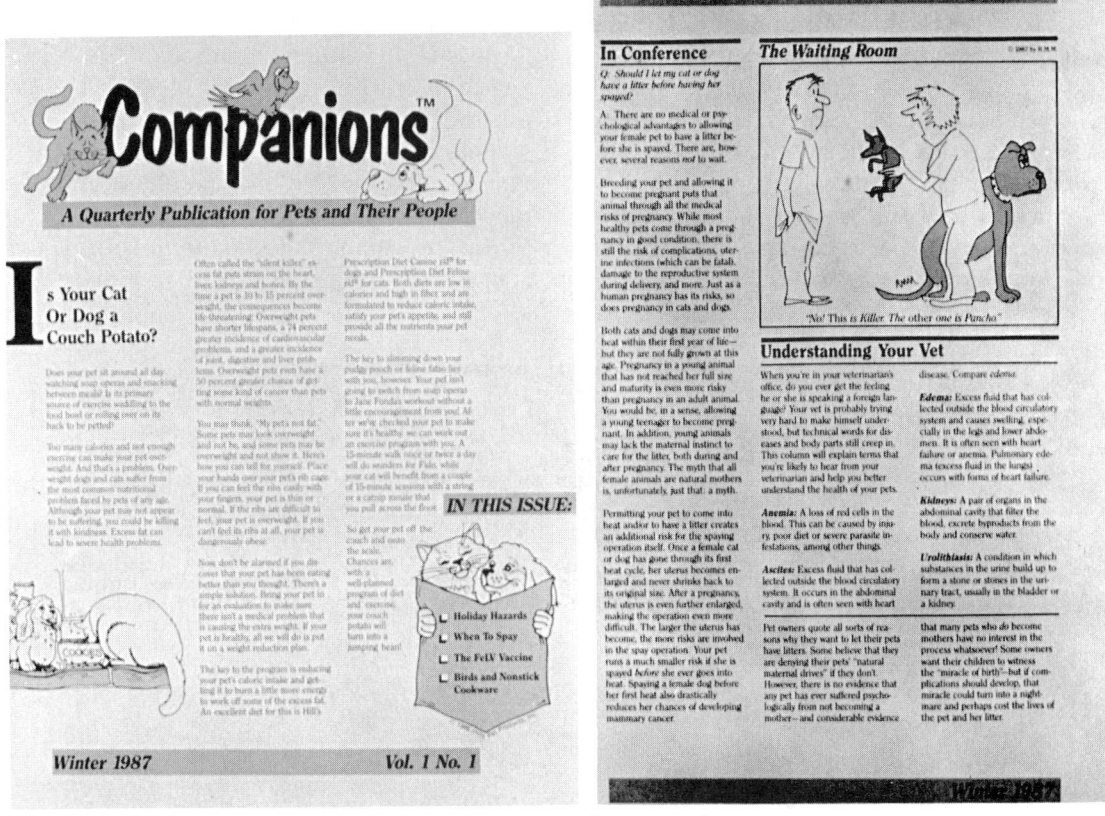

A   **B**

Figure 6-6. Example of commercially prepared newsletter. (A) Front page; (B) inside page (Courtesy of Hill's Pet Products, Inc, Topeka, Kansas)

Handout materials

Marketing with handout materials has been done for a number of years; however, the quantity of commercially available handouts is continually increasing. Most commercial companies realize the value of client-oriented professional literature (Fig. 6-7). These pieces should be carefully reviewed by the practice so that only the acceptable material is made available to clients. Once the material has been reviewed and useful pieces selected, all staff members must be made familiar with how and when they should be used. A professional rubber stamp can be purchased with the practice name, location, and phone number on it and used to mark all handout materials.

In addition to commercial handouts, material may be purchased from organized veterinary medicine. The AVMA, American Association of Equine Practitioners, and American Animal Hospital Association, all have useful client handout materials.

Practices may also produce their own informational material. Handouts on whelping, ovariohysterectomy, cystic calculi, colic, mastitis, and so forth can be prepared on the word processor or typewriter. Practice information brochures can also be produced to more fully explain practice hours, services, equipment, facilities, and staff function (Fig. 6-8*A* and *B*). Other forms of handout materials used on a regular basis are business cards and letterhead stationery. These have become so commonplace that they are also forgotten. They are, however, very effective forms of marketing. Business cards should be made available to clients from both veterinarians and key support staff. Handout materials are more effective when presented to the client rather than having the client just pick them up.

Specialty services

Practices can expand services or add new services to increase their market share. Some services to consider for a food animal practice are nutritional consultation, small ruminant care (llama, goats), prepurchase evaluations, integrated reproductive management, milking machine evaluation, facility evaluation, and so forth. The equine practice might consider an acute care facility, pediatric intensive care

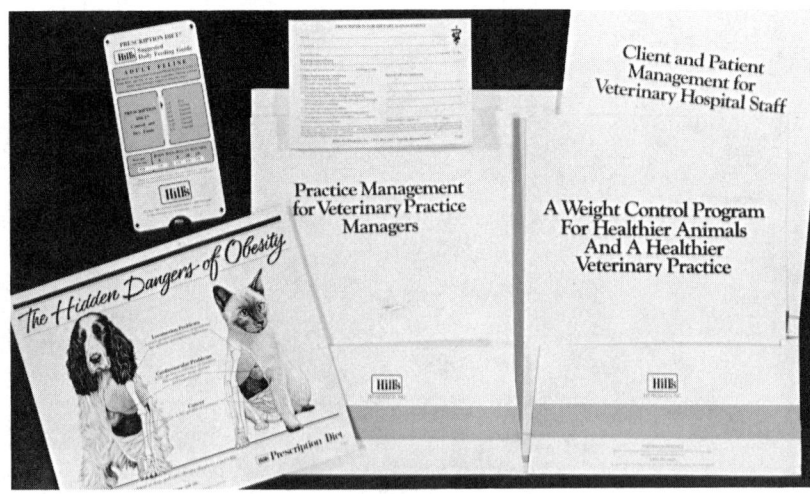

Figure 6-7. Example of commercially prepared handout material (Courtesy of Hill's Pet Products, Inc, Topeka, Kansas)

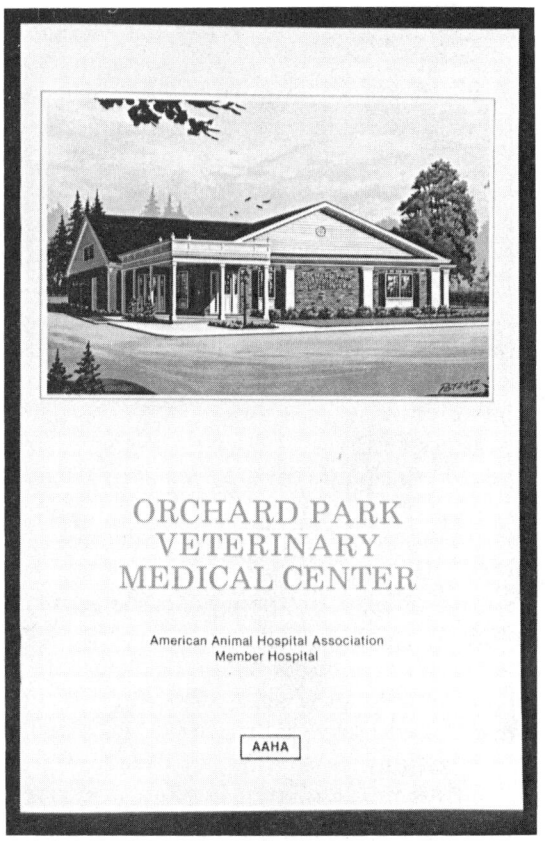

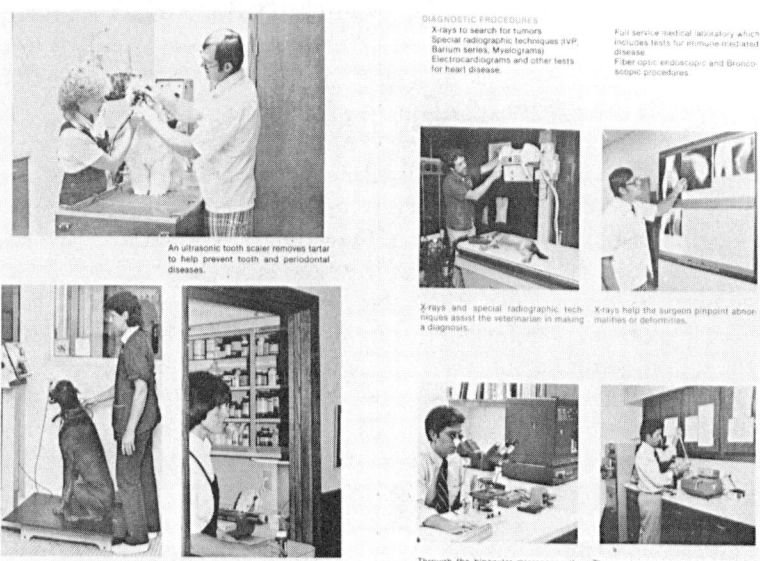

Figure 6-8. Practice information pamphlet. (A) Cover; (B) inner page example (Courtesy of Orchard Park Veterinary Medical Center, Orchard Park, NY)

unit, nutritional consultation, prepurchase evaluations, and lameness evaluation, with referral if needed.

In small-animal practices, market expansion might be in the areas of birds and exotic service, bereavement counseling, prepurchase evaluation of pets to determine suitability for family, nutritional counseling, dental care (i.e., endodontics, periodontics, orthodontics), cremation service, emergency care, and intensive care unit. Because most small-animal clinics cater to dogs, many cat owners do not feel welcome or comfortable in an environment of dog pictures on the walls and barking dogs in the reception area. Practices who want to increase feline clients might be well rewarded by considering the needs of cats and cat owners when remodeling. Having a separate reception area for cats and keeping cats in a separate ward should be a starting point. Our own attitudes about feline care may be the primary reason for serving only 47% of the cat owners with professional veterinary care.

Sales point displays

Until July 1986, the AVMA's *Principles of Veterinary Medical Ethics* stated: "It is considered unprofessional for veterinarians to display leashes, collars, meat, foods, and other nonprofessional products in their offices, hospitals, and waiting rooms." In 1986 the foregoing statement was removed from the *Principles*. This change resulted in the AVMA's Judicial Council stating: "The display of nonprofessional products is undesirable but is permissible if such nonprofessional products are generally unavailable or are difficult to obtain in the general vicinity of the client being served. It is permissible to display professional veterinary products in the waiting room."

The *Principles of Veterinary Medical Ethics* defines professional and nonprofessional products. A professional product is one in which professional veterinary knowledge is indicated whether in the administration of or in the giving of instructions for the safe, proper, and prudent use of the product. Professional veterinary products include but are not limited to biologicals, pharmaceuticals, parasiticides, and prescription diets. A nonprofessional product is one that is considered safe for use by the public without professional instruction. Such products include but are not limited to nonprescription commercial diet foods, grooming aids, and restraint equipment.

Attitudes about in-house displays have changed during the past 10 years. In a recent survey, 64% of the practitioners surveyed indicated they were more favorably inclined than in the past to display products.[5]

When displays are being considered as an internal marketing technique, several important points must be contemplated if they are to be maximally successful. First, the practice must define the client's needs. The specific products must be carefully selected and priced. An appropriate location must be established in the clinic or hospital that may be monitored at *all* times by the support staff. The products must be attractively arranged and kept neat and clean. Prices must be clearly marked on all products.

The most important difference between a hospital or clinic display and a retail store display is the *professional* advice that goes along with each item sold. Professional advice is not available at the feed store, grocery store, department store, or mail order outlets. The support staff should play the key role in product information for the client (Fig. 6-9).

Professional displays may be very limited product lines confined to an examination room (Fig. 6-10) or may encompass a specific area of the reception room (Fig. 6-11), or products may be displayed in a special room adjacent to the reception room (Fig. 6-12).

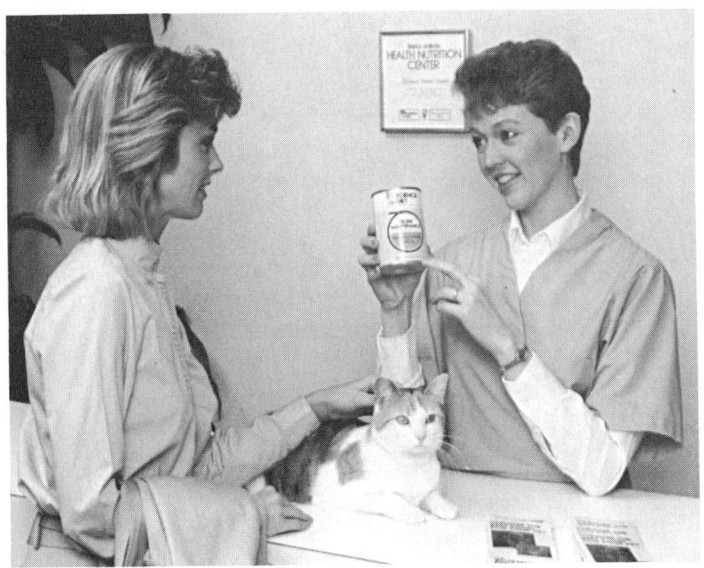

Figure 6-9. *Veterinary technician discussing dietary management with client*

External marketing

Most external marketing activities are aimed at expanding practice activity through identification of new consumers in need of veterinary services. External marketing can be carried out by an individual practice, a group practice, organized veterinary medicine, and commerical companies.

Individual practice and group practice

Some types of external marketing are currently being used in many practices. The use of newsletters, telephone yellow page listing, building signage, producer and client education nights, community service activities, and National Pet Week materials all expand the image of the practice to clients and nonclients.

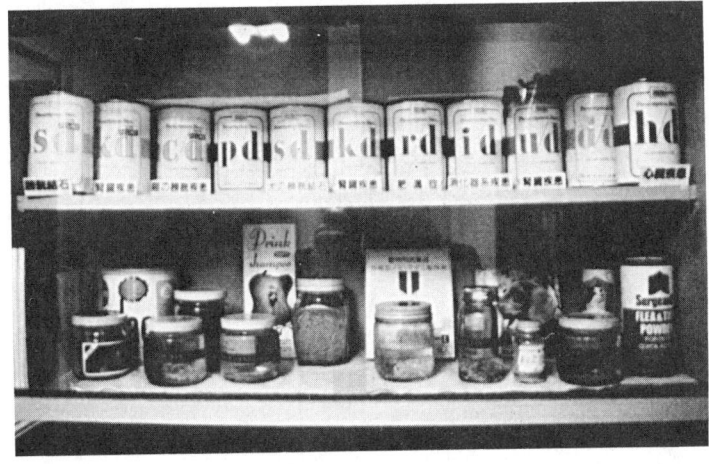

Figure 6-10. *Examination room display area*

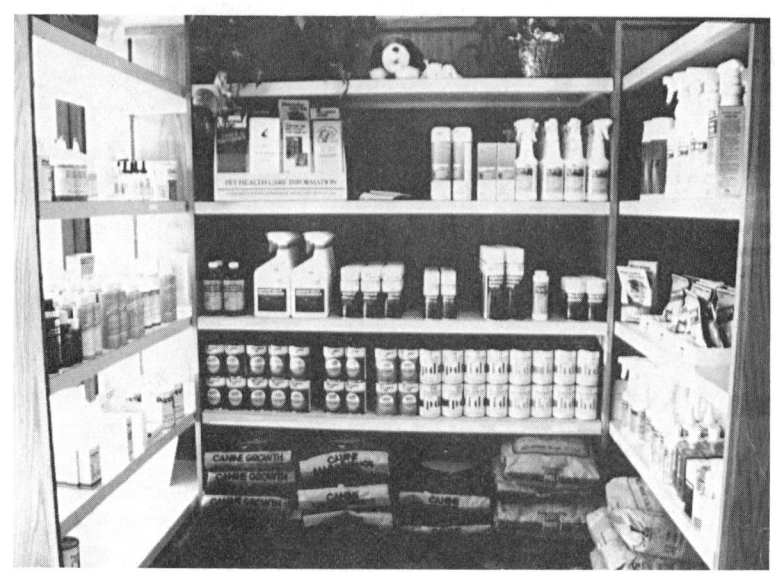

Figure 6-11. Extensive reception area display

When a practice wants to penetrate into the nonclient base, it is essential to make use of advertising.

Professional advertising

Advertising and marketing have been confused by many people. As has been discussed in this chapter, advertising is only one small piece of the total marketing picture, but a very important one. Professional advertising includes hospital signs, telephone book listings, practice newsletters, vaccination reminders, professional business cards, and so forth. The focus on advertising in this discussion, how-

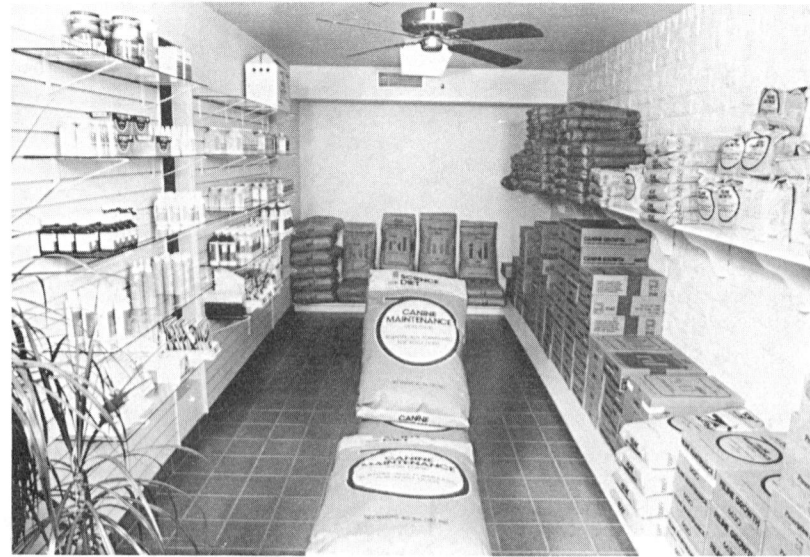

Figure 6-12. Specialized display room

ever, will center on the more "hard-core" forms of advertising: yellow pages of the telephone book, newspapers, magazines, radio, direct mail, and television.

Attitudes about advertising differ between the professional and consumer. A great majority of professionals (physicians, dentists, attorneys, veterinarians) are against advertising for a variety of reasons: it is unprofessional and unethical and lowers status, credibility, and sense of dignity.[6] Just as professionals feel strongly negative toward advertising, consumers feel strongly positive. Consumers generally feel advertising by a professional would not compromise that professional's credibility, status, image, or dignity. In fact, most consumers believe advertising by professionals would help them make a more intelligent choice.[6]

The 1867 United States Veterinary Medical Association's *Code of Ethics* stated in section 5: "In advertising, the veterinary surgeon shall confine himself to his business address. Advertising specific medicines, specific plans of treatment, advertising through the medium of posters, illuminated bills, newspaper puffs, etc., will not be countenanced by this society."[7] The *Priniciples of Veterinary Medical Ethics* now state that the professional shall not make false, deceptive, or misleading statements or claims when advertising. The question is one of *how* we should advertise not *whether* we should advertise.

Telephone Yellow Pages. Veterinarians have been strongly encouraged by yellow page sales staff to market their practice through increasingly large telephone advertisements. Many major metropolitan area telephone books now carry a variety of quarter-, half-, and full-page advertisements for individual veterinary practices. Investing in a larger and larger telephone advertisement is not the long-term solution to market expansion. Unfortunately, some practitioners have not considered other forms of practice marketing. When most practitioners in a specific area are using quarter- or half-page telephone advertising, the consumer impact is the same as when practitioners were using one-line listings. The only difference is the increased cost of the larger listings, which must eventually be passed on to the client.

When developing a new practice, a larger telephone listing is effective, but using an ever-increasing size listing does not replace a multiapproach marketing plan. If a particular practice area is in need of greater client exposure, the individual practitioner cost can be reduced by group advertising. As an example, the local VMA could sponsor a "practitioner locating service" by using a full yellow page listing that groups practitioners by location within the area. These location guides are very helpful to the consumer and represent a savings to practitioners, yet provide a full page of veterinary advertising.

Another approach might be to have specialty groups develop listings. The American Animal Hospital Association has area member hospitals join together for a block listing of all members. Equine and food animal practitioners or large multilocation practices could also form groups to pool resources for larger, more informative, professional telephone listings. One of the most important points about marketing is not to have practitioners compete among themselves but to have them compete for a larger market.

Newspapers. Newspaper advertising, as telephone yellow page advertising, is useful for initial impact when opening or expanding a practice. Many professionals will have a newspaper listing when opening a new practice, relocating an existing practice, or when adding new associates to an existing practice. The continual use of newspaper advertising by veterinarians has been largely prohibited by cost.

In large multilocation practices, newspaper advertising might be used effectively if professionally prepared. The cost–benefit ratio, however, would need careful monitoring.

Probably the best form of newspaper advertising for veterinarians is the "animal care information" format. Weekly animal care information columns are a public service, and newspapers are always seeking interesting material. Pet columns have become popular reading as the public begins to acknowledge the human–animal bond. To address the need for weekly newspaper columns, several private column services have sprung up that will provide the practitioner with 52 professionally written stories on animal care each year. This service can be purchased by individual veterinarians or through associations.

In the larger metropolitan areas, newspapers can become very restrictive about the stories they print. If a veterinarian (or association) is unsuccessful in obtaining an agreement for publication of a regular column, then one should explore the neighborhood papers in the area. These weekly local neighborhood papers are usually well read and circulated and are always open to new material.

Radio and Television. Two of the most powerful advertising mediums are radio and television. Both are expensive and are generally out of the financial consideration of most veterinarians. Consumers are being exposed to increasing numbers of commercials for services provided by attorneys, dentists, opticians, physicians, and chiropractors as professional competition increases.

A few large, multilocation veterinary group practices advertise services on television. If a large practice is considering radio or television media, an advertising consultant should be retained and the cost–benefit ratio closely evaluated.

Veterinary associations can obtain "air time" essentially free by participating in talk shows. The subject of animals, animal care, and animal behavior is a fascinating subject to most listening and viewing audiences. A number of the larger radio and television markets have regularly scheduled talk shows (some hosted by veterinarians) that have question-and-answer formats devoted to animal care. The talk show format is an excellent opportunity for those veterinary associations who have articulate and knowledgeable veterinarians to sell veterinary medicine for the profession as a whole.

Magazines. Advertising in national magazines has not become useful to the individual practitioner or to veterinary associations. The cost–benefit ratio is too low. Certainly, animal supplies are widely advertised in specialty magazines, and some suppliers have included in their advertisements reference to obtaining veterinary care. Most suppliers, however, have attempted to market their products over the products of veterinarians through price promotion.

Political Action Committee. During the past several national elections, political action committees (PACs) have become quite active. Veterinarians have been slow to become politically involved as individuals or as a group. The AVMA formed a PAC in the early 1980s. By the mid-1980s many veterinarians became aware of the political influence necessary to remain competitive in today's marketplace.

Individual veterinarians can be effective at the local level, but groups and associations can be more effective. Veterinary practitioners and associations must become more politically aware and financially support the political process to maintain and improve the veterinary practice market.

Advertising is difficult for most individual practitioners to use on any kind of a regular schedule due to cost; however, using local shopping directories and neighborhood shopping magazines can produce local practice exposure on an irregular basis. The neighborhood paper pet column can also be used. These types of advertising produce limited results and have very little long-term value.

The multilocation group practice may be able to establish a marketing budget for regular exposure in newspapers and magazines. A large yellow page advertisement may also be justified through listing several practice locations in the group practice. A few group practices may be able to afford radio and television spots when advertising for ten or more locations. Television has been successfully used in several large consumer markets when the advertising has been on a regular basis to provide the consumer with information reinforcement.

The bottom line for all individual practices and most smaller group practices is that advertising is too expensive to be carried out on a regular basis. The only medium that has consistently been used to attract nonclients is the telephone yellow pages. Other forms of advertising (i.e., television, newspapers, magazines, radio) must be supported by organized veterinary medicine and commercial companies. Increased interest in promoting veterinarians and veterinary practice has come from commercial companies upon the realization that individual practice expansion results in commercial expansion.

Animal care talks

Both veterinary technicians and veterinarians can become involved in providing veterinary medical care talks to grade school and high school students. These presentations can provide information on routine animal health care, first aid activities, signs to look for when an animal is ill, and general information on educational requirements for becoming veterinarians and technicians. These presentations can help change the established "norms" about animal care.

When a presentation has become polished, service clubs in the community make excellent audiences. Talks to service clubs are helpful to the individual practice and the profession. A slide presentation that features both veterinarian and technician in their "team" roles is quite effective.

Producer or client education night

To enhance client education efforts within the practice, special evenings can be set aside during the year to discuss specific topics. In food animal practice the topics might be integrated reproductive management, preconditioning programs, nutrition, or housing. The practice would invite, by personal invitation, clients along with some nonclients. Speakers could be veterinarians and technicians within the practice or guest speakers from industry or the university sector. These programs could be held in the practice or at a local hotel or motel.

Equine practices could discuss reproduction, nutrition, colic, lameness, exercise physiology, or any other subject that needs client education and attention. Equine owners would benefit from programs covering training, behavior, first aid, and foaling.

The small-animal practitioner could present information on care of the new puppy or kitten, information on exotic pets and birds, first aid, whelping and queening, hip dysplasia, nutrition, parasite control, pet obedience training, and pet selection. Client education programs should be given on a regular basis and offered at convenient times. Attendees should be provided handout material to take home for future reference.

When the education program is held at the practice, a complete tour of the facilities should be planned. Clients are very interested in seeing hospital equipment and understanding more about hospital care. Hospital open houses are an excellent image builder to clients. Having a "behind-the-scenes" tour is something most clients have not had an opportunity to experience. Children are especially impressed with show-and-tell demonstrations.

By providing client education opportunities, the client becomes more bonded to the practice. When veterinary problems arise, the client is more apt to contact the practice that has provided the inside look and veterinary medical information.

Community activities

Veterinary practices that are engaged in community activities have a much wider client contact base. Veterinarians and technicians both can become involved in community service through girl scouts, boy scouts, school board, humane society, breed club, country club, Rotary, Lions, and church activities. Potential client contacts are made in the course of "being involved."

One should *not* join a community activity only to make client contacts. Practice is too time consuming for both veterinarian and technician to become involved in too many activities or activities that are not personally rewarding. However, these activities are an important marketing tool, in addition to being necessary services in the community.

Organized veterinary medicine

External marketing can be made affordable to all veterinarians through group efforts of organized veterinary medicine. National, state, and local professional associations can play a key role in the overall marketing efforts of the profession. The American Association of Equine/Bovine/Swine Practitioners, AVMA, American Animal Hospital Association, State VMAs, and local/regional VMAs can provide funding and personnel support for broad-based marketing activities.

A good example of an external marketing program is the AVMA's National Pet Week, which was initiated in the early 1980s. This program has been helpful to many companion animal practitioners through increased pet awareness on a national and local scale.

State VMAs have become quite active in promoting veterinary medicine on behalf of their members. These programs have involved the following areas:

1. Marketing seminars — to provide educational information to members concerning various marketing techniques
2. Direct mail — to provide members handout materials and form newsletters for clients
3. Spokesperson training — to provide training to a few key veterinarians who will accurately represent the profession to the media
4. Community relations — to foster improved community relations with service clubs, junior and senior high schools, and other community groups
5. Media relations — to provide personal contact with all media in an open and informative manner
6. Public awareness — to inform the general public of veterinary services available in the community
7. Co-op programs — to encourage improved relations and cooperation with humane societies, pet clubs, animal breeders associations, racing groups, and so forth
8. Paid advertising — to educate the potential market of consumers so as to allow them to make animal care decisions based on medical care information rather than price alone

The aforementioned programs can be accomplished through the efforts of organized veterinary medicine. If individual practices attempted these programs, the effects would be much more limited or totally negligible due to time and money. The effectiveness of organized veterinary medicine's marketing can be greatly enhanced when coupled with industry.

Commercial company and industry support

Commercial companies in industry are becoming more active in providing direct support in veterinary marketing activities. Most companies have recognized the symbiotic relationships between practitioners and industry. When practitioners are doing well, industry is doing well. To this end, industry has developed audiovisuals, handout materials, national advertising, and public service announcements to support the individual marketing efforts of practitioners. Industry has also supported the profession through student scholarships, continuing education, educational displays, and national veterinary awards.

Commercial companies have the resources and personnel to develop and support national marketing efforts on behalf of the entire profession or specific segments of the profession (i.e., small-animal, equine, food animal practices). When organized veterinary medicine and industry team up to externally market the profession, the results can be highly successful.

The AVMA and state VMAs must keep communication channels open to maximize efforts. External marketing efforts using advertising can become affordable when industry and organized veterinary medicine cooperate.

Summary

Professional marketing is a rapidly expanding area of interest within the profession. As veterinarians understand the scope and power of marketing techniques, utilization of such techniques in individual practices will rapidly expand. The potential unserved market for veterinary services is approximately 50%. Tremendous opportunity exists for expansion of the entire profession by attempting to attain a portion of the untapped market. Rather than internal competition for the existing pie (as we slice it into smaller and smaller pieces), why not enlarge the whole pie so everyone has a larger piece? Enlarging the pie can be achieved through effective use of internal and external marketing.

Practitioners who aggressively use *professional* marketing techniques will attain improved client services, upgraded levels of patient care, and increased net income. Marketing must become a special interest area of the profession just as herd health, reproductive management, nutrition, and avian medicine have become in recent years. Marketing requires time, energy, and money to be carried out successfully. We all must become involved.

References

1. Troutman, CW: The Veterinary Services Market, (A 161-page report prepared for AVMA). Overland Park, KA, Charles, Charles & Associates, 1983
2. Wise JK, Kushann JE: Synopsis of U.S. Veterinary Medical Manpower Study: Demand and supply from 1980 to 2000. J Am Vet Med Assoc 187: 358–361, 1987
3. Wood E: Personal communication. Breese, IL, Veterinary Services Ltd. 1986
4. Geier D: Personal communication. Topeka, KA, Hill's Pet Products, Inc, 1987
5. Gridley D: Practitioner's attitudes changing toward in-house merchandising. DVM Magazine, 17, No 8, August 1986
6. McCurnin DM, Thompson A: Professional advertising. JAVMA 188, No 12: 1387–1389, 1986
7. Tannenbaum, J: Personal communication. Boston, School of Veterinary Medicine, Tufts University, 1986

Chapter 7

☐

How to buy or sell a practice

Ross D. Clark
Ronald K. Patrick

You have decided to buy a practice. This was the easy part; now come the questions. What can you afford? What should you look for in a practice? What are the liabilities? Which items of the agreement are negotiable? How can you tell whether the asking price is fair?

Or maybe you have decided to sell your practice. When should you begin planning? How can you establish an equitable market price for your practice? To whom should you sell the practice? What is needed to close the deal?

Whether buyers or sellers, the people involved want to achieve certain goals in the transaction. A buyer wants to finance the price, but a seller would prefer all cash. A buyer wants to be sure the net receipts will cover all bills and allow a comfortable income, but the seller wants to be sure there is ample security to replace the cash flow. Each party wants something a little different. That is why it is important for both parties to be as knowledgeable as possible before entering into any buy–sell arrangement.

☐

Buying a practice

When making a decision to buy a practice, one needs to understand that several different factors are involved. Buyers must select the right practice, paying particular attention to location, and must know what they are paying for: inventory, equipment, real estate and improvements, and goodwill and client records. The liabilities and tax considerations need to be examined, as the question of whether restrictive practice covenant can be negotiated.

All of these factors must be reviewed before any kind of buying decision is made.

Select the right practice

Anyone in real estate will confirm that the first three principles of the trade are location, location, and location. These three principles must be used when selecting the right practice. An existing practice is committed to its location, which can make it a little vulnerable. As a buyer, one needs to know what factors affect the right location.

Residential areas

Choose a practice in a city that seems to be experiencing population growth. Better yet, search for a practice that is located on a road servicing a popular residential area. Convenience is very important. Most clients do not like taking their pets long distances in the car.

Exposure and accessibility

In most cases, a freestanding clinic has better exposure than a shopping center clinic. Parking is often better, and location is nearer the street. Shopping center clinics, however, often attract clients who are visiting other shops in the center. A good compromise is a location in a neighborhood convenience center.

Household count

Survey the neighborhoods surrounding the practice and try to estimate whether there are more single-family dwellings or multiple-family dwellings (apartments and condominiums). Pet restrictions often apply to multiple-family dwellings, which limits the client base. Choose a location that has the majority of access to single-family homes.

Across America about 52% of households have either a dog or cat. When all pets are considered, 61% of households have dogs, cats, birds, hamsters, or horses.

Draw a 3-mile circle around the proposed practice site and count the veterinarians within that circle. Divide the total number of veterinarians into the number of households within the circle. Our studies indicate that a practice needs a potential client base of at least 1500 pets. Each veterinarian would need a minimum of 2000 households that use veterinary medical services.

Those households having pets will each have an average of 1.5 to 1.6 cats or dogs. In more affluent neighborhoods as high as 85% of households will seek veterinary medical services. In less affluent neighborhoods there may be less than 50% seeking service.

Assuming 50% of households have 1.5 pets and 66% will seek veterinary medical service, we would like to see 3000 households per veterinarian in the 3-mile area. Of that 3000, 1500 households would likely have pets. One thousand (two thirds) households would seek services. One thousand households would own about 1500 pets. If one can gross $100.00 per pet per year (the national average is $60.00 per year), then this practice location would have a potential gross of $150,000 per year.

Of course, many practices are succeeding with demographics that are not as favorable as suggested here. Just be aware that increased competition may soon change the demographic ground rules. The role of marketing is having an impact on practice growth. Additional information on marketing can be found in Chapter 6.

Household income

The mean income of an area is another indicator of the potential revenue for a practice. Search for a middle-income neighborhood with a large number of school-age children. Enrollment records from community schools can provide this information unless private schools or busing are factors. Look for a community income of at least $75 million per veterinarian.

Traffic count

Clients need easy access to a practice. A practice located on a major six-lane highway with a center median and no access may have less business than a practice on a two-lane road with easy access. And remember those intersections: when traffic slows down, drivers notice the practice more easily.

How to set the price

Once the practice and location have been evaluated, the next step is to establish a price. Both buyer and seller need to value the tangible and intangible assets of the practice. Tangibles include inventory, equipment, and real estate and improvements. Intangibles are goodwill and client records.

Inventory

Included in the inventory are items held for resale (prescription diets, vitamins, flea spray, topicals) and single items held for hospital use (injectables). These items are usually priced at *replacement cost.* The seller should list and price all inventory items with a form similar to that shown in Figure 7-1.

Price adjustments should be made for partially used or damaged items. The buyer should review the items to see whether any-

Description	Remarks	Quantity	Price	Discount	Extended Price

Figure 7-1.   Inventory list

thing is incompatible with the new practice. For example, if the seller stocks drugs used on large animals but the buyer intends to practice only on small animals, he may not want to purchase the large-animal items.

The actual inventory varies daily, so the inventory list should be prepared on the closing date of the sale. During negotiations, estimates are used. On the final inventory, the buyer should perform or at least observe the inventory audit.

When taking the inventory, be systematic to avoid deletions or duplications. Start at one end of the clinic and count all items in the room. If a particular item is in more than one room, list all the items found in that room, then add in similar items from other rooms. During the physical count, one person should list the items and another should count the items. The inventory team can check itself on counts and can also note the condition of the items.

Equipment

Equipment should be listed just like inventory. This category includes large and small medical equipment including instruments, office furniture, fixtures, vehicles, cages, computers, and anything else that is not permanently affixed to the building or land.

Equipment is valued differently than inventory. Inventory is normally sold or used within a short period after purchase, but equipment may last for years.

One method for valuing equipment is *discounted replacement cost* (Fig. 7-2). This method values an item at what it would cost to replace, less any loss in value as its useful life decreases. In other words, it assumes all equipment will be used only a certain number of years. As time passes, the remaining useful life becomes shorter, so the method reduces the replacement cost of the equipment proportional to its remaining useful life.

This method is especially useful for medical equipment and other items of limited marketability. Office equipment can be valued by using the cost of comparable used equipment. As with inventory, review the equipment list for obsolete items or items that are not needed. The average value of equipment is about 75% of current replacement cost.

Real estate and improvements

A complete discussion of real estate is included in Chapter 4. In general, though, if the real estate is included in the sale, it should be valued by an independent real estate appraiser. Be sure to select someone who is familiar with the practice's location and the local economy. Appraisers often value property differently, so a second or third opinion is a good idea.

If the practice is located on leased property, the seller must place a value on the lease and improvements. If the rent is below the fair rental value of the property, the lease has value to the buyer. But if the rent is above the fair rental value, the lease is actually a liability, and the purchase price should be reduced accordingly.

One way to adjust a lease is to multiply the difference between actual rent payments and fair rental value by the number of months remaining in the lease. The result is the adjustment (up or down) in the selling price.

Goodwill and client records

Goodwill is the value of the past business of the practice and the accumulation of clients, hired employees, and start-up activities necessary for any new business. It can be valued simply or derived from complicated formulas. Whatever the method, when valuing goodwill, one should consider the current condition of the practice. Potential improvements are left to the buyer and cannot add any value for the seller.

One simple method of valuing goodwill is as a percentage of 1 year's gross income. The

Description	Condition	Replacement Cost	Total Useful Life	Life Remaining	Percentage of Useful Life Remaining	Current Value
(Item)	(Good fair poor unusable)		(Estimate for new item)	(Estimate for this item)	(Divide column 5 by column 4)	(Multiply column 3 by column 6)

Figure 7-2. Equipment discounted replacement cost

percentage could vary from 50% to 125% of 1 year's gross income depending on practice age, condition, and demographics. Gross income would be the average of the last 3 years' cash receipts from services and product sales. Under this method, goodwill would be the amount left over after subtracting the value of inventory, equipment, and other assets (excluding real estate).

Another simple method is to negotiate a value for each patient record and then buy the records at their value. This is especially good if the practice will be relocated or merged into an existing practice because the newly purchased practice will lose its identity, and its only intangible value will be its client base.

An example of the formula method was presented by McCafferty.[1-3] This method adjusts the net income of the practice by adding back unusual or personal expenses and subtracting normal expenses that a new owner would expect to incur. From this adjusted net income, a fair salary for veterinarians is subtracted as well as an amount for the cost of the buyer's investment. Any amount left over is capitalized over several years.

The underlying assumption in this method is that goodwill is only present if the net income exceeds certain normal expectations. It is difficult to apply the method to new practices because of the lack of historical data.

As was mentioned earlier, employees are also part of goodwill. The buyer "purchases" these individuals' talents and expertise. Existing employees can have intrinsic value because they are acquainted with the clients, and they are trained, which releases the buyer for other business. Existing employees also work together as a team, which can help smooth the rough transitional time; however, the buyer may decide to "clean house," and if so, be sure to adjust the goodwill figure accordingly.

Calculating client or patient records

A quick method of calculating patient records is to count all the patient records whose owner's names begin with "S." Multiply this total by 10 to arrive at the estimated total numbers of patients. (Note that if the hospital in question keeps more than one patient on each client's card it is important to multiply the number of client cards by 1.6 to get the total number of patients.)

A court case in California in 1977 determined that veterinary medical records do have value. At that time IRS accepted $7.50 per record as a proper value. Currently, $20.00 to $25.00 is a fair value depending, of course, on the annual gross per patient. The gross per patient can be calculated by dividing the total current records (all clients who have been in at least one time in the last 36 months) into the annual gross. Our studies indicate $60.00 per pet per year is average. A gross of $150.00 per pet per year would justify a higher value per record. Client records can be depreciated over a 7-year period.

Liability

Normally, the buyer does not assume any old liabilities; the seller pays them. The buyer might, however, inadvertently become liable when purchasing shares of stock in an existing corporation. The corporation is usually liable for all debts, regardless of change in ownership.

Another potential problem is that one might buy assets without knowing there are liens that exist against those assets. Ask the seller about debts owed and to whom they are owed. Then call the creditor to be sure the liens are released.

The buyer may also specify that a portion of the purchase price be held in escrow for a certain period of time to handle any liabilities or claims that may be asserted against the practice. Whatever the plan of action, the buyer must be sure to clear any unnecessary debt.

Tax considerations

Many details of the sale can result in conflicts between the tax situations of the buyer and the seller. Let us say buyer X pays seller Y $100,000 for an existing veterinary practice to be allocated as follows:

Inventory	$10,000
Equipment	60,000
Goodwill	30,000
Total	$100,000

The $30,000 goodwill could result in favorable capital gains tax treatment to the seller, but the buyer would not receive any tax deduction for his $30,000 payment until he sold the practice.

However, if the $100,000 were allocated as follows:

Inventory	$10,000
Equipment	90,000
Goodwill	0
Total	$100,000

Then the buyer would be able to depreciate the higher equipment value and receive a tax deduction. The seller might have to recapture a greater portion of depreciation as ordinary income.

One way to achieve tax advantages for both the buyer and the seller is to set a price for the practice medical records and shift an amount from the value of goodwill. The buyer may be able to depreciate the value of the records and receive a tax deduction, and the seller will continue to receive favorable capital gains treatment.

Another tax consideration is how the purchase price of the practice will be paid. If it is paid all in the same year, the seller may be forced into a higher tax bracket. By spreading payments over 2 or more years, this problem may be avoided or reduced.

The transfer of titles to assets may be structured in a way to obtain maximum tax benefits without affecting the negotiations process. If the buyer plans to operate the practice as a corporation, money might be saved by holding some assets personally and transferring others to the corporation. The personal assets could be rented to the corporation. The corporation would receive deductions for rent payments, and the new owner could report the rent as income. The new owner would then receive depreciation deductions on the assets to partially or wholly offset the rent income. The net result is that the corporation receives a tax deduction and the new owner can take money out of the corporation without being subjected to income or payroll taxes.

A nontax reason for not transferring all assets to the new practice would be if the buyer retains control of the asset. As new veterinarians are allowed to buy into the practice, either as partners or shareholders, the personally held assets do not need to be transferred. This results in a lower purchase price for the new veterinarians and lets the senior partner maintain control of some of the assets.

Tax planning should be an integral part of the negotiation process. Seek competent tax advice before finalizing any sale because the tax laws are continually changing.

Restrictive practice covenant

Any buyer is rightfully nervous about the seller's plans once the agreement is consummated. What prevents the seller from moving a couple of blocks down the street, hanging out their shingle, and stealing all those dearly paid-for clients the buyer just purchased as part of goodwill? The restrictive practice covenant helps solve this problem.

The restrictive practice covenant, written into the final agreement, places limitations on the seller. The buyer may want to limit the location where the seller may practice or set up a particular number of years before the seller can practice again in the area. These restrictions help the buyer become established in the marketplace without competition from the seller.

The only problem with restrictive covenants is the enforcement. Even though agreements in all 50 states include such clauses, some lawyers indicate the restrictive covenant is illegal because a person's right to make a living cannot be limited. Still, try to include the clause for as much protection as possible. When money is paid for goodwill, it has been the authors' observations that covenants not to compete are almost always enforced.

□
Selling a practice

The value of a practice is the amount somebody is willing to sell it for and what someone else is willing to pay. Many veterinarians, however, sell their practices too cheap. If you find yourself in the seller's seat, try following these guidelines to come out ahead.

Plan the sale in advance

Time

The seller should plan ahead to allow plenty of time to prepare for the sale. Some experts recommend up to 5 years of advance planning. Why so long? Long-range planning provides the seller a chance to build the practice into a salable item as well as the time to prepare for a career change, retirement, or transfer.

Annual appraisals

Be sure to have the practice evaluated yearly. Being able to show the buyer what has been done to increase the worth of the business over the past 5 years will help during negotiations. If one can demonstrate that the practice is growing, a higher price can be negotiated.

Growth curves

The seller should monitor increases in growth as well as in value. Graph out how the patient load has increased. Note the peak and slump times of the year. Show the impact fee increases had on receipts. Illustrate the impact of adding a new partner or technician.

Improvements

Building improvements should also be made. About 2 years before the anticipated sale, decide what kinds of improvements would increase the value of the business. These improvements can be taken as depreciation benefits while increasing the value of the property for the upcoming sale.

Cash flow

Finally, go all out to strengthen the cash flow. Be sure the financial statement is as sound as possible. The seller's banker, the buyer, and the buyer's banker will be impressed, and the seller will be able to walk away from the sale with more funds in his pocket.

Establish a price

The years of planning have now elapsed, and it is time to affix a price to the practice. Review the steps and guidelines in the section of this chapter "How to Set the Price." Complete the inventory and value the equipment, know the worth of the real estate and improvements, and establish a price for goodwill and client records. When the seller has accounted for every item of value and has given it fair yet full market value, the seller is ready to look for a buyer.

Sell to a known buyer

When selling, look from within first. If the seller knows the buyer and they have worked together for a few years, one can feel more confident that the practice will run smoothly after the seller is gone (and the seller is more assured of receiving any rental payments or note payments that are due).

This is where preplanning comes in. When sellers know they want to retire or move within 5 years, they should hire an associate who is interested in buying a practice down the road. This way, the owner and the potential buyer know each other and will have a chance to change plans in case the relationship does not work out. It is equally good for potential buyers because the clientele knows them, which helps to ensure a smoother transition when the owner sells out.

□
Gradual method of buy/sell

The gradual buy/sell method lets the senior veterinarian owner (the eventual seller) benefit from the junior veterinarian's additional income (by increasing the senior's income). It also helps junior associates gain advantages by deducting a portion of client records and equipment from their income tax. Let us use an example and see how this works.

A young veterinarian has an opportunity to buy into a growing practice and will be paying little or nothing down. Both parties can benefit in this type of arrangement. The new partnership pays the junior partner, who has ac-quired 1% to 50% of the practice, a fair wage based on experience (a fair wage for 1987 is shown in Fig. 7-3) plus a percentage of profits after all expenses have been paid (including a fair wage to all veterinarians and fair building rent). As an example the junior partner could make $100 more and the senior partner, therefore, takes home $100 less. That saves the senior partner $38.00 in taxes based on a 38% tax rate. The junior partner pays taxes on his addi-

DVM COMPENSATION		
No. Years	Base Salary	Pay 8% of All Individual Gross Over: (Doesn't Count Boarding)
0 to 1	$22,000.00	$10,000.00
1 to 2	26,000.00	12,000.00
2 to 3	30,000.00	14,000.00
3 to 4	34,000.00	16,000.00
4 to 5	38,000.00	18,000.00
5 to 6	42,000.00	20,000.00

Figure 7-3. *DVM compensation*

tional $100 at his 15% tax bracket. Then he pays the $100 back to the senior partner in the form of a note. The senior partner pays capital gains taxes on the $100 at 28% because he sold part of an asset.

Put another way, the senior partner gives the junior partner $100 additional income and receives the money back in the form of capital gain when the junior associate makes his note payment. Income tax advantages for both parties help make the transaction even more worthwhile.

Another advantage for the junior associate is that he can deduct a portion of client records and equipment from income taxes. He can depreciate client records and equipment over 7 years. So for that $25,000 in assets he purchased, he can depreciate (under the 1987 tax rules) roughly $3,500 each of the 7 years.

Negotiable items

Naturally, the buyer and seller have different goals in the purchase, but there is room for negotiation. Purchase price is one area.

The purchase price comprises the down payment, the interest rate, and the term, which is in turn affected by the age of the seller. If the buyer must finance the purchase price, that price goes up because the seller is now losing money that could be earning income or interest elsewhere. Both parties have to be willing to give and take so they can arrive at a compromise.

Another area for negotiation is old inventory. The buyer may have inventory that will probably sell, but the items may not sell for a year or more. These could be special-order items that were never picked up or that were returned or items that just do not move quickly. The buyer can offer the merchandise lower than their replacement cost to compensate for the long holding period.

Closing the deal

The buyer and seller have settled on a price, negotiated the terms, and agree to follow through with the transaction. It is time to close the deal. Be sure to draw up the appropriate documents from those listed here:

1. Partnership agreement (Fig. 7-4) (if applicable)
2. Partners' cross-purchase agreement (Fig. 7-5) (if applicable)
3. A promissory note from the purchasing partner and his executors, administrators, and heirs. The debtor assigns and guarantees payment to the seller, his administrators, and his heirs (if applicable).
4. A purchase agreement (Fig. 7-6)
5. Collateral pledge (if applicable)
6. Equipment lease agreement for tax purposes (if applicable). The buying partner might buy, under a separate agreement, a percentage of the oldest equipment. This could be in addition to the portion of the practice purchase. The buying partner can then redepreciate this equipment. Each partner in turn leases his or her equipment to the partnership. Again, check current tax legislation to learn whether this is a good benefit.
7. Real estate lease agreement (if applicable)

Seeking professional help

There are four major areas where both parties can seek professional guidance: finding a buyer or seller, setting the purchase price, tax planning, and obtaining legal services.

PARTNERSHIP AGREEMENT

This is an Agreement for a partnership made on the   th day of 19   , by and between

D.V.M.,   D.V.M.,

D.V.M., AND   D.V.M.

I. Formation

and   hereby enter into a partnership for the practice of veterinary medicine. Dr.

Dr.   , and Dr.   have been

partners practicing veterinary medicine since   , 19   , as

Dr.   , Dr.

Dr.   , and Dr.

have been practicing veterinary medicine as partners since the 1st day of   ,
19   , and now desire to execute a formal agreement reflecting the basis of their partnership. This Agreement is made for the continuation of the partnership business as partners, and all the parties hereto agree that the terms of the Agreement shall operate retroactively to the commencement of the partnership business on the 1st day of   , 19   .

II. Business

2.1. The parties hereby form a partnership to engage in every phase and aspect of the business of rendering the same professional services to the public that the veterinarian, duly licensed under the laws of the State of   , is authorized to render, but such professional services shall be rendered only through the partners, employees, and agents who are duly licensed under the laws of the State of   to practice veterinary medicine therein; to invest the funds of the partnership in real estate, mortgages, stocks, bonds, or any other type of investment, and to own real and personal property necessary for the rendering of professional veterinary services; and to do everything necessary and proper for the accomplishment of any of the purposes for the obtaining of any of the objectives or the furtherance of any of the purposes enumerated in this Agreement or any amendments thereof, necessary or incidental to the protection and benefit of the partnership, and in general to carry on any lawful pursuit necessary or incidental to the accomplishment of the purposes or the attainment of the objectives or the furtherance of such purposes or objectives of the partnership.

2.2. *Partnership Name and Principal Office.* The name of the partnership shall be   and the principal office of the partnership is to be located at

, or at such other place in   ,
, as the parties may agree.

III. Term

The partnership shall begin on the 1st day of   19   and shall continue until the 1st day of   19   and from year to year thereafter until terminated as herein provided.

IV. Capital

The capital of the partnership shall consist of the following items:
(a) All drugs, supplies, expendables, and equipment as set in exhibit ''A'';

(Continued)

Figure 7-4. Partnership agreement

(b) Records and clients; and

(c) Accounts receivable.

V. Profits and Losses

5.1. *Determination of Net Profits.* The net profits of the partnership shall be computed by deducting monthly from the partnership's gross income the total monthly expenses of the partnership including, but not limited to, rent, telephone, salaries of employees, malpractice and other professional insurance premiums, subscriptions to professional journals, dues in professional associations, the cost of disability insurance and life insurance purchased by the partnership pursuant to this Agreement, appropriate reserves, and such other items as the partners deem appropriate.

5.2. *Division of Profits.* The partners shall be entitled to a monthly draw in the following amounts:

(a) Dr.   , $ a month plus % over $;

(b) Dr.   , $ a month plus % over $;

(c) Dr.   , $ a month plus % over   on any given month.

(d) Dr.   shall receive $ a month as a consultant to the partnership for veterinary medical procedures and administration of the Clinic.

The above-enumerated amounts will be withdrawn from the partnership accounts only after the payment of all operating expenses. Monthly profits if any shall be distributed on or before the 30th of each month.

Yearly, after the deduction and payment of all operating expenses and above-enumerated monthly draws and consulting fees, any monies remaining in the partnership accounts as profits will be divided by the 30th of the month on the following basis:

(a) Dr.   ,   %;

(b) Dr.   ,   %;

(c) Dr.   ,   %; and

(d) Dr.   ,   %.

The partnership will not maintain separate drawing accounts. The partners will make their monthly draws simultaneously, and in the event funds remain in the partnership accounts after the payment of monthly operating expenses and draws, the amounts remaining in the partnership accounts will be distributed simultaneously to the partners in the amounts described above. It is the intent of the partners that the compensation for each individual partner shall not exceed   % of their individual gross production. If this occurs, Dr.   as managing partner may review and adjust the compensation of that partner.

VI. Management Duties

The parties to this agreement agree that   shall be the managing partner.

(a) Day-to-day management shall be shared, except in a case where an absolute impasse exists. Should an absolute impasse occur, the final decision shall be made by   , who shall give so much of his attention and time to the conduct and supervision of the partnership business as he thinks necessary or advisable, provided that   shall devote a minimum of thirty-eight (38) eight-hour (8-hour) days per year to the partnership business.

(b)   ,   and   , shall devote as much time as necessary for the day-

(Continued)

Figure 7-4. Partnership agreement (Continued)

to-day management of the partnership. However, Dr.
Dr.   , and Dr.   may, during
the continuance of this Agreement, engage in any other business for their profit, personal
benefit, or advantage, provided that they notify all their partners in advance and provided
that they shall devote a minimum of thirty-nine (39) hours per week and every fourth Saturday
to the partnership business. If in the judgment of the other partners the additional business
enterprises conflict in any way with a partner's performance of duties as set out herein at
the   Hospital, the partner performing those additional business activities
agrees to terminate those activities three (3) months after notice is given him by two of the
parties to this Agreement that in their opinion the extra business activities are impeding,
limiting, or affecting the performance of his partnership duties as required by the terms of
this Agreement.

VII. Books and Records

7.1. Full and accurate accounts of all financial transactions and affairs of the partnership shall be kept in proper books of account, and each partner shall enter or cause to be entered therein a full and accurate account of all financial transactions relating to or affecting the partnership. The partnership books shall be maintained at the principal office of the partnership, and each partner shall at all times have access thereto.

7.2. The books shall be kept on a cash basis for the calendar year and shall be closed and balanced at the end of each year. At the end of each year, a statement shall then be prepared by a certified public accountant, to be employed by the partnership, showing the result of the year's operations. Each partner shall receive a copy of such statement. The annual statement shall be approved by the partners before final distribution of profits is made in respect to the closed fiscal year. The partners agree that   is currently the certified public accountant employed by the partnership and that said accountant shall continue to serve the partnership until the partners mutually agree on other certified public accountants.

7.3. The partnership books shall be kept on a cash basis.

7.4. The fiscal year of the partnership shall coincide with the calendar year.

VIII. Bank Account

The partnership funds shall be kept on deposit in the name of the partnership at such bank as the partners agree upon. Withdrawals from the partnership account may be made by any of the partners singly or by such other partners as the partners agree. Funds shall be withdrawn from the partnership account for partnership use and benefit only.

IX. Mutual Fidelity

The partners shall deal with each other in all matters relating to or affecting the partnership with the highest degree of good faith, and each partner will give to the other full information as to all professional work being done by him on behalf of the partnership and of all matters that he has knowledge affecting the partnership business and affairs.

X. Leasing of Equipment

10.1. The parties acknowledge that some of the equipment, furniture, and furnishings (herein called "Equipment") to be used by the partnership is owned by Drs.   and   . The partnership shall continue to use said Equipment. An Equipment List is attached hereto and marked Exhibit B, and it

Figure 7-4. Partnership agreement (Continued)

(Continued)

sets out the items of Equipment that are owned by Drs.   and
                                                    and that are leased to the partnership.

10.2. This leasing arrangement shall continue for the life of the partnership or the useful life of the Equipment.

10.3. The partnership shall maintain all said Equipment in good working order at its cost and shall purchase and continue in force complete casualty insurance for all risks, with Drs.   and   named as the insured. The cost of said insurance and the cost of repairs and maintenance of Equipment shall be deemed an expense of the partnership.

XI. Leasing of Partnership Premises

The partnership operations of Dr.   , Dr.   ,
Dr.   , and Dr.   are presently carried on in offices
at   ,   . The improvements, fixtures, and building
at that address are owned by Dr.   and Dr.
                    . The partnership created herein will continue to lease the partnership premises from
Dr.   and Dr.   . This lease will continue during the duration of the partnership Agreement.

XII. Negligence

Except to the extent that the partnership is insured against liability, a partner guilty of negligence or wrongdoing shall reimburse, indemnify, and hold harmless the partnership for damages sustained by the partnership as a result of the negligence or wrongdoing of an individual partner.

XIII. Actions Affecting the Partnership

None of the partners shall perform any of the acts hereinafter noted without the prior written consent of the other partners:

(a) Borrow money in the name of or on behalf of the partnership.

(b) Pledge, hypothecate, or in any way transfer its interest in the partnership, property, or profits thereof.

(c) Compromise or release any of the claims or debts owed to the partnership, except for routine adjustments of the bills of patients.

(d) Bind the partnership as surety, guarantor, or accommodation party.

(e) Lend any partnership funds.

(f) Sell, transfer, encumber or otherwise dispose of the equipment, instruments, furniture or fixtures of the partnership.

(g) Execute a note containing a provision for confession of judgment.

(h) Use any partnership funds or property for any purposes other than those relating to the affairs or business of the partnership and in the ordinary course of partnership business.

(i) Perform any act likely to adversely affect the practice or good name of the partnership.

XIV. Withdrawal

14.1. Should any partner desire to withdraw from the partnership, he shall serve upon the other partners at the principal office of the partnership written notice of his intention to withdraw. Such notice shall be served three (3) months before the effective date of such partner's withdrawal. The value of the partnership shall be determined annually on February 1, based on the profit-and-loss statement from the preceding year. The modified veterinary economics formula as outlined in

(Continued)

Figure 7-4. Partnership agreement (Continued)

Exhibit C attached hereto for the value of a practice will be used. There are two variables in the formula: capitalization and interest rate. Their partnership shall use a capitalization rate of five (5) and an interest rate of ten percent (10%). Such sum shall be paid as set out in Article XVII, paragraphs (a) and (b).

14.2. Should more than one partner desire to withdraw from the partnership and partnership cannot agree as to which partner or partners shall continue the partnership business, a partner or partners shall submit, within thirty (30) days from such date, sealed bids to the accountant currently serving the partnership. The partner or partners submitting the higher bid shall remain as sole partner and continue the partnership business, and the other partner or partners agree to sell his or their partnership interest for the amount of the higher bid. If one partner refuses to submit a bid within the thirty-day (30-day) period, it shall be agreed that this failure to do so shall constitute a bid of one dollar.

14.3. A withdrawing partner agrees to refrain directly or indirectly from carrying on a business similar to that of the partnership for a period of five (5) years from the date of his withdrawal in a radius of ten (10) miles from the principal place of business of the partnership. A withdrawing partner further agrees that he will not call on or serve any of those persons or entities who are clients of the partnership as of the date of the dissolution within the period specified above.

XV. Disability

15.1. *Permanent Disability Defined.* A partner shall be deemed permanently disabled if

(a)   The partner is affected by a disability such as he is unable to give to the partnership practice at least ninety percent (90%) of the work time that would normally be given by him during a continuous four-month (4-month) period; and if

(b)   At the expiration of said four-month (4-month) period the partners agree that sofar as can be reasonably foreseen the disabled partner will thereafter be unable to give the partnership practice at least ninety percent (90%) of normal effective working time.

15.2. *Permanent Disability Payments.*

(a)   If a partner is disabled, then after the expiration of the four-month (4-month) period of disability, the disabled partner shall have the right to receive his share of drawings and profits as if he were subject to no disability whatever, provided, however, that the payments a disabled partner is entitled to receive pursuant to the foregoing provision of this subparagraph shall be reduced by an amount equal to the disability payments that the disabled partner receives or has the right to receive during said four-month (4-month) period under any insurance disability policy purchased by the partnership pursuant to this Agreement.

(b)   After the end of the initial four-month (4-month) period of disability as defined herein, if the partner is still disabled, the disabled partner will be entitled to draw his share of partnership profits for a period not to exceed an additional eight (8) months. A partner deemed disabled under the terms of this Agreement shall not draw their share of the partnership profits for a period exceeding twelve (12) months.

(c)   In the event that it is determined that the disabled partner shall be disabled for a period of more than twelve (12) months, then the partnership shall be deemed to have terminated at the expiration of the twelve-month (12-month) period of disability and the disabled partner deemed to have voluntarily withdrawn, and the provisions of paragraph 14.1 shall be used to determine the value of the disabled partner's interest in the partnership.

15.3. *Interest of Disabled Partner After Termination.* If a partner is permanently disabled for a period of twelve (12) consecutive months, then upon termination of the partnership by reason of such disability, all the rights, title, and interest of the disabled partner in the partnership practice after

(Continued)

Figure 7-4. Partnership agreement (Continued)

payment under the provisions of Article XVII shall be deemed transferred and assigned to the active partners. Payment under the provisions of Article XVII of this Agreement shall constitute compensation in full to the disabled partner's interest in the partnership practice that the active partners are acquiring.

XIV. Disability Insurance

The partnership may hereafter purchase disability insurance covering each of the partners. If such insurance is purchased, then the amount of disability insurance paid to the disabled partner during the aforementioned twelve-month (12-month) disability period (plus the amount of disability insurance that the disabled partner has the right to receive during said twelve-month [12-month] disability period) shall be deducted from the amount that the partnership is required to pay to the disabled partner in respect to the twelve-month (12-month) period. The parties intend that, as provided above, during the twelve-month (12-month) period of disability the disabled partner shall have the right to receive an amount equal to the share of drawings and profits he would have received if under no disability whatsoever, but the partnership shall be required to pay to the disabled partner, in respect to said twelve-month (12-month) period of disability, only the difference between the disabled partner's share of drawings and profits and the amount of disability insurance that the disabled partner receives and has the right to receive during said period.

XVII. Obligation to Purchase

If a partner dies, the interest of the decedent shall be purchased by the surviving partners. The value to be paid to the deceased partner's estate is determined by the same method as outlined in paragraph 14.1 for a voluntary withdrawal. Such sum shall be paid at the election of the surviving partners in either of the following manners:
- (a) The entire sum within one hundred twenty (120) days after the death of such deceased partner, or
- (b) Ten percent (10%) of such sum within one hundred twenty (120) days of the death of such deceased partner and the delivery to such deceased partner's legal representative of a promissory note for the balance of such purchase price that shall be payable in ten (10) equal, annual installments with interest on the unpaid balance at the rate of ten percent (10%) per annum.

XVIII. Purchase of Life Insurance

For the purpose of funding the obligation of the surviving partners to purchase the partnership interest of the deceased partner, the partnership intends to purchase life insurance policies as follows:
- (a) On Dr. _____ , the partnership will purchase $_____ term life insurance and; (b) On Dr. _____ , the partnership will purchase $_____ term life insurance.

The policy shall provide for waiver of premiums in the event of disability. The partners acknowledge that additional insurance may be purchased on the lives of the partners from time to time hereafter, as the partners may agree.

The life insurance policies to be purchased shall be owned and kept in full force and effect by the partnership and shall be deemed an asset of the partnership.

XIX. Dissolution

The partnership may be dissolved at any time by the agreement of the partners, in which event the

(Continued)

Figure 7-4. Partnership agreement   (Continued)

partners shall proceed with reasonable promptness to litigate the business of the partnership. The assets of the partnership shall be used and distributed in the following order of priorities:

(a) To pay or provide for the payment of any partnership liabilities and liquidating expenses and obligation;

(b) To equalize the income accounts of the partners;

(c) To discharge the balance of the income accounts of the partners;

(d) To equalize the capital accounts of the partners; and

(e) To discharge the balance of the capital accounts of the partners.

XX. Vacation and Personal Days

shall be entitled to twelve (12) working days vacation and sick leave.   and   shall be entitled to thirteen and one-half (13½) days vacation.

XXI. Continuing Education

Dr.   , Dr.   , and Dr.   shall be entitled to five (5) working days for continuing education. The partnership shall pay registration fees only at professional meetings attended by the parties hereto.

IN WITNESS WHEREOF, the parties have signed this Agreement the day and year first written above.

_____

_____

_____

_____

_____

Figure 7-4. Partnership agreement (Continued)

PARTNERS' CROSS-PURCHASE AGREEMENT

This Agreement, made this   day of   19   by and between,   D.V.M.,   , D.V.M., D.V.M., and   , D.V.M., partners in the   partnership of Tulsa, Oklahoma, hereinafter called the "Partners".

WHEREAS, the Partners are presently active in the partnership and own the following interest in it:

(a)   ;   %;

(b)   ;   %; and

(c)   ;   %; and

(d)   ;   %; and

Figure 7-5. Partners' cross-purchase agreement   *(Continued)*

WHEREAS, the Partners believe it to be in their best interest and in the best interest of the partnership to provide for continuity and harmony in management of the partnership; and

WHEREAS, it is the Partners' purpose to provide for the purchase by the remaining Partners of a deceased Partner's interest, to provide for the purchase of a withdrawing Partner's interest, and to provide the funds necessary to finance those purchases;

NOW, THEREFORE, it is mutually agreed that:

1. Upon the death of a Partner, the partnership business shall be continued by the surviving Partners. The surviving Partners shall purchase and the personal representative of the deceased Partner shall sell to the surviving Partners the entire interest owned by the deceased Partner at the time of his death at the price and under the terms and conditions hereinafter provided.

2. The value of a deceased Partner's interest in the partnership shall be determined by paragraph 14.1 of the Partnership Agreement. The value so determined is hereby deemed to include each Partner's share of partnership goodwill as a capital item. The Partners shall redetermine the value of each Partner's interest in the manner provided for in the Partnership Agreement.

3. If the surviving Partners should be obligated to pay as the purchase price for the deceased Partner's interest an amount in excess of the proceeds from any life insurance policies referred to in Article V, the surviving Partners may, at their option, pay such excess in full or pay any portion of it as soon as the amount thereof is ascertained as per the terms of paragraph 14.1 of the Partnership Agreement.

4. For purposes of this Agreement, life insurance has been purchased and is owned by each Partner on the life of the other Partners from an insurance company and is recorded on Schedule A attached hereto and made a part hereof. Each Partner shall be the beneficiary of the life insurance he owns on the other Partners. This agreement shall extend to and include any additional policies procured hereunder and they shall be set forth on such Schedule A.

5. In the event a Partner should sell his interest during his lifetime, or in the event of the death of a Partner or the termination of this Agreement, the withdrawing Partner or the remaining Partners, as the case may be, shall have the option, exercisable within ten (10) days, to purchase any life insurance policies on his own life subject to this Agreement. The Partner shall give written notice of his intention to buy such policies to the other Partner or the personal representative thereof. The purchase price for any such policy shall be the terminal reserve and any dividend credits outstanding as of the date of purchase, plus the proportionate part of the premium last paid before the day of the purchase that covered the period extending beyond that date, and minus any indebtedness outstanding. If the option is not exercised within said ten-day (10-day) period, the policy shall no longer be subjected to this Agreement.

6. This Agreement shall terminate upon
    (a) The written agreement of the parties
    (b) The bankruptcy, receivership, or dissolution of the partnership or a Partner or
    (c) The death of all four Partners within a period of thirty (30 days)

    If this Agreement terminates under 6(c) above, its purchase provision shall be inoperative with respect to the interest of each Partner, and the partnership shall be liquidated as required by law.

7. This Agreement may be altered, amended, or modified by written agreement signed by the Partners.

8. This Agreement shall be binding not only on the parties hereto but also upon their heirs, personal representatives, successors, and assigns, and the parties agree for themselves

(Continued)

Figure 7-5. Partners' cross-purchase agreement   (Continued)

and their heirs, personal representatives, successors, and assigns to execute any instruments in writing that may be necessary or proper in carrying out the purpose of this Agreement.

9. When appropriate in this Agreement, words used in the singular shall include the plural and words used in the masculine shall include the feminine. The law of the State of Oklahoma shall govern this Agreement.

IN WITNESS WHEREOF, the parties hereto have executed this Agreement the day and year first written.

_____

_____

_____

_____

WITNESS:

_____

_____

Figure 7-5. Partners' cross-purchase agreement (Continued)

Finding a buyer or seller

Often the buyer and seller find each other without too much search. The seller may be a retiring partner who is selling his share, and the buyer may be an employee being offered a partnership interest. Many times, though, the buyer and seller may need a third party to get them together. They can turn to a practice broker for help.

Practice brokers are much like real estate brokers in that they contact sellers and buyers. Brokers charge a fee for this service, usually a percentage of the sales price.

The broker can help the seller determine a reasonable asking price for the practice and can offer suggestions that may make the practice more attractive to a prospective buyer. The broker will also actively promote the seller's practice and search for buyers.

Remember that a broker represents the seller's interests. A prospective buyer should listen to a broker's sales pitch with caution.

Setting the purchase price

There are two aspects to setting a purchase price. One is an objective appraisal of the practice's assets, liabilities, and goodwill. This is usually performed by someone hired by either the buyer, the seller, or both. The independent appraiser values the business by using objective sources such as tax returns or audited financial statements, physical counts and inventories, and industry information. The appraiser should not be biased toward either the buyer or the seller. One example of this type of appraiser is a certified public accountant experienced in veterinary practice sales.

PURCHASE AGREEMENT

This Agreement is made this   day of   19   , between
                              and   (hereinafter known
as "Sellers") and   (hereinafter known as "Buyer").

The Buyer agrees to buy and the Sellers agree to sell a percent (%) interest in the
partnership of   and   otherwise
known as the   . For purposes of this sale, the
partnership is valued at $. It is the intent of this
Agreement and the parties hereto that the Sellers will sell and the Buyer will buy percent
(%) of the value of the partnership or $. It is not the intent of this Agreement
that Buyer is by this Agreement purchasing any interest in the real estate owned by the practice.

Buyer agrees to buy   percent (%) interest in the partnership of
and   for $. The Buyer agrees to
pay to the Sellers $ for   percent (%) of the partnership
practice secured by a Promissory Note given by the Buyer to the Sellers.

It is the intent of the Sellers to sell Buyer   percent (%) of the records of
                              or   ,   records and   percent (%)
of the   .

For the purposes of valuation of the practice for the sale of a   percent (%) interest
to   , Appendix A is attached hereto and included herein the same as if copied at
length herein, which is a statement of the valuation of the practice.

_____

_____
                                               Sellers

_____
                                               Buyer

Figure 7-6. Purchase agreement

Another aspect of setting a purchase price is the negotiator. Someone needs to get the best price, terms, and conditions for whomever they represent. An attorney could represent either the seller or buyer; a practice broker could be a negotiator for the seller.

Both of these phases are critical to ensure that a practice is sold as quickly as possible and that each party receives fair treatment. Any fees are minimal compared with the cost of a mistake.

Tax planning

Normally the results of tax planning will not change the basic sales agreement. What it may change are the structure, timing, and method of the sale.

Buyers and sellers can have conflicting desires when it comes to tax planning. Therefore, both parties must know all the consequences of the sale. Both the buyer and the seller should hire their own tax advisor and consult him before finalizing the agreement.

Legal services

This is yet another area where each party should have its own counsel. An attorney advocates his client and should not be expected to do anything but maximize his client's position.

The attorney draws up the proper documents and provides advice on how to structure the sale to avoid costly legal problems in the future. So always obtain legal assistance before finalizing any terms or conditions. Selection of an attorney is covered in Chapter 15.

□
Summary

Both buyer and seller should educate themselves before entering into any kind of agreement. The buyer should research the practice and try to evaluate its value. Learn whether there are outstanding liabilities, and examine the tax considerations. Sellers should plan well in advance of the venture, establish an equitable price, and try to sell to someone they know. As the deal is closed, negotiate items to arrive at a compromise, and be sure to include all the necessary documentation. Above all seek professional help. If buyers and sellers follow these guidelines, the sale or purchase of a practice will be much smoother and more trouble free.

□
References

1. McCafferty OE: How to price your practice. Part I. Veterinary Economics July, 1983, pp 38–51
2. McCafferty OE: How to price your practice. Part II. Veterinary Economics August, 1983, pp 56–64
3. McCafferty OE: How to price your practice. Part III. Veterinary Economics August, 1983, pp 68–70

Chapter 8
☐
Welcome to the world of malpractice

Jack R. Dinsmore

In today's era of consumerism, statements of intent to perform a service are generally taken to imply a guarantee of good results. Although professionals in the health fields cannot guarantee the results of surgical, diagnostic, and medical procedures or the use of drugs or biologic agents, legal decisions in recent years increasingly have put veterinarians, like other professionals, at risk of being sued for malpractice. There will always be variables that compound a health problem, confuse the client, and create a potential claim-producing situation. A thorough knowledge of such incidents can help a veterinarian guard against situations that predispose to malpractice claims.

There appears to be a close correlation between the understanding and confidence a client has in a veterinarian, or the lack of this relationship, and the client's decision to file or not to file a malpractice claim. It would be impractical to compile a list of all factors that can lead to misunderstandings. To avoid misunderstandings, however, the veterinarian should always manifest concern for the owner, obtain either oral or written consent, and keep accurate records to document all procedures. Claims related either to procedures or drugs often result from failure to give a full explanation of the treatment and from failure to forewarn owners about potential risks inherent in treatment.

☐
Cause and effect

The definition generally attributed to malpractice by veterinarians is one that has been attached to physicians through many years of litigation. This includes the statement that veterinarians possess and exercise such reasonable skill and diligence as may ordinarily be expected of careful, skillful, and trustworthy persons in the profession. If veterinarians do not possess and exercise these qualities, they are answerable for the results of their lack of skill and care.

Malpractice as a legal concept may be defined as professional misconduct or unreasonable lack of skill or fidelity in the performance of professional or fiduciary duties. It encompasses careless, ignorant, and intentionally improper treatment and conduct.

Professionals are looked upon as having knowledge or skill superior to that of the average layperson and are legally required to use their professional abilities. This does not mean professionals will be judged on the basis of personal ability, but rather against a standard with reference to the profession in general.

The last consideration obviates the application of the *Locality Rule* in determining the standard of care a veterinarian can be held to in comparison with others. The prior application of the Locality Rule has been that veterinarians would be judged by professional standards in their own or similar localities and under the same or similar circumstances. In recent years, the rule has drawn considerable criticism in that it does not take into account the current level of veterinary education, continuing education seminars, publications, and other means of communication within the reach of virtually every member of the profession.

Responding to such criticism, courts in a number of states have restricted or removed the Locality Rule as a defense in malpractice lawsuits. The courts are expected to remain reasonable in that a veterinarian in general practice in a small community or rural area should not be judged by the standards of a university hospital. Similarly, the general practice veterinarian should not be judged by the standard applied to a specialist; however,

all veterinarians will be held responsible to avail themselves of facilities or specialists within some reasonable proximity to their locations. The courts also recognize the obligation of veterinarians to refer patients when equipment or services may not be adequate. At the very least, the owner should be given the opportunity to make decisions for the welfare of the animal.

Recognition of the term *professional negligence* as a replacement for malpractice or negligence has occurred in professional liability lawsuits. This modernization of dissimilar terms has brought a more definitive understanding of the older term *malpractice,* particularly as it applies to veterinarians.

It has been stated that medical malpractice cases fall within one of the following two categories:

1. Cases where an accepted procedure was not followed
2. Cases where the expected good result did not occur

Circumstances that affect veterinary malpractice claims not only encompass liability for negligent practices but extend to negligent animal handling and restraint procedures as well. Included with claims related to the physical control of a patient are custodial claims related to stall or cage injuries, injuries from other animals, parasite control, and disease control.

Specific causes of malpractice claims are many and varied although the following are in the high-risk category:

1. Inept, improper, and erroneous information by veterinarians and employees
2. Lack of proper consent for euthanasia
3. Error in application or dosage of drugs
4. Shipping certification in violation of destination requirements
5. Failure to provide specific service as requested

6. Professional fees not fully explained
7. Follow-up treatment not carried out
8. Injury to a human—either client or bystander
9. Inappropriate remarks regarding prior service
10. Admission of error without evaluating cause from the malpractice standpoint

□
Malpractice—a changing scene

The impact on the veterinary profession of the medical malpractice crisis has been confirmed in recent years by the numbers of claims (claim frequency) and by the costs of defense and judgments (claim severity). The combined effect of these increases is reflected in premium costs to maintain coverage.

Claim frequency

Information regarding the number of claims reported per year in a group of veterinarians insured in a national professional liability insurance program shows a steadily rising number of claims. From 1976 to 1984 the claims reported increased from one claim per 25 veterinarians insured to one claim per 16 veterinarians insured. This increase parallels the claim frequency reported in medicine where one claim per eight physicians is not uncommon in recent years.

Claim severity

It is not as easy to outline increases in severity because claims with high value tend to require long periods of litigation to settle, thus distorting recent years (2 to 5) by understating the paid claims for those years. It is apparent, however, in the last decade that dollars paid including legal expense to settle claims have more than doubled, with claims paid for human injuries totaling 15% of all claims paid.

The increase in malpractice claims during the last decade is not confined to physicians and veterinarians but includes accountants, architects, attorneys, dentists, engineers, psychiatrists, and others. No professional is immune, as is evidenced by the ever-increasing frequency of claims.

Malpractice concept

In reviewing the general concept of veterinary malpractice actions, there are a number of factors that must be considered:

1. An increased public awareness of the use of litigation to recover losses, real or imagined. The American system of justice provides everyone their "day in court," and the backlog on court calendars is proof.
2. An increased awareness by plaintiffs' attorneys of the veterinary profession. This awareness has become more evident as practice economics have improved. As attorney Michael A. Coccia has noted, "We are a nation of laws and a nation of laws is, perforce, a nation of lawyers. Thus, given a specific complaint, and with attorneys ever eager to remedy a grievance, lawsuits in increasing numbers are inevitable."[1] The ease with which a lawsuit may be filed is directly related to the desire of an attorney to accept a lawsuit on a contingency fee basis and a share of the anticipated judgment.
3. An increased level of professionalism expected by animal owners that has been described as a "revolution of rising expectations." Veterinary medicine shares with medicine many of the sophisticated techniques, miracle drugs, and medical knowledge to the extent that the public expects results often beyond any realm of possibility. It is at this level of client communication that veterinarians or em-

ployees can ill afford to leave an impression of guaranteed results.

4. An increase in economic value attached to a loss. The values of individual animals or the values of groups of animals have increased markedly due to inflationary and other market pressures so that in the event of a loss real dollars become a factor of economic recovery to a plaintiff. Many investors are part of a corporate or syndicated venture with large sums of money at risk and in the event of a loss will look to a source to recapture these dollars. This source is often the veterinarian who is defending an allegation with no basis in fact.

Areas of malpractice

To gain a perspective one needs to look at examples of problems involved in litigation.

1. *Money charged* is contested without the results of a procedure or service being considered. A disagreement as to charges may raise the first contention in the mind of the owner. From that point on, all manner of allegations, real or imagined, take place. Add to this a consultation with an attorney knowledgeable in professional liability litigation, and one sees an immediate lawsuit on a contingency basis.

2. *Value of animal* refers to an attempt by an owner or owners to claim value beyond reasonable appraisal for the loss of an animal. This category does not take into account any claim for emotional value but would look only at monetary value as related to chattel or property. The variables encountered include registered or purebred animals, loss of breeding or reproductive value, costs of care and feeding (multiplied by the numbers of animals involved), loss of market value (slaughter vs. sale for breeding), costs of transportation, loss of income due to quarantine, and others ad infinitum. All or any of the aforementioned would require legal services to arbitrate or try

a claim in court to conclusion against a veterinarian if reasonable value cannot be established.

3. Litigation after *admission of responsibility* by veterinarians who in their minds feel they have done something wrong is not always as it seems. Wrong in your mind and wrong insofar as a definition of liability from a legal standpoint may not be the same. For instance, death of an animal may have been accidental, and even though a veterinarian was involved by rendering a professional service, the death may have been beyond the control of the attending veterinarian. Also, drug-related losses, even though apparently directly caused, may have been the result of an individual idiosyncracy rather than negligence of the veterinarian.

On the other hand, an admission of negligence when no attempt was made to treat the animal or an actual abandonment takes place after a mishap leaves little to defend in a court of law.

4. *Bodily or physical injury to a person,* usually a client, is a constant threat in all types of practice. An infinite number of variables affecting risk to a client result from the design of physical facilities, experience of employees, types of services performed, and types of species managed. An innocent bystander, adult or child, can also be involved with the same degree of liability as an animal owner. The responsibility of a veterinarian for a human injury should not be taken lightly because the legal system is directly concerned with pain and suffering, loss of income, and costs of medical and surgical care. All of these are essentially without a ceiling as to damages. The resulting settlement depends totally on the negligence of the veterinarian and the position a judge or jury may take.

The usual position assumed by a plaintiff's attorney is that the veterinarian has been negligent and has failed to exercise the necessary standards for the protection of others. There are remote instances where a position of contributory negligence provided a defense, but this is usually difficult if not impossible to prove.

5. *Personal injury* as opposed to physical injury refers to a veterinarian or other professional who in some manner as defined by law intentionally interferes with another person. These so-called intentional acts include assault and battery, libel and slander, defamation of character, false arrest, and unlawful detention. Personal injury coverage is not always a part of professional liability coverage. Attention should be given to the inclusion of this special coverage because litigation involving any of the aforementioned acts is exceedingly expensive and, if determined by court that damages have occurred, the amount awarded could be in excess of the coverage in the policy.

The involvement of a veterinarian in a manner to induce a personal injury suit is somewhat remote as long as one's deportment remains above reproach. There have, however, been occasions where the best judgment did not prevail and an open commitment was made that brought a threat of suit or an actual court filing.

Another circumstance that causes veterinarians to be involved in personal injury lawsuits occurs as a result of serving in a professional capacity on boards or committees that bring disciplinary action against veterinarians. Such involvements can result in complicated and expensive lawsuits that, in considering the good intentions of dedicated veterinarians, are not warranted.

6. *Collection suits* bring countersuits for malpractice or negligence as surely as night follows day. For whatever reason an owner did not pay for the service rendered, after the usual attempts to enforce payment, the filing of a collection suit more times than not ensures the veterinarian of a countersuit for malpractice. After all, what better way to forestall, embarrass, and possibly even win a settlement for alleged or real malpractice or negligence than a countersuit for malpractice?

The rightful assessment would be that the service was rendered within all normal standards and limits. No guarantee of results accompanies medical care unless someone inadvertently makes such a promise. The veterinarian, having performed a professional service, has the right to request payment.

The amount of money involved in the nonpayment may vary from as little as an office and vaccine charge to as much as a full year of farm or ranch service charges. Once the veterinarian assumes a serious position relative to the attempt at collection, an attorney for the client will enter the picture. When this occurs, a serious evaluation of the situation should be undertaken. Attorneys trade information in sufficient depth to determine a real threat or a running bluff. The situation calls for a cold, unemotional evaluation to determine whether a lawsuit is "worth a day in court." Professor William O. Morris, Law School of Virginia, states a flat "No."[2] He refers specifically to the dental profession where a dentist can ill afford to close a one-person office to testify in court. Any results from that court hearing would be a losing proposition.

Let it be understood, the veterinarian has the right to collect. The practitioner can file a lawsuit on advice of counsel and, if there is no countersuit, determine whether winning is worth the effort. In the event a countersuit for malpractice or negligence is filed, professional liability coverage will defend and pay costs and judgments. The veterinarian will need to assess the time involvement. A customary conclusion to most suits is a compromise during the court procedure. The plaintiff drops the malpractice charges, and the veterianian drops the collection suit. Who wins? Only the attorneys! The veterinarian, client, and the insurance company carrying the policy all lose. The legal expenses for this type of claim cover a wide spectrum from a few hundred dollars to several thousand dollars, with only the attorneys winning. If one is concerned with the cost of insurance coverage, bear in mind, there are no "free lunches." All costs, and specifically legal costs, are charged against the case. Someone must pay for these expenses.

Malpractice policy coverage

To explain malpractice coverages further, there are several other premises of professional liability insurance that are not always understood. The following are usually a part of the insuring agreement of the policy:

1. The coverage agrees to pay on behalf of the insured such costs of damages for malpractice, error, or mistake as may occur in rendering or failure to render professional services.
2. The coverage will defend and pay damages even if groundless or false, but the company can make such investigations as necessary and, with the consent of the insured, settle a claim or suit.
3. The coverage does not apply to illegal acts but does cover acts of employees unless such acts were committed jointly.
4. The coverage does not apply to advertising, broadcasting, or telecasting activities.
5. The coverage does spell out certain conditions naming limits of liability, notice of claim or suit, and other matters including one that states the insured shall assist and cooperate with the company and attend hearings and trials, secure and give evidence, obtain witnesses, and aid in the conduct of the suit.

There have been numerous instances where item 5 was not considered important by the insured veterinarian. This lack of cooperation prevents the development of an adequate de-

fense and can result in an expensive compromise to escape an adverse lawsuit.

☐
Limiting malpractice claims

The following five areas suggest ways to limit the number of malpractice claims against a veterinarian or veterinary practice.

1. The question of veterinarians practicing quality medicine vs. defensive medicine is one that is more academic than realistic. It is true that defensive medicine may be a method to cover an indefinite approach to solving a clinical problem; however, the economic constraints governing most practices reduce the opportunity to load a diagnostic problem with a series of unwanted and unnecessary procedures. The object, then, is to provide a quality of medicine with full disclosure to a client in keeping with the demands of the case.

2. Regardless of the philosophy of the practice and the veterinarian, an adequate medical record system is a necessity to protect against the allegation of an owner regarding procedures and results of those procedures. These allegations would be impossible to refute in the event of a law suit without complete medical records to substantiate the procedure. State examining boards, by virtue of their responsibilities to protect the consumer, have incorporated statutes governing the contents, quality, and retention of medical records. The question, then, of the existence of medical records is not only for defense of malpractice but is also mandated by statute. Veterinarians should be aware that owners and attorneys representing owners are well aware of these requirements and present demands for all existing records as a part of the preparation of a lawsuit. Complete and accurate records should contain not only all procedures but also the results and evaluation of those procedures. Above all, do not erase, mark over, or delete records in any manner because an opposing attorney will

destroy a defense by showing a lack of credibility.

3. Consent forms that are always a part of human medical and surgical procedures are not in common use in veterinary medicine. The many and varied excuses for their nonexistence are not plausible in the face of a mistaken surgical procedure authorized or not understood by an owner. Consent forms that are lengthy and complicated with a profusion of legal terms not only confuse an owner but will also negate their use in the practice. The forms should be relatively easy to read and understand. It should be noted that consent forms are not an escape from a malpractice lawsuit but only an added measure of defense. Gross negligence on the part of the hospital or veterinarian essentially destroys the protective value of "informed consent."

4. Dealing responsibly with an animal's owner is a major factor in limiting malpractice claims. Thus, the behavior and attitudes of employees can be a great threat to a practice. All aspects of hospital management, telephone courtesy, receptionist response, involvement of veterinary technicians, nursing care, and other such activities, are factors that can function as "trigger" mechanisms, raising an owner's doubts and concerns about the level of care provided. Above all employees must maintain consideration and compassion for the patient and the owner under all circumstances. A staff member's (or veterinarian's) unfeeling or callous attitude combined with an unfortunate result will establish grounds for a lawsuit in the mind of the owner. Detailed information concerning client management can be found in Chapter 2.

5. Veterinary technicians have become an integral part of well-managed veterinary practices. The actions of a veterinary technician are the legal responsibility of the veterinarian on the basis of an employer–employee liability relationship. Technicians should not hold themselves out as veterinarians, should not diagnose or alter treatments, and should not sign documents or otherwise perform duties that are the responsibility of a licensed veterinarian.

Malpractice actions against veterinarians that include allegations of negligence on the part of a technician will be defended under the insurance coverage for the veterinarian. Proof of a technician performing services that are legally the responsibility of a veterinarian reduces the defense of a malpractice suit significantly. Chapter 12 outlines the duties and responsibilities of the veterinary technician.

Anatomy of a lawsuit

As has been stated many times, one does not have to be guilty to be charged. It is only necessary to be accused to be welcomed into the court system that guarantees every person their day in court. The adversarial contest guarantees equal rights in a court of law to both plaintiff and defendant and is the basis of the legal proceeding in a malpractice lawsuit. To continue one step further, it is also the court's concern for "due process of law" that dictates the total involvement of a defendant once a court summons is served. Relief comes only from the lawsuit being dropped, from acquittal, or from a judgment against the defendant.

Members of nearly every profession are faced with increasing numbers of malpractice lawsuits. No professional is immune, and those who ignore the possibility of being called to defend their practices are, at best, naive.

One of the principle explanations for the increase in veterinary malpractice actions relates to the public's greater willingness to take its problems to court. More specifically, the doctrine of rising expectations based on the knowledge and understanding of the general public as applied to their own medical services constitutes an increasing demand for results without failures in veterinary medical service.

Even though accused of professional misconduct or lack of skill in performance of professional duties, one should not leap to the conclusion that the threat of a claim by an owner or a letter from an attorney threatening dire consequences will lead directly into a court room. There are many steps and several avenues to be considered before a court appearance will take place. It might be well to review the procedures that will be used.

First, there is of necessity the act of notification of a claim by the veterinarian (i.e., the insured) to the insurance company. The policy that is issued to the veterinarian will state in the insuring agreement that written notice shall be given to the company or its authorized agent as soon as practical. Further, if claim is made or suit is brought against the insured, all demands, notices, summons, or other processes shall be forwarded immediately. Admittedly, this does not set a fixed time for notification but makes clear that upon becoming aware of any alleged injury covered in the policy, written notice shall be sent to the insurance company. Timely notice is an important factor for the company to consider in providing an adequate defense to protect the veterinarian as well as its own position. Failure to notify causes problems for the defense including but not limited to the following:

1. Any span of time causes memories to fail and details to fade.
2. Records are lost or not completed.
3. Witnesses move or disappear.
4.. As has happened on occasion, notification will arrive just before a court date, thereby preventing any preparation and leading to a default judgment.
5. Lack of notification on a timely basis under extreme circumstances could lead to a denial of coverage.

Second, investigation by trained personnel from the insurance company takes place as soon as possible after notification to record the facts as reported by the insured. You can be assured these investigators are well trained and experienced in reporting facts as presented and in being objective in the interpretation of those facts.

Investigators' reports are not only in written form but may also include tapes, fully transcribed, of interviews with veterinarians, office personnel, and other staff. Full cooperation of veterinarians and staff who may be involved is the key to the success of this part of the operation.

Third, on completion of the investigator's report, the findings, including a summary, are forwarded to the claims adjustor for evaluation. To ensure uniformity and consistency in claims management, evaluation usually occurs in a central office once the information is complete.

Several steps take place to administer the file at this time.

1. A dollar reserve is established to protect the claim.
2. A letter to the plaintiff or plaintiff's attorney acknowledges the report and the status of the inquiry to date.

The investigative report may be positive enough at this time to show that the veterinarian is not at fault. If this is the decision, the letter takes the form of a denial. If the claim is not clear, then usually further investigation is needed. In the event that a summons has been served or an answer to substantiate a legal opinion is necessary, an attorney is appointed, and the required answer to the summons is prepared.

These procedures are concluded in as reasonable an amount of time as is possible on behalf of the veterinarian at the expense of the company to protect the insured and establish a claim file for defense. Further, the insuring agreement states that the company will defend any suit against the insured that alleges injury and seeks damages on account thereof, even if the suit is groundless, false, or fraudulent, but the company may make an investigation and negotiation and, with written consent of the insured, a settlement of any claim or suit as the company deems expedient. The requirement for written consent from the insured protects the veterinarian from a settlement without knowledge of the decision to make a settlement. A veterinarian can assist this relationship by reviewing claims and advising the claims adjustor on difficult decisions.

With the establishment of the respective positions of the principles in a malpractice claim, we arrive at the question: pay or defend?

H. W. Hannah, professor of law at the University of Illinois, observes that any settlement, however small, though there is no malpractice, creates the impression that the veterinarian did something wrong.[3] It is his opinion that despite cost, loss of time, and some risk of defeat, cases should be defended when there is clearly no negligence on the part of the veterinarian.

The question, then, becomes how to arrive at a decision of "no negligence" on the part of the veterinarian. First, the claim form reports the incident to the insurance company. The same claim form states that the veterinarian agrees or does not agree to a settlement. Second, the report of the insurance company investigator and the accompanying summary provides background information. Finally, with the appointment of an attorney by the company to defend a possible court case, there is the advantage of a pretrial hearing upon which to base an opinion.

When courts are crowded, many lawyers and judges try to clarify issues and thus shorten the trial through pretrial hearings. There are advantages to both sides. Frequently, pretrial proceedings show the lawyers that the case has no merit or there is no defense. The result is an agreed settlement, or the judge and attorneys will agree on a dismissal.

After the pretrial hearings, if the issues are not resolved, then a court date is set. As an example, let us assume there has been no malpractice and no negligence by the veterinarian, the associates, or the employees of the practice. Then, to ensure a favorable verdict, every effort is expended to educate the judge and the jury, if one is present, regarding the problems of practicing veterinary medicine.

All the ground rules, all the bases for legal opinions are founded in medical malpractice. To win lawsuits where there is little case law to reference veterinary malpractice, an all-out effort has to be made to educate those who hear the trial. The ground rules in veterinary practice may differ from those in medical practice. Therefore, there is a need to educate both judge and jury in presenting trial evidence. Attorneys play the game of court room evaluation of the opposition every day, and any slight chance that the opposition's effort has fallen short is capitalized upon immediately.

Expert witnesses from many disciplines are necessary to aid in the defense of difficult court cases, thereby resulting in a battle of the experts — often with unpredictable outcomes. Expert testimony will ordinarily be required by the plaintiff to prove that the treatment provided by the defendant veterinarian was negligent.

Good attorneys are great judges of the impact of a witness. This was most significant in a recent acquittal of a veterinarian being sued for the loss of a valuable thoroughbred after a drug reaction. The veterinarian for the defense was the most convincing witness. This was a jury trial, and credibility was a major factor in dismissal.

It is significant to note that most claims related to a professional service, such as those involving a medical or a surgical procedure, are defensible on the basis that acceptable procedures have been followed. There are some situations, however, that speak for themselves—for example, surgery performed in error or on the wrong patient. There is little to discuss when one of these situations arises. The same is true of the classic case of a "surgical sponge in the abdomen." No defense.

There is another group of claims of an accidental nature where the premise of "no negligence" is difficult to argue and impossible to defend. Examples are fatal injuries to a hospitalized dog by other hospitalized dogs, head injuries or fractures from falling, cage accidents, and other similar situations. These claims are usually paid.

The insuring agreement states that the insured shall cooperate with the company and shall assist in securing evidence and obtaining witnesses and in the conduct of suits. Unfortunately, lack of cooperation does occur, not often, but if it happens, a lawsuit will be lost.

Insurance companies are concerned about a segment of potentially expensive claims that follow human injury, a hardship physically and mentally to the person injured. These cases are difficult to defend and can result in large settlements in or out of court.

It has been said that using an attorney for small problems is like watering plants. It only makes them grow. The need for attorneys to defend claims is the reason for increased legal costs, and it is the cost of defense that protects the veterinary profession. To pay or defend is always a difficult decision. The aforementioned guidelines do achieve a balance between good judgment and economic and professional considerations.

☐
Professional liability insurance: what it is and what it is not

The following statement by Dr. Vyrle Stauffer is a fitting conclusion to this chapter:

Professional liability insurance is not meant to be used as a public relations vehicle by which a veterinarian purchases the continued good will of a client by having the insurer pay for damages which are not due to the veterinarian's negligence. There have been instances where sympathetic veterinarians personally have paid a client for losses of animals and then requested reimbursement from the insurance company. This should never be done. The insurance policy clearly states that the insured shall not, except at this own cost, make any payment, assume any obligation, or incur any expense. To do so, in effect, negates the insurance policy. Payment of a claim is an admission of negligence on the doctor's part, and should be authorized only when the claim is meritorious as to both cause and amount of damages. Payment of nuisance claims for no other reason than to be rid of them is an unwise policy. It is probably one of the main reasons why professional liability insurance has become so expensive for other health-related professions.[4]

☐
References

1. Coccia MA: Personal Communication. Chicago, IL, Baker and McKenzie, 1976
2. Morris WO: Personal Communication. Charlottesville, VA, University of Virginia, 1974
3. Hannah HW: Personal Communication. Champaign, IL, University of Illinois, 1982
4. Stauffer V: Insurance note. J Am Vet Med Assoc 180, No 11:1291, 1982

Chapter 9
☐
Starting a practice

Robert E. Lewis

It has never been easy to start a practice; however recent changes in the labor force and the relationship of veterinary medicine to the various communities have made it even more difficult. During the golden era of veterinary medicine, which has been described as the 1950s and 1960s, veterinary practices could be started almost anywhere in the United States with little effort and be almost guaranteed to succeed. In today's delivery of veterinary medicine the opportunities are still quite diverse; however, there is the realization that practices are becoming closer to each other and today tend to be in competition for the same client base.

Anyone considering starting a practice must be willing to devote considerable time and effort to the enterprise. This time and effort demand more than just the delivery of quality veterinary medicine. This extra time often necessitates a change in the life-style of individuals starting practices. With the different allocation of time, individuals must temporarily alter their efforts toward some of their own goals, particularly those related to family and leisure activities. This will provide sufficient time for the management and start-up efforts required in a new practice.

Monetary reward is a big consideration when starting a new practice. The idea is that a greater compensation can be generated for the starter and owner of a new practice. One of the principles not fully understood and certainly not well used in the veterinary profession is maximization of capital investment. This principle demands that capital investment must be used to its greatest extent to give an excellent return on investment to the investor. In veterinary medicine, with many solo practitioners, maximization of capital is poorly used. If a new practice can be started, one may want to consider the goal of multiple veterinarians working within the practice to make maximization of capital possible and convert the practice into a profitable business.

Individuals starting a new practice will find themselves with many frustrations brought about by the management challenges of operating a small business. Some individuals have the background and training to be able to provide top management skills. These skills and knowledge are not usually taught as part of the veterinary curriculum. Those individuals with a family background of a small business operation are going to be much better prepared than those individuals raised in a family unit where the family primarily lived on a set salary each month. Most veterinary students are more interested in learning about medicine and surgery; therefore, little time and effort are given to practice management that could be learned in the teaching hospital. The principles of operating a teaching hospital often do not seem to apply to a private practice. The major difference is that personal financial reward is one of the driving forces of maintaining a profitable private business.

This discussion will provide an outline for anyone who has the personal resources in time and effort as well as accessibility to the financial investment necessary to develop goals for starting a practice.

□
Who should start a practice

There are three classifications of veterinarians who may consider starting a practice. The first type of individual is the new graduate who has limited experience other than short-term employment during veterinary school. Such individuals are often trying to develop a job in an area they have chosen to locate but cannot find employment as an associate veterinarian.

The second type of individual is an associate veterinarian of an existing practice who has experience from 1 to multiple years, working in a practice as well as observing and possibly participating in the management of the business. These individuals may be doing the same thing as the new graduate but more often cannot find a suitable practice in which they can be allowed to either purchase entirely or as a part-owner.

The third type of individual who may consider starting a practice is a current owner of an existing practice. These veterinarians may wish to add an additional practice to expand their current business or start a new practice that eventually could be sold to an associate or another veterinarian. Such individuals may be looking only to protect their territory (client base) from someone starting a practice or may be interested in increasing their net worth by starting a new business with investment capital.

The disadvantages to the new veterinarian starting a practice upon graduation are that unless the location is in the individual's hometown, there may be a lack of understanding of community, traffic flows, and ability to design, finance, and manage a new practice. These deficiencies can be overcome through obtaining training, showing diligence to details, and seeking assistance of other individuals in developing the new practice.

Associate veterinarians, if starting a practice in the same community in which they have previously practiced, may face the problem of a covenant not to compete and the ill will of their previous employer. The associate has had time to study the community, make decisions on a practice site, and study the management techniques and philosophy of the current employer.

The individual who is in the best position to start a new practice already owns at least one practice. This individual has not only had experience but usually has had a longer time period to study the community and determine where the growth potential will be located. This individual may also be well recognized within the community and be able to purchase land, obtain zoning, and obtain a better bid in the construction process than someone who is not familiar with the community. Another advantage for current owners is their existing business; they may be in a better position to either already have financing available or to be able to secure financing for development of the practice. Current owners have cash flow to support the growth of a new practice.

When to start a practice

When planning a new practice, a comparison should be made between starting a new practice or purchasing an existing practice. There are advantages to each of these endeavors, and each needs to be weighed very carefully.

The advantages of buying a practice are (1) an immediate cash flow, (2) current clients who will continue their animals' medical service at the current location, and (3) somewhat less time commitment because the facilities, equipment purchases, and general management have already been established. The disadvantages of buying a practice are (1) acceptance of the current practice philosophy and general operation of the practice, (2) limitations on equipment and facilities, (3) acceptance of current personnel, and (4) monthly payments that may restrict upgrading the quality of service as rapidly as desired.

The new graduate starting a practice will devote a large amount of time to (1) doing the planning, (2) overseeing construction, (3) developing management procedures, and (4) establishing a client base. The time required will affect the life-style of the individual and may not be compatible with financial rewards early in the development of a new practice. The veterinarian starting a practice may find it

difficult to even draw a salary for at least 6 months after opening the practice. This may be a burden that many veterinarians cannot handle without extra financial planning and support.

Associate veterinarians who start new practices oftentimes have an urge to "be their own boss." The associates feel owning the practice gives job security that can never be accomplished as a long-term employee. Another advantage to ownership is related to financial planning and growth of net worth. Growth of net worth is more difficult to accomplish as an employee.

Many practices are started by associate veterinarians as well as new veterinarians because they could not negotiate partial purchase or ownership within an existing practice. The reason partial purchases or partnerships cannot be formed is usually because fair compensation to the original owner as well as the new partial owner cannot be determined.

Where to start a new practice

Several considerations should be made in determining where the new practice will be located. The first consideration should be geography. Several factors affect the geographic decision-making process. The first step is to determine in which region of the country to establish the practice. Second, determine the type of community. Once these requisites are determined, then the specific community within the region may be selected. After the community is determined, the absolute location of the practice must be evaluated and selected.

Secondary considerations of where the practice will be located often revolve around the climatic conditions. The owner must decide the importance of everyday climatic conditions versus those desired for leisure and recreation. For example, if the owner wishes to be in an area where snow skiing is readily available on a weekly basis, he must be willing to accept the influence of that type of weather on the business and facility design.

Many times location is influenced by spousal desires and goals. There is often difficulty in trying to satisfy the job opportunities for two spouses with different employment needs. The spousal needs have to be taken into account to arrive at a common region, community, and specific location that will accomplish the goals of each spouse.

The species of animals served by the veterinary practice will determine to a great extent the location. If a 100% small-animal practice is to be initiated, a sufficient population and client base is required. If the practice is to be 100% equine, the veterinary practice must be located within a sufficient equine population. The more urban the community, the more likely the practice will be small animal with perhaps some equine. The more rural the community selected, the more likely the practice will be mixed with both large and small animals.

The client base necessary to support a practice must be examined. This client base is determined by evaluation of the population, the households, the economic level of those households, and the ownership of animals. Some of these data can be obtained through the local chamber of commerce. The farm animal data can be obtained through U.S. Department of Agriculture reports. There must be sufficient clients and animals to provide the financial base for the practice. This financial base must be able to provide the owner-veterinarian with a suitable compensation to allow the chosen life-style. Table 9-1 shows an estimate of the small animal potential within a given population. It must be realized that all calculations used in this determination are estimates, and to provide accurate data, these numbers and types of households must be determined for the community in which the practice is to be established.

Table 9-1
Estimate of animal potential

Total Population	19,200
2.0 People per Household	
Total Community Households	9,600
50% Households Own Pets	
Total Pet-Owning Households	4,800
50% Seek Veterinary Care	
Total Pet-Owning Households	2,400
Receiving Veterinary Care	
1.25 Animals per Household	
Total Animals Receiving Veterinary Care	3,000
1.50 Visits per Animal	
Total Animal Visits per Year	4,500

As an example of how the values will vary, if the community is primarily single-family residential, then the number of people per household will be higher due to the number of children in each family unit. If the community is primarily made up of apartments, there may be more single-member family households, and the number of people per household will decrease. Relative to the number of households owning pets, the more families with children and the more single-family housing, the higher the ownership of pets will be. The ownership of pets will tend to be lower in condominiums and apartment dwellings due to restrictive clauses within the housing community.

□
What type of practice to start

Several considerations concerning practice type must be taken into account. For example, it is usually easier and requires less outlay of capital to start a small outpatient clinic than a practice providing full medical services. The primary difference between these two is the lower investment necessary for outpatient service versus the higher cost of both facilities and equipment if complete medical care is to be provided.

Another decision is whether the practice will provide primarily medical and surgical care or complete medical and ancillary animal services. The latter concept would require additional areas for boarding, grooming, and merchandising and other ancillary animal care services in addition to the primary medical and surgical management of the animals. The purchaser will also have to decide whether the facility is going to be a freestanding building with the opportunity to expand as needed or whether the service will be provided in a shopping center complex where space may become a premium. Chapter 4 discusses in detail the factors concerning the practice site.

□
Outline of how to start a veterinary practice

Several general considerations must be made in developing the plan for starting a new veterinary practice. Each of these will be dealt with specifically relative to the area of the hospital involved. General considerations of each topic will be presented before the details of planning.

Before anything else is undertaken, the goals of the practice need to be specifically outlined and written down. A mission statement should be written that will represent the philosophy of the practice. The objectives need to be specific in relation to the veterinarians, the support staff, the clients, and the animals. The goals as to the number of personnel needed, training of personnel, practice business policies, list of services, philosophy of delivering these services, and financial base necessary to make the business a profitable operation need to be written.

The facilities have to be designed so that the physical plan will be an efficient functional unit. This function must take into account all the specific goals that are already written. The number of people to be involved in the practice must be estimated. The number of people in the building may have the following ratio:

two to four support staff per veterinarian and 15 to 20 clients with animals per day per veterinarian. These ratios can help determine the square foot requirements for the various areas of the hospital. For increased efficiency, various activities can be grouped into one room versus having separate rooms for each activity. As an example, the clinical laboratory and pharmacy may be combined, or the radiology and patient/preparation areas could be together.

The shape of the room has an effect on the efficiency of the use of floor space. Often with square rooms, space is poorly used in the center of the room. If more wall space is needed, long narrower rooms provide greater usable space per square foot.

In addition to having an architect complete the design to assist in making a functional unit, there are other regulations that must be followed. Many states have facility design codes for veterinary hospitals. Both federal and state regulations control the use of x-ray equipment and radiation safety. Specific requirements as to the amount of shielding necessary as well as the design of the rooms to minimize personnel exposure are requirements that must be reviewed. Regulations concerning waste disposal from medical facilities are being planned. Another hazard that is currently being examined and that must be evaluated is the hazard of anesthetic waste gases. The anesthetic gases must be controlled and exhausted from the building in some acceptable manner. Fire regulations may also influence the design of the building, including the number of exits and the way the doors must function within the building. These are areas where an architect can be of assistance in guiding the planning of the facility.

Another general consideration is balancing the cost of construction against the cost of cleaning and maintenance over an extended period of time. Some floors and wall surfaces that are low maintenance and easy to clean will be much more expensive in the initial construction. There will be trade-offs of these types in designing the facility.

The building design should give consideration to making additions for expansion or later remodeling. Therefore, when designing the original layout of the building, consideration must be given to how easy it will be at a future date to add on space that will be tied in functionally to the current structure and make it easy for expansion of the business. This may require that very few internal walls in the structure be weight bearing and that the plumbing be designed so that floors will not have to be torn up at a later date to rearrange the drainage.

The construction of walls and doors is important not only to segregate various functions but to provide sound and odor control within the building. Most sound is controlled by the density of construction material, so the greater the density of the walls and doors, the less the sound transmission.

The layout of the building on the piece of land takes special ingenuity and preplanning to make for convenient parking and accessibility of clients and animals into the facility. If possible, parking for hospital staff needs to be separated from client parking. Consideration should be given to the security of escaping animals being brought from the client's car or truck into the facility. Fencing and distancing from high-traffic roads help with this problem.

Decisions must also be made regarding whether equipment will be owned by the practice or whether equipment will be leased. This becomes a financial decision in that leasing can often provide a greater amount of equipment initially with less capital outlay. Leasing or purchasing needs to be considered not only for capital outlay but also for the tax advantages; a period of years must be taken into account.

Should all equipment be purchased new, or can some used equipment be found to serve the needs? In many cases, used equipment will work well and may be obtained at a lower cost. However, used equipment has a greater risk of failure after it has been moved and may not function as a new piece of equipment. Some equipment has undergone considerable technological change during the last few years so that the used version of this equipment may not be as adequate as a new piece in providing quality service.

The specific items of equipment purchased during the original establishment of the practice relate to both a judgment of the quality and quantity of service to be provided. If two examination rooms are designed for the facility, initially only one examination room may be equipped until adequate cash flow allows the second room to be equipped. Other items that may be limited are specialized diagnostic and treatment equipment. These may not have sufficient justification for purchase early in the establishment of the practice. A new practice may find that in the beginning it must refer some cases when equipment is limited. The referrals may then decrease as additional equipment and quality of service within the practice can be increased.

The following outline for planning a new hospital will hopefully align one's thought process in an organized manner. The outline provides information about various work/service areas of a practice as follows: (1) a list of objectives, (2) facilities recommendations, and (3) a list of equipment needs. The outline is oriented more toward a small-animal practice, but the same concepts will apply to starting a large-animal practice.

The list of objectives give a feeling for what has to happen in the area for the practice to provide service to clients and their animals. The specifics of how each objective is accomplished will vary considerably depending upon the training, personality, experience, and resources of the individual starting the practice. They will also be influenced by the clients' animal care education, relationship with their animals, and financial and accepted standards of the community.

In facility requirements, specific space needs are not outlined because this will vary with each practice. Relationships to other areas, maintenance, air handling, people and animal flow, as well as some general considerations for design are given.

The equipment needs are not considered to be mandatory but are found in most practices. A greater number of practices are installing central communications central anesthetic gas system and central wet-dry vacuum system. This type of equipment adds convenience to the practice at a minimal investment.

I. Client Reception Area
   A. Objectives
      1. Easy view and accessibility to the receptionist
      2. Comfortable seating
      3. Pleasant and open environment
      4. Client education
      5. Separation of animals
      6. Point-of-sale displays
   B. Facilities Recommendations
      1. Entrance from client parking area should be easy.
      2. Entrance should directly view business reception area.
      3. Seating arrangement or walls should provide some client and animal separation.
      4. Anteroom entrance should prevent animal escape and permit climate control.
      5. There should be space for seating a number of people. It may be calculated by multiplying the number of examination rooms × 1.5 (number of clients with each animal × 3:, one client late, one on time, one early). For example, with two exam rooms, one should have nine seats.
      6. There should be separate doors for exiting.
      7. Wall space should be provided for passive client education materials and product displays.
      8. Access to restrooms is required.
   C. Equipment Needs
      1. Comfortable seating—ease of cleaning is a major consideration.
      2. Seating may be wall hung, which prevents rearrangement and aids floor cleaning
      3. Platform scale for weighing animals is needed.
      4. Display shelves/cases for products and client education materials are necessary.

II. Business Reception Office
   A. Objectives
      1. Telephone communication with the client
      2. Personal greeting of the client.
      3. Initiation and storage of medical records
      4. Cashiering
      5. Management of a recall/reminder system
   B. Facilities Recommendations
      1. Primary view of entrance and client reception area seating
      2. Counter for greeting clients and admitting animals
      3. Counter for cashiering, near exit door
      4. Desk/work area for writing
      5. Work area for computers/cash registers/peg boards
      6. Secure cash drawer
      7. Medical record files
      8. Accounts receivable files
   C. Equipment Needs
      1. Pegboard/cash register/computer
      2. Typewriter

3. Telephone(s)
4. Intercom system
5. Chairs/stools
6. Medical record file cabinet
7. Credit card imprinter or credit card sales terminal
8. Cash drawer

III. Examination Rooms
  A. Objectives
    1. Comfortable environment for client and animal
    2. Animal examination and sample collection
    3. Client education
    4. Treatment of animals
  B. Facilities Recommendations
    1. Square footage table to allow two staff members, 2 clients, animal
    2. Two doors — one to client reception area, one to lab-pharmacy
    3. Sink, optional
    4. Writing surface
    5. Storage for equipment/supplies
    6. Individual room exhaust system
  C. Equipment Needs
    1. Examination table, counter
    2. Oto-, ophthalmaloscope
    3. Stethoscope
    4. Magnifying loop
    5. Examination lights
    6. Client education devices, film/TV
    7. Double-radiographic viewer

IV. Pharmacy
  A. Objectives
    1. Storage of medication and vaccines
    2. Repackaging of medications for dispensing
    3. Use of medications for in-hospital treatments
    4. System of maintaining supplies
  B. Facilities Recommendations
    1. Easy access to examination rooms

2. Easy access to treatment room
3. Counters and storage
  C. Equipment Needs
    1. Typewriter for labels (computer)
    2. Refrigeration

V. Laboratory
  A. Objectives
    1. Process samples for diagnosis
    2. Prepare samples for sending to outside labs
  B. Facilities Recommendations
    1. Proximity to examination rooms, treatment/work area
    2. Counters and storage
    3. Sink
    4. Exhaust system over sink
    5. Extra power outlets
    6. Limited traffic area
  C. Equipment Needs
    1. Microscope
    2. Tube centrifuge
    3. Microhematocrit
    4. Refractometer
    5. Hemocytometer/differential counters
    6. Auto cell counter (optional)
    7. Automatic chemistry unit (optional)
    8. Microbiological incubator (optional)

VI. Treatment/Work Area
  A. Objectives
    1. Treatment of animals
    2. Preparation of animals for and performing special examinations
    3. Preparation of animals for surgery
    4. Observation of animals recovering from anesthesia
    5. Observation of acute care patients
    6. Dentistry
    7. Medical baths and dips
  B. Facilities Recommendations

1. Proximity to animal holding
2. Proximity to pharmacy, laboratory, surgery
3. Sinks, counters, storage
4. Anesthetic gases, central or individual tanks
5. Tub for baths and dips

C. Equipment Needs
1. Work tables—one with perforated top
2. Cages for intensive care unit/anesthesia recovery
3. Counters/storage
4. Clippers
5. Dental equipment
6. Endoscopic equipment (optional)
7. Intravenous (IV) stands/ceiling hooks
8. Anesthetic machine
9. ECG/cardiopet
10. Cage dryers

VII. Radiology
A. Objectives
1. Performing radiographic examinations
2. Processing radiographs
3. Viewing radiographs
4. Storing and retrieving radiographs

B. Facilities Recommendations
1. Square footage for x-ray machine, control area, and film storage
2. Ease of access to surgery
3. Light-proof developing area
4. Radiation barrier walls (floors if basement or machine on second floor)
5. Adequate isolation from high-traffic people areas
6. Capability of dimming lights for collimator light visualization

C. Equipment Needs
1. X-ray machine
2. Processing equipment, hand tanks, automatic processor
3. Lead aprons
4. Lead gloves
5. Apron/glove storage devices
6. Identification systems/photoprinter
7. Safelights
8. Hangers and racks if hand processing
9. Unexposed film storage
10. Cassettes
11. Positioning devices
12. Measuring calipers
13. Viewers

VIII. Surgery
A. Objectives
1. Performing various surgical procedures
2. Maintaining correct environment
3. Controlling health hazards to personnel
4. Monitoring animals during anesthesia

B. Facilities Recommendations
1. Easily cleaned surfaces
2. No sinks or counters
3. Positive-pressure air flow
4. Single door entrance
5. Wall storage for supplies (may be through wall)
6. Windows to treatment/work area
7. Anesthetic gases, central or tanks
8. Emergency lighting
9. Cabinets/storage, sinks for:
   Cleaning Area (not in surgery room)
   Sterilization area (not in surgery room)
   Surgeon scrub area (not in surgery room)
   Gowning/gloving area
10. Electric outlets $4\frac{1}{2}$ feet from floor

C. Equipment Needs
1. Hydraulic tilt surgery table ("V" optional)
2. Ceiling-mounted surgery lights
3. Instrument stands
4. IV stands/ceiling hooks
5. Surgical suction
6. General packs
7. Special packs (orthopaedic, eye, thoracic) optional
8. Clock with a second hand
9. Monitoring equipment
10. Ultrasonic cleaner
11. Packing, sealing equipment
12. Steam autoclave
13. Gas autoclave (optional)
14. Electrocautery (optional)

IX. Animal Handling Area
A. Objectives
1. Housing animals under medical and surgical care
2. Feeding of animals
3. Providing for exercise and rehabilitation of animals
B. Facilities Recommendations
1. Separate cage vs. run (exercise area)
2. Hose-down cleaning in runs (high pressure)
3. Multiple wards
4. Isolation area (preferably outside door only)
5. Floor drains
6. Negative air pressure
7. Feed/prep area
8. Heavy-duty exhaust
C. Equipment Needs
1. Cages of various size
2. Cage racks for some cages
3. Cleaning equipment

X. Ancillary Areas
A. Objectives
1. Area for boarding
2. Area for grooming
3. Offices for veterinarians/staff
4. Storage of animals for disposal
5. Lounge
6. Restroom (may separate client/staff)
7. General Storage

To determine the supplies necessary to start a practice, each work/service area must be considered. A list for each area would need to be made. In each area categories of supplies will help make the list more complete; that is, in the pharmacy, there should be a separate list for (1) injectable products, (2) oral products, (3) eye medications, (4) ear medications, (5) heartworm medications, (6) cardiovascular medications, (7) anesthetics, and so forth. In the business office, there should be lists for (1) printed materials, (2) client education materials, (3) computer supplies, (4) general office supplies such as pens, pencils, note pads, message pads, staples, clips, rubber bands, and so forth.

Particularly with pharmaceutical and medical supplies, it is easy to overpurchase both in the sense of too many duplications of similar products as well as in the quantity of products. With modern delivery systems, most supplies can be obtained in 24 to 48 hours, so do not invest more capital into expendable supplies than is absolutely necessary. Just because volume purchasing reduces the unit cost does not necessarily mean it is a good buy. Inventory and equipment control is discussed in Chapter 18.

Chapter 10

□

Practice and personal protection

John W. Judy, Jr.

The practitioner must find financial security or protection through financial planning involving the use of insurance, investments, and pension or profit-sharing plans. Little help is provided to guide people through the decision-making process of selecting from the large number of options available. This chapter is designed to provide some guidance and leave the final choice to individuals and their advisors.

Most people are skeptical of representatives offering both advice and products. Combining this with a lack of understanding causes many people to postpone a choice until it is too late. One needs to provide protection for contingencies either through a product sold in the marketplace or through a well-conceived financial plan.

Losses can occur in many forms. The veterinarian must be concerned about and plan for the loss of key employees (including himself) through death, sickness, and disability; changes in the economy; fire, wind, flood, and business interruption; escape of patients; and bad debts, theft, fraud, and embezzlement to mention a few.

Protection against these potential losses can be acquired at a cost. Each person must analyze the costs and benefits of getting or planning for protection. Insurance premiums can be reduced by increasing the deductible (amount one must pay) and by having coinsurance (copayment) up to a set level of loss.

□
Insurance

Insurance is the first thing that comes to mind when thinking about protection in case of a loss. Life, medical, disability, liability, property, and other insurances may be needed. The questions that must be answered are how much and which ones.

Life insurance

Life insurance is sold as term insurance, annuity, or a combination of these under a multitude of names. *Term life* insurance provides only protection. The person is betting they will die next year, and the company takes the bet for the premium. No cash value is generated. *Level term life* insurance means that for the term of the policy, the protection dollar amount remains the same. A $50,000 level term policy will pay that amount on the first or last day of the term of the policy. The premium of the policy will rise as the age of the policyholder increases.

Declining or *decreasing term life* insurance has the protection dollar amount go down over the life of the policy. A $100,000 decreasing term policy will pay $100,000 if you die in the first year of the policy term. At the middle it will pay about $50,000 and toward the end may be only $10,000. During that time the premium paid remains the same. This provides $100,000 of protection early at a premium only slightly higher than the $50,000 level term policy. These decreasing term policies are used to pay off loans in the event of death before the end of the payment cycle. The choice between the level and decreasing term life is made on the basis of the protection needed over time.

Annuity policies are saving programs with a guaranteed payout at the end. These are used in retirement to ensure a flow of income. They accumulate cash value that can be borrowed against or withdrawn. The rate of interest paid or return on investment makes these a poor investment but good for providing a level income during retirement.

Ordinary or *whole life* insurance is a combination of decreasing term and annuity policies. The protection or risk to the insurance company is high in the early years and nothing in the last years — the same as decreasing term insurance. The annuity portion provides a growing cash value over the years. A whole life policy is thus all cash value at the end. This cash can be used as part of a retirement program or borrowed during the life of the policy for other investments. As with the annuity policy, ordinary life insurance is not a good investment but may be needed for protection.

Life insurance companies are organized as *stock* or *mutual* companies. A stock company is owned by stockholders who receive the profit earned by the company. Mutual companies are owned by the insurance policyholder. The profits in mutual companies are paid as dividends to the policy owner as cash or by reducing the premium. The initial insurance policy premium (cash out of pocket) from a stock company is lower than that of a mutual company for the same protection. This is the least costly protection for someone who thinks he is going to die soon. If one expects to outlive the policy, then the initial higher out-of-pocket premium for the mutual company is the best choice. Research reports prepared by independent agencies provide a listing of the top ten least-cost companies. One should shop for life insurance as for a car or home.

How much life insurance is needed? The first step is to develop a plan or budget. Each person needs x dollars for burial. If this amount is in the bank, then no life insurance is needed to cover this contingency. Next, plan to cover all debts. Usually decreasing term life insurance is purchased. A term policy purchased separately from the lending institution will usually be less expensive. Additional dollars may be needed to cover raising and educating children. One must also consider the potential income of the spouse when planning a budget to determine insurance needs. Include in the plan the amount of support provided through social security. Income is paid to the surviving spouse as long as the children are of school age. That standard may change, as will the level of support over political time.

Do not purchase more insurance than is needed. The premiums can consume your entire income and leave your family with a poor life-style. If your family members have been insurable and your health can be expected to remain good, use term insurance for the needed protection. Group insurance policies usually offer the lowest premiums, but remember to shop. If the insurance company plans to collect $12,000 in premiums before you reach the age of 65, the sooner the policy is started, the lower the payments will be. By delaying the option to purchase, the premium will become higher "because you are older." The company still collects about $12,000 whether it is short- or long-term. Do not be rushed into the purchase of life insurance.

Medical insurance

The largest potential outlay of cash during life is for medical care. Family coverage is needed. If funds are limited, consider purchasing major medical insurance to cover the very large medical or surgical bill. One may be able to borrow money to pay the costs up to where the insurance coverage begins. Total medical coverage is desirable if the premium is affordable. Group policies (like the American Veterinary Medical Association [AVMA]) can save money. Always read the policy to determine what is and is not covered. Do not rely on the brochure describing any insurance policy. Ask for a specimen policy to read. An example of the problem is the fact that Blue Cross has a large number of different levels of medical coverage — all called Blue Cross.

Disability insurance

The practice of veterinary medicine requires seeing patients to have a flow of income. Should you become ill or unable to work, that income stops, but bills still need to be paid. One cannot afford to not have disability income insurance to cover these contingencies. Premium savings occur as the waiting time before being paid increases. A policy providing income at the end of the second week off work will cost more than one that waits a month. Shop for these policies as for life insurance.

Read the specimen policy to determine when they pay, how much they pay, how long they pay, and how they define disabled. Some policies define a disabled hand as "loss at or above the carpal joint." A veterinarian needs the words "loss of use of the hand" to be protected. Determine what the policy defines as being permanently disabled. Permanent disability from being able to practice veterinary medicine is much different from being able to be trained in another career. Retraining in another career may then allow all payments to stop.

Social security also provides some minor benefits when one has been disabled. Obtain these figures as the budget is being developed to provide the total picture.

Business interruption insurance

Disability income insurance is usually based on take-home pay. This will not be sufficient to meet the payroll, business loan payments, and taxes. Therefore, business interruption insurance was designed to meet that contingency. Other causes of business interruption covered by this type of insurance are fire, wind, flood, and explosion. For example, the generation of gross income stops when the clinic burns down, but the taxes and mortgage continue to require payment. Business interruption insurance provides the funds to pay these.

Business fraud insurance

Protection is needed against employee embezzlement—one of the main reasons for failure of small businesses. Numbered receipts and other accounting checks and balances are deterrents to this kind of loss. For this reason veterinarians usually do not carry this insurance. This insurance will pay if one is embezzled, robbed, or given counterfeit money or bad checks, or a check is altered. The premium is usually low and should be considered in the overall insurance plan.

Liability

The largest cost of liability exposure is the legal defense and not the payment of claims. Professional liability is the first thing that comes to the mind of a medical person. See Chapter 8 for a discussion of this major insurance need. Other liability exposure is almost unlimited. This includes liability for injury to another person, damage of tangible property, slander and libel, errors and omissions, failure to inform an employee under a right-to-know law, sexual harrassment of an employee, and any of the aforementioned when caused by the employee performing a task for the veterinarian.

The "umbrella" liability policy is a low-cost approach to protection. These policies will provide liability protection from a minimum dollar amount (i.e., $300,000) up to 1 or 2 million dollars for all liability exposure, except professional. The umbrella protection will be provided at a much lower premium than having all other policies extend to 1 million dollars. The policy will state the minimum liability coverage that must be carried on the home, office, and vehicles.

Liability protection is available as a part of homeowners, tenant, automobile, truck, and office insurance policies. As a renter, there is some liability exposure, so this protection should be obtained in a tenant policy.

Include medical payments as part of any liability policy. This provides medical payment to an injured person even if it was not your fault. This may reduce hard feelings and does not require friends to sue to get paid for medical care. Be certain the liability policy protects against claims resulting while serving as an officer or board member of an association. If it is not provided, the association should purchase liability protection for anyone serving in any official capacity.

Property insurance

Property losses occur through theft, fire, wind, explosion, deterioration, flood, and obsolescence. Deterioration and obsolescence cannot be insured. The other causes of loss can. *Coinsurance* and *deductible* are means to reduce the cost of this type of insurance. Coinsurance means the policyholder will pay a percentage (20%) of the loss up to a stated maximum amount ($200). Deductible means payment is made for any loss up to the deductible amount.

Be certain the policy uses the term *all risk* when referring to types of losses. This statement usually expands the coverage to losses related to the occurrence. As an example, a fire in the back room of a veterinary clinic is reported by the police on a routine check. The first department arrives and must chop down the front door to gain access. The fire hose is turned on as they move through the reception room, the water sweeps the chairs into the corner, and drug bottles are broken on the floor. The fire in the back is successfully extinguished. The fire insurance adjuster advises that the company will pay for the fire damage in the back room but not the rest of the damage. The damage to the door, furniture, and drug bottles was caused by the water from the hose and not the fire! An all-risk policy will pay for all related damage.

Buildings should be reappraised on a 3-year basis for replacement cost. The property insurance should be increased to cover the new value. Most property insurance policies today have a built-in inflation provision to provide for replacement coverage. The policy inflation clause should apply to the contents of the building as well.

Animals in the building are usually not covered by a standard property insurance policy. Coverage for them may be acquired as part of the AVMA's insurance program and should protect against escape and death.

Automobiles or trucks are also property items. Collision insurance provides protection for loss to the aforementioned insurable risks. Liability and medical coverage should be a part of this policy. Be certain that trailers, boats, and other vehicles are either a part of this protection or are insured individually.

Workman's compensation

This insurance is required by law and varies from state to state. Check the local state law for the coverage required and companies offering protection. This insurance provides medical payments and income to an employee injured in the course of work. Employee claims against this coverage must be monitored closely because any claim (founded or unfounded) will affect the premium rate.

Pet insurance

Medical insurance on animals is an important part of veterinary medicine today. The practicing veterinarian must be the salesperson because it is unlikely that this will become a fringe benefit to most employees. One will need to be aware of insurance companies providing coverage within the state and the process to gain reimbursement for services. When unfamiliar with the company that a client indicates will pay for services, insist they pay for the service and collect directly from their company.

Life insurance policies on animals provide some challenges when recommending euthanasia. Be certain to inform the insurance company and gain permission before euthanatizing the animal. Some companies must be advised before any general anesthesia because the animal could die during the procedure.

□
Financial planning

Some people have great interest in and success at managing their own money. Most veterinarians are not adept at investment fund management because they do not have the time to read and follow the markets. Most busy professionals should obtain the services of a knowledgeable and professional financial planner. The selection of a financial planner is not an easy task.

The financial planner will need a set of personal life and professional goals. Personal goals include how much do you want to earn? When do you plan to retire? What do you want to do in retirement? How large a family will you have? Do you expect to pay for their college education? Do you prefer free time to money? What size of a home do you want, including vacation residence?

Professional goals are equally important. They must not be in conflict with your personal goals. Stating all goals on paper helps avoid this conflict. Questions needing answers include the following. Do you always want to practice? Are there other careers in veterinary medicine that would better meet your personal needs? What size of a practice do you want, solo or several-person practice? Do you want the largest, best-equipped clinic in the area or something more modest? Do you want to spend time with the client and patient, or do you want to be more efficient in the use of your time? There is room for all types of practices, and only you can make the choice. Your advisers will listen to you and direct you in the best way to attain your goals.

A tax adviser is needed before opening any practice. This person should be a certified public accountant (CPA), manage other medical or veterinary practices, and attend a tax school each year. Time must be set aside to provide advice on at least a quarterly basis. The practice should not employ an accountant and then only use him at tax time. This person can and should be used for advice on purchase and building decisions before actions are taken. The bookkeeping system or computer system should be acquired only after using the accountant's advice.

An investment adviser is the most difficult to identify. Start the search for this person the first day of practice even though investment funds will not be available for several years. People who can help in this search include bankers, contractors, lawyers, doctors, other veterinarians, and friends from the community. Obviously there will be a long list of advisers after this initial inquiry. Talk with those people who are on more than one person's list. Over the next few years listen to their advice and take action based on that advice by buying stock or mutual funds on paper. By this I mean have a small notebook to record the purchase without actually buying. Follow the advice and sell on paper at a later date. Record who provided the advice on each transaction. After several years a log of good, better, and best advisors will become established. When money finally becomes available to invest, the people to use will be identified. Start early and listen well. There are no sure things, so do not invest all available funds in one item.

Investment decisions are important, and no one will provide for your own retirement but you. Invest well or have a good investment counselor to provide sound advice.

Investments

Many investment advisers recommend splitting investments half and half between the *fixed stable* type and the more volatile *growth* investments. Stable investments include a savings account, government bonds, and other interest-earning accounts in banking and land. Common stock, some mutual funds, corporate bonds, and the commodities market are examples of growth or volatile investments.

Industries have cycles that the price of their stock go through. Invest in businesses that you know or are interested in reading about. The most interesting business should be your own practice.

The economic value of the practice business must be maintained. This is done by applying good management including a frequent analysis of fees and the use of labor. Remember that one must have a good return on the money invested in the practice if it is to be salable in the future. No one would buy stock in a company that is losing money, so do not expect someone to purchase a veterinary business if it is losing money. This return on investment is the building block of "blue sky" or goodwill.

The land and building used by the practice should be selected to be marketable. A realistic rent for the building should be established on the basis of current real estate values in the area. The rent becomes the return on investment, which is paid out of the profits. The amount of profit left after rent is what you earn as a manager and a veterinarian. Most rental property has the rent based on 1.0% or 1.5% of the current market value per month. Additional information concerning real estate management and buying and selling a practice is found in Chapters 4 and 7.

The home you purchase is also part of your real estate investment package. Select the location wisely so that values can be expected to rise in the future. Do not buy the lowest- or highest-priced home in the subdivision. Either one will be hard to sell.

Interest-earning accounts

Depositing money in a savings account is an investment. Other types of savings investments include certificates of deposit (CDs), money market accounts, and treasury bills.

Income in a veterinary practice varies through the year. Practice cash flow management dictates that some cash be carried to meet expenses when income is low. Wise money management dictates keeping excess cash in an interest-earning account and not leaving money sitting in a noninterest checking account. Therefore, the manager must be prepared to move funds to get the best interest given changing circumstances.

Savings accounts permit deposit and withdrawal of money on any banking day. Computerized banking permits movement of money between checking and savings any time of the day. This money is insured by a federal deposit insurance agency in case the bank fails. The rapid availability of money results in a lower interest being paid.

CDs are offered by banks and pay a higher interest because the funds are unavailable until the end of the deposit time without paying a heavy penalty or loss of interest earned. These are good for holding business funds for 3 to 6 months if the money is not needed. If a need occurs near the end of the CD term, borrow money by using the CD as collateral. The interest on the note should be less than the penalty for early withdrawal. Calculate the difference when deciding on the best option. Also, remember this when selling US bonds if an interest payment is about due.

Money market accounts are offered by brokerage firms and insurance and investment companies. These require a large minimum deposit to open and pay interest at a rate usually higher than money market certificates.

Some offer checking service if checks are written for set amounts such as $500. These money market funds are only as secure as the company offering it. Federal deposit insurance does not protect these investments. Thus with more risk, there is a higher interest. Remember that when an interest rate far above the market is offered a higher risk of losing the money is involved.

Stocks and bonds

Stocks and bonds are sold to finance a business when those owning the business are not able or do not desire to borrow money from the banks. Because many companies use this system, markets have been established that trade stocks and bonds. Usually these sales are not between the company and the buyer but between owners of the stock or bond. A veterinarian may elect to incorporate his practice to gain capital for growth and expansion; however, the stock will never be sold on the big markets that are listed in the *Wall Street Journal*. Therefore, incorporation of the practice may produce capital but may become difficult to sell when the veterinarian retires. Numerous excellent references are available on the management of an investment portfolio. Specific reading recommendations can be made by a financial planner.

A young investor should be interested in *growth stocks*. These are stocks of companies that reinvest their profit in research and expansion. They usually have little or no dividend payment record. The price change in the stock value is the only return to investment that can be observed or expected.

Older investors are interested in income for retirement. They shift from growth companies to ones that pay dividends on a regular basis. They might even be seen moving to bonds or treasury bills for the same reason. Investment advice from or for an older person is thus different than that for a young person.

Important factors needed for investing in stocks are knowing the industry, its economic condition and that of the company, the level and direction of sales and profit, dividend expectations, the quality of management, and the level of research and development they are doing. What new products are they or the competition coming out with, and how will this affect profit? Dividends are a distribution of profit by the company board of directors to the stockholders. *Preferred stock* has a set dividend rate that is paid before common stock dividends. If the company loses money for several years and has not paid a preferred dividend, they may have to catch up on these payments when profits return before paying common stock dividends.

Information is available through brokers and libraries concerning companies. *Standard and Poor's, Moody's,* and *Value Line* publish bulletins or notebooks that provide a history of the company and industry performance. Computer programs and services are also available to help research companies. They may even provide a recommendation of how they expect the company's stock to perform.

The future price of stock is not predictable. Newscasters always have a reason why the market went up or down. Never invest more in the stock market than one can afford to lose. This permits the investor to ride out rough times and not be forced to sell low.

Bonds are also sold as a means to raise money for the government or corporations. They have a set interest rate that will be paid annually or at the end of the term. Because the interest rate is fixed, the price of bonds goes up when interest rates fall and drops when interest rates go up. More money is therefore made in the bond market by predicting changes in the interest rate, which determine when to buy or sell. The prudent investor must become a student of the Federal Reserve Bank whose board sets interest rates to control the money supply and thereby the economy. An understanding of the use of money to control the aggregate economy is helpful in forecasting interest changes. An adviser might indicate a rise or fall in interest rates that could help in corporate bond investments.

Municipal bonds are tax-exempt at the federal level. The higher the personal income tax rate, the more desirable these become. Always investigate a state or municipal bond offering before purchasing. Some have defaulted or not paid in the past. *Standard and Poor's, Moody's,* and *Value Line* publish bulletins that provide a history and performance of the company.

Mutual funds

A means of gaining expert stock investing advice is by purchasing it in a mutual fund. The managers of the fund have a full-time job studying and investing in the market. *Standard and Poor's* and *Moody's* have analyses and recommendations concerning most of these funds. Take time to study the investment opportunities in *growth funds*, which are invested in stocks of companies that are expected to increase in size; *income funds*, which are invested in high-interest bonds or high-dividend stocks; bonds, either corporate or municipal; and treasury bills.

There are *load* and *no-load* mutual funds. Load funds mean they charge a management fee for their services each quarter or year. *Front-end load* means that the first purchase may have a commission and management fee subtracted. No-load funds do not charge a management fee, but it is an expense that reduces the earnings of the funds. A no-load fund may still charge a commission up front.

Real estate

In addition to one's home and practice, an opportunity exists for real estate investment in farms or other rental properties. During rapid inflationary times, the increase in value of the land more than makes up for the low rental return. During the early 1980s land values dropped, and rental income became the important investment objective. A change in federal tax laws also resulted in a reevaluation of real estate investments. Remember this history when looking to a tax benefit as a reason to do anything unless it is within the current tax year.

Rental property should earn 1% to 1.5% of the current market value per month to be a good investment. This is true as long as the prime interest rate is below 15%. A practitioner may have the opportunity to lease a practice site rather than purchase. If a site can be leased for less than 1% of the sale price per month, it is probably better to lease than buy. The decision to purchase rental property in good condition can be based on these percentages. An example is a property with a monthly rent of $1,200. The rent divided by 1%, or 0.01, equals $120,000. If the property can be purchased for less than that amount, it is a good investment assuming there are no legal problems related to the land.

Other investments

To get rich quick is the desire of everyone! Many investors are tempted by gold, silver, other precious metals, diamonds, art, and antiques. As with other investments, these require an excellent knowledge of the industry. The investor must know when to buy and when to sell. A knowledgeable person can make good money in any of these by "buying low and selling high," as in the stock market.

Commodities—cattle, wheat, corn, sugar, as examples—are sold on the futures market. This market was established to provide producers with a means of ensuring the sale price of their product at some date in the future. At the same time the manufacturer could also en-sure the price to be paid for raw material in the future. Speculative investors play this market during the dates in between. They sell things they do not have (sell short) and buy things they do not intend to have delivered. Through these transactions they make and lose money.

Selling short is done with the intent of purchasing the item at a later date to replace the sale. A sale before a purchase is anticipating a drop in price of the commodity before the delivery date. If the investor sells corn to someone for delivery in 2 months at $3 a bushel and later buys that corn for $2 to deliver, $1 is made on each bushel less the commission. If, however, the price of corn went up to $10 a bushel before the delivery and that is the amount one must pay to cover, then the investor loses $7 per bushel.

Retirement planning

In your personal financial plan you must identify whether and when you wish to retire. Given the age and the style in which you wish to live, a retirement plan is developed. The aforementioned investments are part of this plan. Social security and life insurance will provide a small part. Some veterinarians are employed where a retirement program is part of the benefit package. Be certain to understand completely what benefits are provided. Plan for providing medical insurance during the retirement period. Most people spend 80% of their health care dollars in the last year of life!

The practice can provide a retirement program through a *Keogh plan*, profit sharing, or pension plans. These plans provide some form of federal tax shelter under 1987 tax laws. The current tax provisions for self-employed and corporation retirement plans should be checked before making a decision in this vital area of planning. Some form of a tax-sheltered retirement program is an advantage. The money individuals or corporations place in plans that are tax sheltered is not taxed until withdrawn. Thus, if the individual's tax rate is 35%, for every $100 deposited in the plan, $65 is the individual's money and $35 is the government's. Between that date and withdrawal, interest is earned on the government's money as well as the individual's money. That interest is not taxed until withdrawn.

The *Keogh plan* was passed by the federal government to provide retirement benefits to self-employed individuals similar to those found in corporations. Provisions for tax sheltering in 1987 are about the same for corporations and sole proprietors. The reason for incorporating has therefore been lost. The tax law is continually revised and may be slightly different at the time of reading. Although the provisions have changed over time, the basic way the plan works remains the same. All employees in the business must have the same retirement plan options. The benefits must be extended to all employees after 3 years of full-time employment with the business. This is why many firms only employ part-time people. If an employee is given these benefits before the 3 years, all current and future employees must receive the same benefits at that lapsed time of employment. It is advised that all employees should wait the 3 years.

The funds deposited by the employer for the employee must be at the same percentage of wages as the owner. At the time that money is deposited, it is vested and belongs to the employee. They can collect the money without penalty when they leave employment, or they may leave it in the fund. If the money on deposit in the Keogh plan has been on deposit for less than 10 years, it should be withdrawn.

Profit sharing and *pension plans* are designed for incorporated businesses. Pension plans must be funded (dollars deposited every year) even if the corporation loses money. This is not required in Keogh plans or profit sharing. For this reason many small corporations avoid pension plans in favor of profit sharing. The maximum that can be deposited in 1 year is about the same for all plans under 1987 tax laws. A pension plan specifies a set percentage of the wage that is deposited each year. The amount of income on retirement depends on the investment skills of the fund manager.

A profit-sharing plan also provides a tax-sheltered retirement program. The profit of the corporation is divided and deposited in the plan on the basis of a percentage of the wages up to a set maximum. All profits do not need to be distributed to the plan. No deposit is required when the corporation loses money. This should not be confused with profit sharing used to motivate employees through bonus programs.

Most young people are not concerned about retirement plans as much as they are about trying to reduce their debt load. These plans, therefore, may not motivate employees because of the long time before they will get to use the money. Remember that the earlier a retirement plan is started, the fewer dollars per year are needed to reach the retirement goal. Individual Retirement Accounts provide a minor tax-protected retirement fund. Other retirement plans will be developed by the government, so the retirement issue will need yearly monitoring. The benefit of tax-protected deposits for retirement should be used regardless of the size of the plan.

Chapter 11
☐
Fee setting and collection

William J. Kay
Ronald L. Burk
Edward P. Kerrigan
Carmen Rodriguez

Perhaps no single issue will be responsible for creating or diminishing the success of a veterinary practice more than one's income and net worth. The practitioners' perceptions will be greater when they have the ability to create a reasonable and profitable fee structure and procedure for collection.

Fees are usually based on perceptions, and seldom are statistical data tested in this regard. As a group of professionals, veterinarians have fees that are basically unregulated, and comparative data are scanty. In developing a fee structure, one should consider the following questions and factor in the responses:

- What is my goal in terms of annual income? Be specific.
- Is my goal attainable? What must I do to accomplish my goal?
- How serious am I? How willing am I to achieve this goal?
- Has my goal changed over the years? Will it change in the future? Does it fluctuate too much? Not enough? What are the reasons for its changing?
- What drives or controls my fee? Consider the following: my needs, wants, energy, ethics, my view of service to others, level of skill, training, experience, public perception, fears and anxieties (e.g., "Will people feel I'm not working?"), and ego and arrogance (i.e., "Of course my services are worth it!")

It is important to understand that fees are derived from the aforementioned factors, which are seldom based on objective data. In other words, fees may be structured by a sense of ill-determined factors within yourself and the clientele you attract.

Data on what clients will pay for a particular veterinary service are scanty. The immense range of feelings among clients regarding their responsibilities as pet owners suggests there are variations in the extent to which they will pay for services. You must ask yourself, however, whether you care what people think about the fees you set. This point is critical, for if you *do* care about upsetting clients, you will need to consider this when setting personal and practice goals as well as financial objectives. A magnanimous nature and sliding scales for all services will undoubtedly affect income, expenses, outflow, and net worth. As a new veterinarian, you may not yet know what amount is required to get through life; raising a family, providing for parental support, expanding the practice, planning for retirement, and so forth must be taken into account. Most of us will admit we require more money to accomplish our ever-changing goals, and the more we can make, the better our lives will be. The setting of professional fees will thus determine how we live. The question remains, then, whether we know what we want.

There are as many different views about setting fees as there are individuals engaged in setting them. Both veterinarian and client may operate out of fear: we, fearful of upsetting and angering clients and staff, fearful we are not worth our fees, fearful our practice will fail; our clients, fearful their animals will die, that they will be unable to pay for a desired treatment. Fear is always a powerful motivator and, as such, must be seriously considered in the structuring of fees.

□ The context of fees

Ideally the worth or value of a particular service should be set objectively. More often, however, personal or practice goals will be the overriding determinant. Thus veterinarians generally underestimate costs and therefore undercharge for their services. A personal attitude toward fee structure and revenue can be developed frivolously or after extensive planning and study.

In recent years, the population of practicing veterinarians has increased dramatically, and this perceived glut will likely create the perception that competition is keen and that clients have more choice when they believe the fee is too high. This fear has led to the development of an endless stream of veterinary "boutiques" or "supermarkets" based on who can give the best *rate* rather than who can offer the best *service*. In general, however, clients will pay for what they perceive as optimal veterinary care that is based on mutual respect. If one chooses to practice with high fees or very low fees, what is really being reflected is one's personal view of the publics' wants and needs. In the case of low fees, the client's attachment to the pet or perhaps the veterinarian's skill is held in low regard. Understand that what the client is really paying for is the veterinarian's skill and expertise; the power behind this belief should not be underestimated. To the extent that one is clear about one's own ability, fees will be higher. Conversely, when one is unsure of one's skill, fees will be proportionately lower.

Veterinarians vary dramatically in their interest, skill, training, age, and response to animals. Without judging either on an ethical scale, it appears that three groups emerge: (1) Those veterinarians with a deep love or regard for animals or for the relationship between veterinarian, owner, and animal establish a fee structure that will enable maximal opportunity for the animal, its health, prognosis, and well-being. (2) Those who hold the view that animals are owned and their primary responsibility is to the client may provide a fee structure based upon the client's worth, interest, and concern. (3) Finally, those who are focused on themselves, family, or profession will have a fee structure that reflects these realities and perceptions. It is safe to say most of us do not neatly fall into one or another of these categories but rather combine aspects of all three.

Among the *objective* factors that drive the fee structure are the following: (1) fees set or charged by colleagues (i.e., "the going rate"); (2) payment of salaries, equipment, and debts; and (3) clients' response to fees and perceived satisfaction, as evidenced by practice growth. *Subjective* factors are as follows: (1) How long have I been in practice? How many hours per day, days per week will I work? (2) Must I work harder to live the way I wish? Am I willing to? For how many years? (3) What percentage of income must be derived from the practice? Have I made full use of investment opportunities?

Veterinarians operate from the aforementioned objective and subjective factors, yet few have analyzed the market. For instance, in a telephone survey of clients' attitudes toward The Animal Medical Center, we surveyed nearly 1000 current or former clients. We were interested in their feelings, views, and attitudes because our practice volume in the period between 1974 and 1985 was in decline. An important factor was made clear to us: Although a high percentage of pet owners viewed our services as good or excellent, an equal percentage viewed our fees as high or very high. What should we conclude from such confounding data? Can we survive with both realities? Which reality will dominate? Can we continue to raise our fees, and if so, how high can we go?

The oft-cited quote "Quality is remembered long after the price is forgotten" should be our guide. Most veterinarians will regard the service they provide as quality service. Less frequently analyzed, however, is what constitutes quality service, how it is perceived, and by whom.

□
Fair fees

Philosophy

The concept of what is "fair" will be different for any two persons and is certain to vary among clients as a group, veterinarians as a group, and between individuals. *Practical* is a better key word. Practical is what clients as a group can afford. Practical is what must be charged to be competitive with other veterinarians in one general location (as each practice will define the boundaries of such location). Finally, but not the least important, practical is what each practitioner wishes to have and can reasonably expect from a "practice." Inasmuch as the definition necessarily involves the client, other veterinarians, and yourself, the following points must always be considered: (1) Are my clients, as a group, able to pay my fee and reasonably willing to do so? (2) Are my fees well below or well above those of my colleagues? (3) Can I and do I wish to continue practicing at these rates?

Every fee set will involve answers to all three questions, with each question having various levels of complexity. Consideration of the client and colleague will be discussed first, and specific fee areas will be considered later in the chapter.

The client

Location and the types of animals in that location will both be factors in setting fees and in administering the practice. A client's ability to pay is affected by his location. Obviously a client living a low-income area of New York City cannot and will not pay the same fee as a client from affluent Park Avenue in the same city. Yet, if the client chooses to go to a veterinarian who practices on Park Avenue, can that client expect to pay less than other clients? The answer, exclusive of other factors such as charity, must be No.

Basically, what price clients as a group can afford to pay must be surmised from the neighborhood in which the veterinarian practices. Clients' income and their expected ability to pay must be considered when alternative methods of treatment exist that vary significantly in cost. In setting overall fees, however, the income level of potential clients is a necessary consideration.

Your colleagues

Veterinarians who offer service in the same general practice area will by necessity compete from the same client pool. Therefore, fees set for common services such as office calls, trip charges, vaccinations, hospitalization, and so forth will affect the number of clients using a specific practice. When one practice charges very high fees, client numbers in that practice may decline. Bankruptcy may ensue if the fees are too low. The definition of what constitutes a fee that is far above or below that of one's colleagues is somewhat complex. For example, a single night in the hospital for an animal at two different hospitals may cost $24 in one and $32 in the other, a significant difference. At first glance, it may seem that one facility is either overcharging or undercharging, but further consideration will reveal that higher charge includes fluids and all drugs whereas the lower charge is for cage care and ordinary pet food (special diet foods cost extra). The fees for fluids and drugs in the second example are added as professional services.

One veterinarian may charge more for office visits than another. A look at the nature of the practice, however, may reveal that walk-ins and emergency visits are standard, whereas a veterinarian whose fee is lower will encourage appointments and treat walk-ins only in dire emergencies. The higher charge, then, underwrites vacant time slots and affords the opportunity for the client to arrive at a moment's notice. In short, the effort to price competitively must take many factors into consideration. Many of these factors go unnoticed at first glance.

At this time, one should be aware that price fixing by written or oral agreement is illegal. Exchange of price lists is usually considered *prima facie* evidence of price fixing. When one's practice fee schedule is similar to another's practice fee schedule, a strong case might be made for price fixing. The Federal Trade Commission (FTC) has taken a dim view of so-called price fixing and has successfully prosecuted several cases.

Piecemeal vs. package rates

A doctor who tries to charge for every item will never be entirely successful. After all, who charges for tongue depressors? On the other hand, package rates are often so narrowly defined that some people feel it is a euphemism for piecemeal pricing.

Every practice will establish its own general policy of package fees or piecemeal and then agonize over when to be generous with certain piecemeal fees or to more narrowly define certain package fees.

For instance, The Animal Medical Center has a general policy of piecemeal rates. This policy is based on the opinion that the cost of a sick outpatient visit or any inpatient visit is more easily explained when a client knows all of the items involved. Nevertheless, we have several routine inpatient elective procedures such as declawing, spaying, and castrations that are priced as packages. The reason is that the hospital stay, surgical procedures, and drugs involved are quite predictable. Nevertheless, great care is taken to explain to the client before the procedure is performed that any complications may necessitate further charges for adjunctive therapy.

Regarding hospital room and board, is it wise to have a daily package rate? Return to the aforementioned example of the $24 and $32 daily rates for hospital care. Some believe clients would prefer a higher rate to avoid being met at the animal's discharge with bills for fluids and drugs that were not expected. Our belief at The Animal Medical Center is that the client will consider the inclusive rate too high without adequate explanation, which can be misunderstood amid the high anxiety that surrounds the hospitalization of a seriously ill animal. Furthermore, after being told the facility has an inclusive fee, the client may find it difficult to understand why a procedure such as cardiopulmonary resuscitation was not included in that rate. We have found that there are few surprises — other than the announcement that food is included in the fee — when clients are given a low fee for cage care only.

An excellent example of a package fee that is *not* a package fee is a vaccination charge that includes an examination. Because good veterinary practice requires a prevaccination examination, some charge for this must be built into the fee. This is reasonable, but because several vaccinations are often given, how do we explain that the first vaccination is more costly than the next? We believe it is simpler to have a charge for a prevaccination examination. On surgical procedures, especially electives, it may be wise to have a package fee when the charges involved are predictable. However, is it wise to include in the package a fee for such items as suture removal and other routine follow-up care? At The Animal Medical Center, we limit the follow-up care, and most important, we advise the client that there is no partial refund if suture removal or follow-up is done in another practice.

Large-animal practitioners are confronted by the question about trip charges to a farm or ranch for inoculation of a large number of animals. Should one set a fee that absorbs the cost of a trip to a ranch 50 miles away (including the cost of potential business that had to be turned away due to driving time), or should one simply add into the total a per-mile or per-hour fee? Although we are engaged primarily in small-animal practice, we suggest a fee be applied for a visit that is higher than the office fee and then a separate fee for vaccinating the group of animals. If one decides to absorb trip costs in a package price for the inoculation, the veterinarian must be prepared to explain to the client on a subsequent visit to the same location to care for one sick animal why the trip costs are now being tacked on as a separate charge. The explanation should include that on the group inoculation visit the cost and time involved were predictable but cannot be closely estimated on a visit for one animal.

In summary, the following points must be considered: (1) The procedures involved in a package rate must be preditable. (2) The client must be told very clearly and precisely what the package includes. A specific statement such as "It does not include any other treatment or procedure" is advised. (3) To be economically feasible, a package rate can be considered only after the charges for all the items and procedures involved have been tallied. Any further discount of the overall price should only occur when more business can be encouraged as a result of this packaging.

□
Fee setting

Fees are a combination of the costs involved added to the expected earnings (profit). To set a fee wisely, the veterinarian needs accurate information on costs and earnings.

Costs

Costs are payments or debts that are acquired for every item used in the practice, from paper towels to the most expensive piece of equipment. The cost of consumable supplies and frequently replaced equipment should be recovered in the same year that such costs are incurred. The cost of very expensive equipment or long-lasting equipment must be recovered over the useful life of such equipment, a process known as *amortization*. For tax purposes, it may be useful to use a shorter-than-normal life expectancy. This aspect, like all tax aspects of practice, should be discussed with the accountant or whomever prepares the tax returns. Monthly rent would be treated as a consumable supply, whereas an owned building would be treated like long-lasting equipment. For example, practice A uses or is estimated to use the following:

Consumable supplies of $25,000 per year
Frequently used or replaced equipment of $15,000 per year
Rent of $24,000 per year
Long-lasting equipment of $100,000, with an average life of 10 years (or $10,000 per year)
Interest, in the first year, of $8,000
Staff salaries (excluding any salary for the owner) of $25,000

The costs for the first year of operation would be approximately $72,000, not including taxes. This example is quite simplified, and your real situation would probably be calculated with the assistance of an accountant.

Profit

Profit is the difference between the revenue generated by the practice and costs, as described previously. Funds from profits reinvested in the practice are still profits that can be subject to tax. The reinvestment then becomes part of the overall costs, as described before. Please understand that this summary of costs and profit is intended only as a background for discussions with the accountant or other financial consultant.

The principle is that, once the costs and the amount of profit necessary to maintain a minimum style of living have been determined, then the sum of both determines what the total fees must be. The most difficult part is to set the specific fees.

Fee list

Total fees, which in the case of most practices means gross revenue, must now spread over all procedures or services rendered to clients. Now is the time to construct the fee list, which should start with a procedure list. No list is going to be all-inclusive, and any list over five pages long is probably too complicated to be very useful.

In a large practice, the procedures might be categorized, e.g., radiology, surgery, drugs, hospitalization, and so forth. In a small practice, we recommend a breakdown by frequency of occurrence, starting with the office visit, followed by vaccination (by type), followed by specialty examination, and so forth.

The next step is to attach a fee to each procedure. Categories — such as fluids, antibiotics, and so forth — should be used wherever possible. When this list is complete, you must estimate how close the total revenue will come to the revenue needed to meet the total of costs and profit. To do this, you must estimate the frequency of each service and multiply that frequency by the charge for that procedure. For instance, if a practice expects 1500 visits per year and charges $25 for each visit, the total revenue for visits would be $37,500. If the practice expects 500 visits at $25, the revenue from visits would be estimated at $12,500.

When the revenue for each procedure and service has been determined, the total revenue for the practice can now be calculated by adding together the revenue from all procedures. By comparing the total revenue to the costs plus profit expected, one attempts to avoid shortfalls or overcharges in the price list. The review of the revenue may also reveal too much optimism for the frequency of one or more services rendered. If the overage or shortfall is greater than 20% the price list must be redone.

The new practitioner should not expect the revenue goals (of cost plus profit) to necessarily be met in the first year. However, in 3 years or less, the expected profit should be achieved. In 5 years the average expected profit should be achieved, or one must reevaluate each aspect of the practice from management to location.

A final note on price lists: they should be reviewed on a semiannual to annual basis. When initially preparing the fee list and in reviewing the fee list, one must always consider the client, the competition, and the needs of the practice.

□
Financial statements

Many veterinarians will not have the services of a full-time bookkeeper or require certified financial statements. The basic financial needs, however, will be for

Tax information (probably prepared by someone other than the practice owner)
Information on how much the practice owes in long-term (over 1 year) and short-term (under one year) debt
General financial information such as assets, equity, cash position, and profit (including cash withdrawn)

All of this information can be obtained by contracting with an accountant who will work 1 or more days per month, as required. Financial management is detailed in Chapter 19.

□
Cash vs. credit
Cash business only

In today's world, cash payment must, as a matter of practicality, include checks. In the case of clients who are known to the practice, returned checks should not be a problem. For new clients or known transients (e.g., clients who visit practices located in a resort area), a check guarantee service should be considered. If the practice decides not to accept checks from new clients (except as a last resort), then the client should be informed when they call for an appointment that payment is by credit card or cash only.

When checks are taken, at least two forms of personal identification should be required. A valid driver's license and a major credit card are good forms of identification. Clients who write checks that are returned for insufficient funds should be charged a bad check fee. This fee should cover the practice's time required to collect and process the bad check.

Credit cards

In general, credit cards carry less risk of being charged back to the practice than checks returned by the bank for nonpayment. They are particularly effective when dealing with a transient clientele because a client cannot charge back a purchase that is incurred more than 50 miles from his home. However, charges over a certain amount must be verified with the card-issuing company. A sales point terminal may be tied to the phone line for automated card verifications.

The various card-issuing companies including MasterCard, Visa, and American Express, all have representatives who would be happy to explain these services. Keep in mind that the cost of this service, which is expressed as a percentage of credit card charges, is negotiable. The monthly rate should be reviewed any time an increase in charges for a period of time is noted on the applicable credit card issuer.

Personal credit

Good advice is not to extend credit; however, this is usually not practical. Credit is best confined only to those whose ability to pay is known personally or to long-standing clients. Outstanding clients receive a personally prepared, typed statement (Fig. 11-1). The total accounts receivable, at any one time, should never exceed 25% of 1 month's gross income.

☐ Methods

There are four basic methods for setting fees: hourly rate, cost plus, colleague based, and client based.

Hourly rate

The hourly rate method is calculated by first determining the total cost (includes both fixed and variable costs) and necessary profit. Next the billable hours are determined and are simply divided into the total cost plus profit to compute a standard rate. In determining the total cost, both fixed (such as rent or payment on a building, salaries, insurance, and so forth) and variable (such items as syringes, needles, fluids, forms, labor, or anything that as a cost would vary with the number of patients treated) costs must be considered. Labor is treated as a variable cost if an increase in clientele would require an addition of either support staff or another veterinarian.

Once the total cost has been determined, it is necessary to determine an acceptable level of profit. Because a practice is a financial investment, a profit factor should be included

above and beyond whatever the owner may pay himself as a reasonable salary. This profit level should at least reflect the rate of return if a similar investment of capital were put into a relatively secure investment such as treasury bills. Once the total cost and necessary profit are defined, the next step is to define the number of billable hours. The hourly rate can then be easily determined by dividing the billable hours into the total cost. Two advantages of this method are that most clients and staff find it easy to comprehend and it is fairly easy to measure whether targets are being met. Disadvantages include the inability to accurately predict billable hours as well as the fact that each veterinarian in a multiveterinarian practice will have a different degree of productivity per unit time. Therefore, one can easily imagine a client ending up with a bill larger or smaller for a particular service depending on whether a recent veterinary graduate or an associate partner had conducted the service. A third factor is that charging by unit time diminishes the doctor–patient relationship and focuses more on the doctor–client relationship. Although this may be appropriate in food animal practice, it is inappropriate in most pet animal practices. An hourly rate is probably appropriate for instances in which the veterinarian goes to the site of service, be it to a client's home for a pet or to a ranch for a herd. In those settings, an hourly rate may be the logical way to cover the costs of transportation by charging a certain amount per hour for going to and from the site of service. This is a common practice in many types of businesses in many areas of the country.

Cost-plus method

This method is similar to the hourly rate method in that it accounts for all costs and a profit factor but differs in that the fee is directly associated with the specific service provided rather than the length of time required to per-

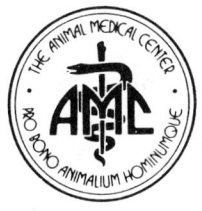

THE ANIMAL MEDICAL CENTER
SPEYER HOSPITAL AND CASPARY RESEARCH INSTITUTE

510 EAST 62ND STREET
NEW YORK, NEW YORK 10021
TE 8-8100

April 1, 1986

Mrs. J. Roth
111 Park Avenue
New York, NY 10028

Acct.# 105767
Case # 46-31-59

February 24, 1986	Visit for Anna	$ 38.00
	Hospitalization	26.00
	Laboratory	3.00
	X-ray	50.00
	Laboratory	17.00
	Laboratory	29.00
	Laboratory	2.00
	Laboratory	3.00
	Drugs	12.00
	Catheter	15.00
	Fluids	12.00
February 25, 1986	Hospitalization	26.00
	Drugs	36.00
	Fluids	36.00
February 26, 1986	Hospitalization	26.00
	Laboratory	17.00
	Drugs	36.00
	Fluids	36.00
February 27, 1986	Hospitalization	26.00
	Drugs	6.00
	Drugs	6.00
February 28, 1986	Discharge Medication	4.75
	Discharge Medication	4.00
	Laboratory	9.00
	Fluids	24.00
	Drugs	24.00
	Balance	$ 523.75
	Total Balance Due	$ 523.75

Figure 11-1. Detailed client statement

form the service. The method consists of determining the total costs (materials, labor, overhead) for each service. Then a profit factor is added. An example of such pricing might be a feline ovariohysterectomy. The costs can be assigned for direct supplies (sutures, scalpel blade, anesthestic, drapes), overhead (lights, heat, surgery instrumentation and sterilization), labor (surgery time, technical support, general labor [kennel cleaning, accounting]), and a profit factor. After calculations the appropriate fee would be apparent.

The advantage of this system is that each client pays those costs directly related to the treatment the animal receives. It is a fairly standard method of developing fees in human medicine, veterinary medicine, and dentistry. The disadvantages are similar to the hourly rate model, and it is difficult to predict with accuracy the types and frequency of services. Furthermore, this method (as well as the hourly method) does not address any competitive issues.

Colleague-based method

With this method you ascertain the fees charged for various services by colleagues in the area and then set fees based upon these findings. You can determine colleagues' charges either by blind telephone surveys, interviewing clients who have seen other veterinarians, reviewing advertised fees, or interviewing other veterinarians. This practice has potential legal complications because it is illegal if the intent of the conversations is to collusively set prices (i.e., price fixing). It is unlikely that there would be a problem if conversations were held one on one or in very small groups and no agreements were made. However, if an organized body determined to review fees for an area and publish the results for the purpose of suggesting fees as a result of their findings, this would clearly be collusion in price fixing and could result in legal action.

The advantages of the colleague-based system are establishing competitive rates for the area and requiring minimal effort in evaluating one's own practice. The major disadvantage is that the system fails to consider the financial needs of the practice. The second potential disadvantage is that the validity of this method is predicated on the premise that price competition is the major factor in the selection of a

veterinarian. Although it might seem likely, there are few data to support this. Previous studies have suggested that location and perceived concern and competence are greater factors than price. Except for commonly performed services such as neutering and vaccination, the applicable fees are rarely obtainable by a client over the telephone. Therefore, the "hassle factor" in obtaining price comparisons for services such as surgery or complicated medical problems decreases the effect of price competition.

Client-based method

This method is difficult to implement because valid data are difficult to obtain. Typically anecdotal tales from happy or disgruntled clients sway decisions on fees. Another variation would be to hire an outside firm to survey the pet-owning public in the area and then use this information to base fees. It would be difficult to derive a valid sampling, however, for few people will provide an answer to the question of how much is a reasonable amount for a certain veterinary service simply because they are not faced with a real situation such as an emergency, major trauma, or fractured long bone.

The advantages of a client-based system are that client complaints are potentially fewer and interaction with clients is seemingly more caring. The major disadvantages are that such a system totally ignores the financial needs of the practice and that there is no valid method of data collection.

Other methods

Superimposed on any of these methods is the use of a *loss leader*, which competes in a focused, limited-price, competitive niche and develops a client loyalty so that the veterinary practice will come to be used for other full-priced services. Ideally, a loss leader should cover the variable costs but probably will not cover the fixed costs (e.g., rent or labor). Animal neutering is a common loss leader because it is frequently performed on a less-than-full-cost basis (i.e., the cost of preparing the pack, suture, and scalpel blades is rarely recovered). Loss leaders require visibility to be effective. It does no good to have a low-cost service that nobody knows about. For a loss leader to be used successfully, therefore, the practice will need to do some marketing, either minimal, as in telephone quotations of fees, or aggressive, in the form of media advertising. Professional marketing is discussed in Chapter 6.

Fee setting — the bottom line

Our recommendations incorporate the cost-plus method as the basic structure. Its advantage addresses the issue of what the service should be worth to the client in a manner that is equitable to the client. The difficulty in developing the first fee schedule is considerable when there is no history of what type and frequency of services will be performed by a particular practice. In this case, contact with local colleagues will be helpful in determining the character and types of service fees that an area uses. Once a fee schedule has been created based on this system, it is relatively easy to modify by reviewing data of what services have been performed and the monies generated. The fee schedule can thus be changed as necessary. Superimposed on the cost-plus method must be an appreciation of both the colleague-based and the client-based systems. Fees must be modified to fit the competitive environment.

With any method there will be client complaints about fees. If the complaints are numerous, one can presume the fees are out of the competitive environment. If fees become a major issue between a practice and its clients, it is necessary to reconsider the fee schedule. The major problem is the difficulty involved in assessing objectively the importance of client complaints. It is human nature to be overly sensitive to the one or two who scream loudly and apply this to an assessment of the overall issue; however, it is important to maintain a proper perspective.

□
Maintaining fees

The practitioner needs to review fees at least annually and preferably twice a year to ensure they are within competitive ranges, generating adequate cash flow, and equitable. By reviewing the price list at least twice a year, the veterinarian can make necessary adjustments on a timely basis. To appropriately assess whether fees are adequate, it is necessary to have an ongoing set of records to determine whether current profitability is meeting preset goals. The practice accountant or financial adviser should be asked for an assessment of the practice's financial position. It is also important to have the discipline of reviewing fees at least twice a year to consider other aspects of how fees must be set. It may be necessary to adjust fees owing to changes in either the macro- or microenvironment of the economy. For example, those practitioners in the Sunbelt may have recently seen an influx of upper- middle-income people such that their environment will allow for a higher fee structure, whereas others in economically depressed areas may notice that any increase in fees will profoundly decrease their practice volume. Another reason is to force reevaluation of expectations. It may be that previously set financial goals are too optimistic and need to be reevaluated. Further, it is important to review fees frequently because costs change in a continuous rather than a discontinuous manner. Finally, the competitive environment is always in flux, and changes in competition, whether based on price, number of practices, or number of pets, must be considered on a regular basis.

At the same time fees are reviewed, a service review—consisting of evaluating services to the client—should also be performed. Are the services up to date, and are they offered in a manner in which the client can readily obtain them? If problems exist, then the fees need to be adjusted or the service level changed. It makes little sense to reduce your fees to create an increased volume of service if the actual problem is that the services are not easily available to the client. The second area to evaluate is client service. Does your staff maintain a good attitude so clients feel well serviced? Do you have methods of contacting clients or potential clients to solicit their business? This might be in the form of a practice newsletter or annual vaccination reminders. These areas should be addressed as a function of the practice income and are appropriate to review on a semiannual basis.

□
Small claims court

Should a veterinary practice pursue an unpaid bill in either civil court or small claims court? The answer involves several considerations. First, what is the likelihood of recovering the fee? Consider not only the likelihood of *obtaining* a judgment but also the likelihood of *enforcing* a judgment. One must also consider the cost of obtaining a judgment at all. Clearly it makes little sense to spend $50 on a court action to recover a $10 fee, regardless of the principle involved. Another factor to be considered is the public relations aspect if a nasty, well-publicized legal battle ensues over the collection of a fee. What is the likelihood the resultant publicity will either aid or harm your

practice? Another matter to consider is how much staff time is going to be required to pursue the matter. Beyond this, one must also factor in the principle. If the veterinarian performs certain services, it is appropriate that he or she receive fair compensation. It may be individually worthwhile to pay to enforce this principle.

Legal actions initiated in civil court are rarely appropriate because the cost is usually significant. On the other hand, small claims courts will, for a reasonable cost, provide a venue. There is usually a maximum value that can be set on actions through the small claims courts, and each jurisdiction varies in the set amount (in New York, it is $1500). Most small claims courts work by having the plaintiff file an action with the court, declaring their complaint, and having that complaint served upon the defendant. Some jurisdictions do not require a court officer for service, so serving can be done by the complainant. There is usually a small fee charged for the service. A court date will then be set and the parties summoned. In many jurisdictions the court will, at this point, ask whether the complainant and the defendant are willing to submit to arbitration rather than insist on a formal small claims court hearing. We recommend that arbitration usually be bypassed because the arbitrator is duty bound to mediate and therefore may hesitate to award a full judgment.

When going before the court, the veterinarian stands as an acknowledged expert. If the defendant claims malpractice, it is the responsibility of the defendant to prove malpractice occurred. Thus, expert testimony must be provided by another veterinarian. When a client is taken to court, however, it must be remembered that there is typically some sympathy for the defendant if anything went unfavorably during treatment. That is not to say one should not proceed, but it is incumbent upon the practitioner to explain fully and clearly to the court the difficulties involved in the treatment regimen so there remains no doubt as to the appropriateness of the therapy rendered. Once the testimony is heard, the court passes a judgment. The next step, enforcing the judgment, varies by jurisdiction and can be unpleasant. In most cases, defendants will pay the judgment in a reasonable manner. When dealing with an unreasonable person, the services of a sheriff or further legal maneuvers may be necessary to collect the judgment.

What if the veterinarian becomes the defendant in a small claims action? Typically the allegation will be malpractice, which may result from the client's perception that the fees were excessive for either the treatment rendered or the result. It is important when explaining a treatment to a client that the veterinarian not suggest a guaranteed result. Assuming the absence of a guarantee, then the response in court is easy. One problem may be that when served with a complaint the insurance carrier would prefer to settle out of court. If this happens the carrier's case information and judgment should be questioned. When a practitioner chooses to defend, it is best to go "by the court" rather than through arbitration because the veterinarian is the established medical authority. If the complainant fails to produce expert testimony, the veterinarian's opinion will stand as the statement of medical fact. This is not necessarily true with an arbitrator.

An important aspect of the legal procedure in either case is to have adequate documentation available of both the medical treatment and the associated fees. When the fee estimate has been raised during treatment, it would be important to document that the client was informed of or agreed to the revised fee estimate. This information ideally should be located in the medical record. Chapter 15 provides a more in-depth view of veterinary medicine and the law.

Communicating fees to clients

Receptionist – client interaction

Communicating the essentials of a fee structure to animal owners requires the involvement of several persons so that it is done harmoniously, all or nearly all fees owed are collected, and both client and practitioner are satisfied without adverse effects on business. Fundamental is the intention of the practitioner in desiring or requiring his staff to be as specific as possible. A set of clear ground rules should be decided on, distributed in written form, and understood fully by the staff members responsible for communicating information on fees.

The successful delivery of information on fees involves primarily the necessity of creating the perception of optimal value, integrity, and clarity. It is one thing to be deliberately vague about the cost of any service and quite another to be faced with estimating a charge over the phone or in casual conversation without the benefit of examination and diagnosis. Support staff must be cautioned *not* to attempt a diagnosis over the phone. The staff must be clear on the specific boundaries of medical information.

Veterinarians must create broad practice guidelines to allow receptionists and telephone assistants to quote fees, estimates, and revisions of estimates accurately. Included in this is the need to explain why certain procedures justify a specified fee. The veterinarian would do well to review with reception personnel a variety of procedures and the steps involved so the receptionist is better prepared to elaborate with a skeptical client. There should be no hesitation on any staff member's part to fully describe the time and number of professionals involved in an animal's care. The general nature of "behind-the-door" practice, which for most owners creates a fear of the unknown, can thus be overcome, and the client will usually be willing to pay for services rendered. The clearer the picture presented, the easier it will be to collect the fee.

Doctor–client interactions

Discussion about fees delivered with power and clarity are easier for the client to accept. Inherent in the successful delivery of fee information is the requirement that the veterinarian be perceived as worthy of his fee. Delivery depends upon such factors as confidence, experience, forcefulness, sincerity, and belief in the value of the services. Written estimates detailing the services involved will further clarify clients' inherent resistance to fees.

Ongoing communication

The frequent and timely delivery of fee information in person or by telephone is critical to the successful collection of fees.

Estimates, estimate revision, and admission agreements

Written and oral fee estimates (Figs. 11-2 and 11-3) and their revision constitute a common component of fee assessment, fee statements, and fee collection. Professional services may be categorized as routine, semiroutine, nonroutine, emerging, planned, or unplanned. The more consistent and predictable the service (e.g., vaccination, nail trim, anal gland expression), the easier it is to establish a specific fee that can be generally adhered to. A less predictable set of circumstances involves services rendered for chronic diseases and disorders with less clear prognoses (e.g., heart failure, renal failure, coma, hindlimb paralysis) and for animals whose owners are willing to attempt limited treatment, commit to only a specific length of treatment, or set financial

ceilings. Unless the lines of communication remain open, ever-changing estimates for ill-defined diseases and those with unclear outcomes will create tension and anxiety among owners who perceive altered diagnostic and prognostic states as somehow dishonest or fraudulent. Clients generally believe and hope for lower fees and a better outcome but become anxious when this is not the case.

Diseases or conditions that do not follow the expected course are the rule rather than the exception. Revising the estimate according to guidelines and before the initial estimate proves no longer valid will create a greater sense of integrity. Estimate revisions should also specify a period of time during which tests and treatments are performed and results observed.

The incremental approach to treatment through financial estimates that are regularly revised is a standard practice at The Animal Medical Center. Fee averaging to account for highs and lows of certain treatments and services is a common technique in human medicine. So-called diagnosis-related groups (DRGs) have established costs for each of hundreds of treatments and diseases. The theory behind the DRGs reflects that nearly all diseases and injuries have a wide range of presentations, courses, outcomes, and complications. The fees are based on averages worked out over long periods of time within many human health care settings. Veterinary medicine does not yet have broad-based third-party reimbursement systems with which to create an accurate portrayal of the high, average, and low costs of sufficient numbers of cases to compose accurate DRGs. Additionally, there is an inherent unfairness in asking people to pay more or less than the actual cost. It must also be remembered that euthanasia is always an option in veterinary practice.

In reviewing a series of 1000 consecutive estimates made for pets hospitalized at The Animal Medical Center during 1985, we found

ADMISSION DEPOSIT WORKSHEET

DATE:_____

SERVICE:_____

DR._____

HOSPITAL PAYMENT POLICY:

1. Payment for clinic services prior to hospitalization must be paid before you admit your pet.
2. Fifty percent (50%) of the initial hospital estimate must be paid when you admit your pet.
3. The balance of the hospital invoice must be paid when you pick up your pet.

(A) OUTPATIENT SERVICES (PRIOR TO ADMISSION):

Examination	$_____
Vaccinations, ECG, Xrays, etc.	$_____
Other	$_____

PAYMENT FOR SERVICES ALREADY RENDERED IS NOT PART OF THE HOSPITAL ESTIMATE

AND IS DUE IMMEDIATELY . . . . $ _____

(B) TRAUMA ESTIMATE or INITIAL IN-PATIENT WORKUP ($350.00) — $200.00 DEPOSIT REQUIRED $ _____

An estimate for additional diagnostics and therapy will be given to the client upon completion of in-patient work-up.

(C) INITIAL ESTIMATE FOR TREATMENT IN THE HOSPITAL BASED ON PRELIMINARY EXAMINATION:

Hospitalization:_____ Ward_____ ICU $ _____

Diagnostics:
Radiology. . . . . _____
Initial Laboratory Screen (SMA, CBC, U/A, Fecal, FelV, Heartworm, Cytology) . . . . _____
Repeat Laboratory Tests. . . . . _____
Other Tests (EKG, EPH, Coag, Bone Marrow, Microbiology, Serology) . . . . _____
Special Procedures (Endoscopy, Special Radiology, Enema, CSF/EEG, EMG,
    Echo, U/O, Skin Test) . . . . _____

NOTE: DIAGNOSTICS MAY HAVE TO BE REPEATED WHILE PET IS IN THE HOSPITAL.

Treatment:
Drugs (Injectible and/or oral). . . . . _____
Fluid Therapy . . . . _____
Jugular Catheter . . . . _____
Surgical Procedure (plus anesthesia and fluids) . . . . _____
Pathology . . . . _____
Consultation . . . . _____
Other . . . . _____

Initial Estimate $ _____

DEPOSIT (Including Fees for Outpatient Services) . . . . $_____

THIS IS AN INITIAL ESTIMATE BASED ON THE ADMITTING DOCTOR'S PRELIMINARY FINDINGS. THIS IS NOT A BILL. ADDITIONAL DIAGNOSTIC STEPS AND TREATMENT PROCEDURES WILL BE ORDERED AT THE DISCRETION OF THE DOCTOR IN CHARGE. THESE ADDITIONS WILL INCREASE THE ABOVE ESTIMATE.

RECORD COPY   _____
Client's Signature

Figure 11-2. Admission deposit worksheet

ORANGEWOOD ANIMAL HOSPITAL, P.C.
7147 N. 7th STREET • PHOENIX, ARIZONA 85020
602/997-6313

JOHN D. CLARK, D.V.M.

OWNER _____

PET NAME/DESCRIPTION _____

CHANGE/NEW _____

DATE _____

CLIENT # _____

PHONE # _____

PROFESSIONAL SERVICES	CD	FEE
CONSULT./EXAMINATION	101	
PEDIATRIC EXAMINATION	102	
GERIATRIC EXAMINATION	103	
VACCINATION EXAMINATION	104	
MULTIPLE ANIMAL EXAM.	105	
AVIAN/EXOTIC EXAM.	106	
EXTENDED CONSULTATION	107	
RE-CHECK EXAM./CONSULT.	108	
REPRODUCTIVE CONSULT.	109	
ORTHODONTAL CONSULT.	110	
CARDIOLOGY CONSULT.	111	
RADIOLOGY CONSULT.	112	
SPECIALIST PHONE CONSULT.	113	
	114	

IMMUNIZATION	CD	FEE
CANINE DA2PL WITH PARVO	201	
CANINE DA2PM WITH PARVO	202	
CANINE RABIES	203	
CORONA	204	
BORDETELLA	205	
FELINE C.R.P.	206	
FELINE RABIES	207	
FELINE LEUKEMIA	208	

MEDICATION	CD	FEE
1. INJECT.	301	
2. INJECT.	301	
	302	
1. Rx	303	
2. Rx	303	
3. Rx	303	
4. Rx	303	
Rx DIETS:	304	

RADIOLOGY	CD	FEE
1st PLATE	401	
ADDITIONAL PLATES	402	
O.F.A.	403	
SKULL/G.I./U.G. SERIES	404	
MYELOGRAM	405	
INTRAVENOUS PYELOGRAM	406	
MEDIA/SUPPLIES	407	

ANESTHETIC	CD	FEE
I.V./INHALANT GENERAL	501	
LOCAL	502	
PRE./POST ANESTH. DRUGS	503	
SEDATION	504	

SURGERY	CD	FEE
1.	510	
2.	510	
3.	510	
SURGICAL ASSISTANT	511	
SURGICAL ROOM	512	
PACKS/SET UP	513	
DISPOSABLES/SUPPLIES	514	
HEART MONITOR	515	

DENTISTRY	CD	FEE
ULTRASONIC SCALE/POLISH	520	
EXTRACTIONS	521	
DENTAL/ORAL SURGERY	522	
GING./PERI. CURETTAGE	522	
ORTHODONTIA	523	
APPLIANCE ADJUSTMENT	524	
SUPPLIES/APPLIANCE	525	

LABORATORY	CD	FEE
SAMPLE COLLECT./PREP./EVAL.	601	
LAB FEE	602	
LAB FEE	602	
CBC/WBC/HT/T.P./U.A.	603	
FECAL O & P	604	
GIARDIA DIAGNOSIS	605	
SKIN SCRAPING(S)	606	
FUNGAL CULTURE	607	
HEARTWORM DIAGNOSIS	608	
FELINE LEUKEMIA ELISA	609	
BRUCELLA CANIS P.T.	610	
SEMEN EVALUATION	611	
VAGINAL CYTOLOGY	612	
ADRENAL-PIT. AXIS PROFILE	613	
T.S.H.-STIMULATION	614	
	615	

MEDICAL SERVICES	CD	FEE
EAR TREAT/CLEAN/FLUSH	701	
EAR TAPE	702	
ECZEMA/CLEAN/TREAT	703	
ANAL GLAND EXP./PACK	704	
ARTIFICIAL INSEMINATION	705	
SPLINTS/CASTS/DRESSINGS	706	
ELECTROCARDIOGRAM	707	
URINARY TRACT CATH.	708	
BONE MARROW ASPIRATE	709	
TREATMENTS	710	
ENDOSCOPY	711	
BIOPSY	712	
NECROPSY	713	
	714	

HOSPITAL CARE	CD	FEE
WARD CARE/SANITATION	801	
DAILY PROF. CARE	802	
NURSING CARE	803	
OXYGEN THERAPY	804	
FLUIDS	805	
BLOOD TRANSFUSION	805	
INTRAVENOUS CATHETER	806	
1. INJECT.	807	
2. INJECT.	808	
ORAL/TOPICAL MEDICATION	809	
GASTRIC ALIMENTATION	810	
SPECIAL DIETS	811	
SPECIAL EQUIPMENT	812	
DISPOSABLES/SUPPLIES	813	
	814	

MISCELLANEOUS	CD	FEE
TICK & FLEA DIP	901	
MANGE: MED. BATH/DIP	902	
MEDICAL GROOMING/BATH	903	
NAIL TRIM	904	
ANAL GLAND EXP.	905	
HEALTH CERT./CLERICAL	906	
EQUIPMENT RENTAL	907	
EUTHANASIA/AFTER CARE	908	
INDIVIDUAL CREMATION	909	
	910	

METHOD	CD		RECORD OF PAYMENT	
CASH	1	5	TOTAL CHARGES	
CHECK	2	6	CREDIT/PREV. B.	
CARD	3	7	TOTAL DUE	
	4	8	PAYMENT	
CH#		9	BALANCE DUE	

Figure 11-3. Fee estimate sheet

that nearly 90% required revisions at some point because the center's staff of nearly 70 veterinarians made estimates that were usually too low. Perhaps we live in hope the disease or injury will improve quickly. A written admission agreement is of value and is used on each of our admissions (Fig. 11-4).

□
Collection

Cash and credit cards

Cash clients constitute the bulk of clinic revenue. For example, we hold a vaccination clinic on Saturday with slightly lower rates for vaccinations and examination. This clinic encourages payment by cash in consideration for the slightly lower fees. These clients are extremely price conscious and will shop around for a private veterinarian or clinician who offers routine outpatient services at a bargain price. In contrast to credit card payments, cash payments do not involve paying a service charge to the bank. On the other hand, clients who pay by credit card will more readily request additional veterinary services. Although the interest rate is high for the privilege of using a credit card, clients do have a 28-day billing cycle between the time the charges are incurred and the bill is received. This enables the client to plan out a payment schedule.

Whenever possible the veterinarian should encourage full payment of all services at the time service is rendered. When full cash payment (cash, check) is not possible, then the client should be encouraged to use credit cards. A credit account should only be used after extensive exploration of various methods of cash payment.

Credit

The Animal Medical Center collects nearly 93% of all fees charged. Clients are extended credit considerations when a large bill is incurred or extensive treatment is required. Each veterinary practice should create a policy for payment to include basic rules and exceptions. Categories of payment, including deferred payment, "gold card" holders, and preferred billing, should be established and the ground rules written for reference.

The center does not encourage credit, but we accept that a client may be faced with a difficult situation when confronted with a large bill of several hundred dollars for a treatment period of 3 to 5 days. Because this is a sensitive subject with clients, we discuss terms and consider several factors (including the amount paid on admission) before determining a payment schedule of 30 to 90 days.

Large-animal practices are often in a position of waiting for payment until livestock or crops are sold. Every effort should be made to prevent the client from delaying payment.

The credit report and payment interview

The complexity of current veterinary practice requires that animals be admitted to the hospital for evaluations, tests, and treatments. The cost of such professional services is routinely high and can reach hundreds to thousands of dollars. The often unexpected nature of the illness or injury and the lack of preparation for payment require great skill in collecting all monies due while also maintaining concern for client and pet.

The credit interview at admission should take place in a quiet and comfortable place under the direction of a firm, knowledgeable, mature credit admissions officer. This person could be a receptionist, technician, administrative person, or other skilled individual who conveys sympathy, concern, knowledge, and firmness. The person responsible must be competent in creating a legitimate basis for hospital fees and the collection of monies from persons who routinely claim not to have

THE ANIMAL MEDICAL CENTER

ELLIN PRINCE SPEYER HOSPITAL ● CASPARY INSTITUTE

510 EAST 62ND STREET
NEW YORK. N.Y. 10021

ADMISSION AGREEMENT

TELEPHONE 838-8100

_____
DATE

_____
WARD/CAGE

_____
DR./SERVICE

DO NOT LOSE THIS AGREEMENT. IT MUST BE RETURNED WHEN THE ANIMAL IS RELEASED FROM THE HOSPITAL.

PERMISSION TO TREAT

The Client authorizes The Animal Medical Center to hospitalize the above-described animal and to render such medical and/or surgical treatment as the doctors deem necessary including diagnostic tests or procedures.

PAYMENT POLICY

The Client realizes that in many cases it is not possible to determine in advance the exact extent of medical or surgical treatment required for an animal. The Animal Medical Center will attempt to estimate the cost of the treatment but it is understood that the final cost may exceed this estimate, depending on the extent of treatment required.

The Client agrees to pay a deposit of at least 50% of the initial estimate ($_____) when the pet is admitted to the hospital.

The Client agrees to pay the balance of the fees due before the release of the pet from the hospital.

LATE CHARGES — In some instances, charges for services rendered in the hospital may still be in the processing stage when you pick up your pet. The Client agrees to pay for these services when a bill is received.

ABANDONMENT OF ANIMALS

The Client agrees to remove the animal within 3 days after a request for removal is made; the request may be made personally, by telephone, or by letter mailed to the Client at the above address. Should the animal not be removed within the specified time, the Client hereby relinquishes all claim to the animal and The Animal Medical Center is at liberty to make whatever disposition of the animal as it may see fit.

In the event of death of an animal, The Animal Medical Center will, unless otherwise instructed by the Client, arrange for the disposition of the body.

DISCHARGE HOURS:
Only Between 12 Noon and 9 P.M.
Every Day

BY _____
Client

FOR _____
Animal Medical Center

Figure 11-4. *Admission agreement*

such funds. Some pet owners assume, imply, or state that an animal as a living thing has a right or privilege to quick, efficient, and highly skilled care by the veterinarian and that such care be delivered irrespective of the owner's ability to pay. The admission officer must create a different reality—one that supports the humaneness in delivering required services but with the understanding that these services cannot be delivered without compensation and that veterinary medicine does not have adequate third-party sources of support. The reality of practice as a business and as a shared responsibility without guilt or fear will lessen the burden of such collections. The key issue is to determine who in the client–veterinarian relationship is responsible for what. As veterinarians and as deliverers of required services, we must be capable and willing to provide such a service—and owner-clients must be able and willing to pay.

Anxiety and fear are common occurrences if people delay or defer treatment. Guilt and anger become associated with the animal. Anger directed at the veterinarian, hospital policy, and credit interviewer is routine. Sympathy and compassion must be elements of the interview without allowing the financial burden to be shifted to the veterinarian. It is often helpful to have available for distribution a printed concise statement of the practice's policy of shared responsibility: the veterinarian provides the skill and care, and the owner provides the financial resources. New veterinarians often are confused about the assignment of responsibilities.

When people "cannot pay"

A daily routine issue in institutional practice is the pet owner who cannot pay or claims he cannot pay. Perhaps it is closer to the truth to say the owner *will* not pay or *chooses* not to pay. It is common for owners to believe professional services should be available regardless of the ability to pay, similar to the human model. Furthermore, such services should be at a high level and should continue for the required length of time. This view, although noble, totally ignores the issue of who must accept ultimate responsibility for the animal's disease or illness.

The veterinarian is usually unable to conduct a "means test" or income survey to gather information on the client's ability to pay. Therefore, practicing veterinarians must establish guidelines that will be applied to all regarding who will receive what services at a less-than-standard fee. Institutional practices are expected and thus routinely challenged to provide free or subsidized services. At The Animal Medical Center, several funds and guidelines for the use of these funds have been established to assist selected groups and individuals who require financial support (e.g., poor, aged, disabled, welfare recipients, clergy, medical professionals). Apart from these guidelines nearly all fees are collected. The policy relieves the veterinarian and credit interviewer from arbitrary decisions to lower fees for one individual over another.

Billing

Client accounts that are not paid as agreed become the responsibility of the center's in-house billing department. The collectors establish telephone contact with clients with 0- to 90- day accounts. The phone call is followed by a form letter or, if necessary, a specifically composed letter that details specific aspects of treatment and the charges involved.

Clients generally fall into one of three categories: (1) those who pay as agreed, (2) those who will not pay until a bill is received, and (3) those who agree to pay and do not.

We attempt to maintain our accounts receivable under 90 days and have been successful in referring accounts to the collection agency on a monthly basis.

Although carrying charges, or interest, can be added to the bill, we do not use this approach.

Accounts for 30, 60, 90 days

Our aging cycle is 90 days. Once the animals are discharged from the center, the records are referred to the in-house billing department. An itemized statement is sent to the client. If the client does not remit payment 15 days after our billing date, a telephone call is made. Often clients will have questions regarding the bills and will call with an explanation as to why accounts are not paid within 60 days. Accounts that are not paid within 120 days are referred to a registered collection agency.

Collection letters

How one communicates with clients by letter reflects the commitment to fee collection. A handwritten note attached to past-due bills will give the client a sense of personal attention. This is time-consuming, especially in a large practice or institution. Photocopies of form letters to past-due accounts will communicate that the practice is haphazard and impersonal. The care and gravity of the collection process reflects directly on the veterinary practice. The collection of practice funds is a professional responsibility.

If the practice has computer capability, using word-processing software will simplify communication. Letters with an increasingly serious tone can be composed and generated as the billing cycle progresses.

At The Animal Medical Center we have used the following communications, all of which can be easily revised:

Reminder notice at 30 days (Fig. 11-5)
Second reminder at 60 days (Fig. 11-6)
Final notice at 90 days (Fig. 11-7)
Payment notice sent on accounts for which we have made payment terms but where the client is slightly late in meeting payment (Fig. 11-8)
Late-charge letter sent after the account has been made passive and additional charges have been posted on the account (Fig. 11-9)
Bad check letter sent when the client's check is returned by the bank (Fig. 11-10)
Itemized statement used to set up all treatment charges and description at the client's request (Fig. 11-11).

Collection services

Unfortunately, an external collection service to collect fees may be required. The center uses two collection agencies to provide a comparison of results. Our results with outside agencies have been moderately successful, a reflection of careful selection, providing updated information, and close monitoring.

When considering the services of a collection agency, the practice should be provided with a sample of the techniques used. The external collection agency staff should be interviewed regarding the techniques, at which time fairness, professionalism, and humaneness should be stressed. Although collection agencies are regulated by law, their skills and techniques vary.

□
Conclusion

We have written a chapter to guide the reader in setting and collecting fees for services. This chapter contains information to enable the practitioner to create a structure within which

(Text continues on p. 216.)

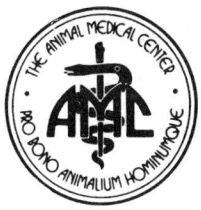

THE ANIMAL MEDICAL CENTER
SPEYER HOSPITAL AND CASPARY RESEARCH INSTITUTE

510 EAST 62ND STREET
NEW YORK, NEW YORK 10021
212 - 838-8100

Dear Client:

    We recently wrote you regarding your delinquent
account. Assuming this may be an oversight on your part,
we are allowing an additional 15 days' grace before taking
further action.

    When making payment, please remit the full balance
shown and mark it to my attention.

AMOUNT DUE   _____

CASE #   _____

ACCOUNT #   _____

                 Sincerely,

                 Ms. Matatha F. Jemison
                 Collection Department

Figure 11-5. Thirty-day reminder notice

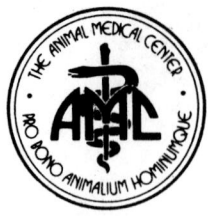

THE ANIMAL MEDICAL CENTER
SPEYER HOSPITAL AND CASPARY RESEARCH INSTITUTE

510 EAST 62ND STREET
NEW YORK, NEW YORK 10021
212 – 838-8100

Dear Client:

    There remains an unpaid balance on your account. Please give this matter your immediate attention.

    When making payment, please remit the amount shown and mark it to my attention.

AMOUNT DUE   _____

CASE #   _____

ACCOUNT #   _____

        Thank you,

Matatha F. Jemison

        Ms. Matatha F. Jemison
        Collection Department

Figure 11-6. Sixty-day reminder notice

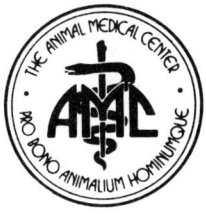

THE ANIMAL MEDICAL CENTER

SPEYER HOSPITAL AND CASPARY RESEARCH INSTITUTE

510 EAST 62ND STREET
NEW YORK, NEW YORK 10021
212 - 838-8100

Account No :
Case   No :
Balance Due:

FINAL NOTICE

Dear Client:

The Animal Medical Center is a nonprofit Animal Care
facility. Our business is not to make money for personal
profit, but rather, to provide a full-service veterinary
hospital open 24 hours a day delivering the highest
standards of veterinary care.

The cost of such a facility is high--much higher
than what our fees can cover. We are asking of you what
is only fair--to pay your long-overdue account. We require
your full payment of the balance shown above. If we do
not receive your payment, we shall have no alternative
but to turn the matter over to our collection agency.

We hope to keep the doors of The Animal Medical Center
open to you for future need. This is why we urge you to
fulfill your financial commitment for services provided.

Sincerely,

Carmen Rodriguez
Collection Manager

Figure 11-7.   Ninety-day reminder notice

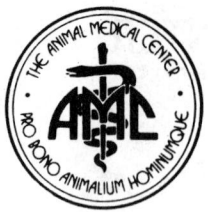

THE ANIMAL MEDICAL CENTER
SPEYER HOSPITAL AND CASPARY RESEARCH INSTITUTE

**510 EAST 62ND STREET
NEW YORK, NEW YORK 10021
212 - 838-8100**

Dear Client,

We have not received your payment for the month

of _____. This may be just an over-

sight on your part. If this is the case, please take care

of this matter immediately.

If your payment has been sent, please disregard

this letter.

TOTAL BALANCE DUE _____

ACCOUNT # _____

CASE # _____

Sincerely,

Matatha F. Jemison

Ms. Matatha F. Jemison
Collection Department

Figure 11-8. Late-payment notice

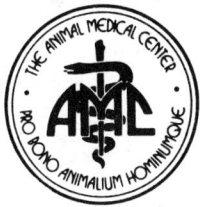

THE ANIMAL MEDICAL CENTER
SPEYER HOSPITAL AND CASPARY RESEARCH INSTITUTE

510 EAST 62ND STREET
NEW YORK, NEW YORK 10021
212 – 838-8100

Dear Client,

    Please be advised that an additional charge has been charged to your bill. The services were rendered to your pet while in the hospital. But, the vouchers were not received by cashiers for posting until a later date.

    We are sorry for any inconvenience we may have caused you.

Amount Due   _____

Charge For   _____

Case #   _____

Account #   _____

Total Amount Due   _____

Sincerely,

Matatha F. Jemison

Ms. Matatha F. Jemison
Collection Department

Figure 11-9. Additional late-charge notice

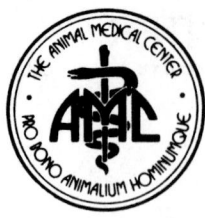

THE ANIMAL MEDICAL CENTER
SPEYER HOSPITAL AND CASPARY RESEARCH INSTITUTE

**510 EAST 62ND STREET
NEW YORK, NEW YORK 10021**

212 – 838-8100

Dear Client:

     Your check of _____, in the amount of

$_____, was returned to us marked _____.

     This is a serious matter. Unless you contact us or

submit $ _____ by money order or certified check

within ten (10) days of this notice, you will leave us no

choice but to refer your account to our collection agency

for immediate action.

Amount Due _____

Case # _____

Account # _____

                              Sincerely,

                   Matatha F. Jenison

                    Ms. Matatha F. Jemison
                    Collection Department

Figure 11-10. Returned-check notice

THE ANIMAL MEDICAL CENTER
ELLIN PRINCE SPEYER HOSPITAL • CASPARY INSTITUTE
510 EAST 62nd STREET
NEW YORK, NY 10021
TEL. NO. (212) 838-8100

Kay   Dr. William,
510 E 62nd Street
New York, NY 10021

Acct. No.: 5225768
Case No.: 35-87-68
Code: Employee

Pet Name: "Stelly"
Species: Feline

Date of Admission: 8/27/86
Date of Discharge: 8/27/86

Clinic Dr. R/X
Hospital Service: O/P

Billing Date: 10/01/86

Posting Date	Service Date	Charge Code	DESCRIPTION	AMOUNT
9/24	9/24	2	Visit	38.00
9/24	9/24	19	Payment Visa	258.00-
9/24	9/24	103	Hospitalization	26.00
9/24	9/24	715	Treatment-urinary obstruction	20.00
9/25	9/25	103	Hospitalization	26.00
9/25	9/25	316	Lab-Feline Leukemia Virus	16.00
9/25	9/25	705	Drugs	6.00
9/25	9/25	708	Intravenous Catheter	15.00
9/25	9/25	710	Intravenous Fluid Therapy	6.00
9/26	9/25	705	Drugs	12.00
9/26	9/25	710	Intravenous Fluid Therapy	12.00
9/26	9/26	103	Hospitalization	26.00
9/26	9/26	305	Lab-Biochemical Profile	29.00
	9/26	710	Intravenous Fluid Therapy	12.00
	9/26	705	Drugs	12.00
	9/27	705	Drugs 02x	12.00
	9/27	711	Discharge Medication	11.20
	9/27	19	Payment Visa	21.20-

(Last Page)

This bill is payable upon receipt.
If there are any charges still in
the processing state, you will
receive a statement in the mail.

ESTIMATE	CHARGES	CREDITS
408.00	279.20	279.20-

BALANCE DUE .00

Figure 11-11. Itemized computer statement

he or she can develop a plan, philosophy, and written materials. All veterinarians — those with extensive practice management experience as well as those with minimal experience — should, if dissatisfied with their practice life as it relates to fee setting and collection, examine their true views toward professional fee setting, and in a larger sense, perhaps toward their professional life. This difficulty could serve to clarify the reality within which practitioners operate their practice. Eventually it will result in happier clients and a more promising and financially rewarding practice.

Chapter 12
□
Utilization of the veterinary technician

Robert A. Taylor

Veterinary technicians can enhance the quality of a veterinary practice. When used properly, they can perform many routine procedures that allow veterinarians to expand their professional services and abilities (Figs. 12-1 and 12-2).

There are now approximately 60 accredited animal technology programs, and they have placed some 9400 technicians in the field.[1-3] Unlike the early correspondence schools for veterinary technicians, the educational programs today are carefully regulated and provide an excellent education opportunity for young people. These programs are carefully scrutinized by the Committee on Animal Technician Activities and Training (CATAT), the official regulatory arm of the American Veterinary Medical Association (AVMA). For a program to be accredited, the same careful site visit, monetary scrutiny, and staff and educational review as provided for veterinary college accreditation are accomplished. The results reflect an increasing number of well-trained veterinary paraprofessionals.

Although some flexibility exists in various training programs, all accredited programs are required to teach an approved curriculum and provide documentation that the student can perform a broad range of required technical tasks. Unfortunately, there are still several mail-order home study programs that do not meet any AVMA accreditation requirements.

Initially when the technician concept was introduced, there was concern they might either displace veterinarians or offer competition. These concerns have not been realized. Most veterinarians recognize the skills and expertise of technicians and use them to augment, support, and enhance their practices. To

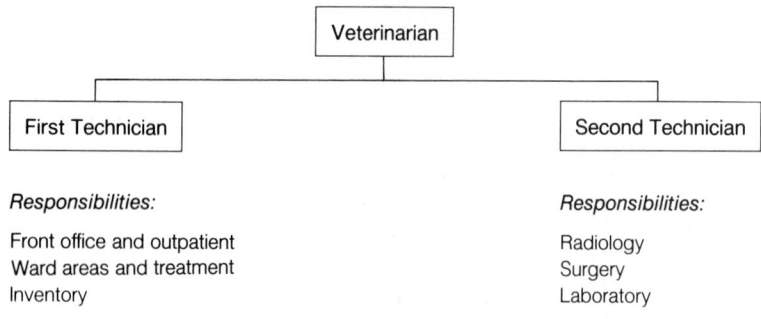

Figure 12-1. Flow chart for technician utilization in a one- or two-person practice

date 15,879 technicians have graduated from AVMA-accredited programs nationwide.[1-3] In spite of these numbers, there exists a growing need for technicians. Most programs are able to place their graduates in practice situations shortly after graduation. In 1985 there were 250 new graduates seeking employment, and there were over 1900 job openings on file with all programs.

□
Education of animal technicians

AVMA has established clear guidelines and educational requirements for accredited programs. It is largely due to these efforts that standardization and quality have prevailed.

The CATAT has established a list of required

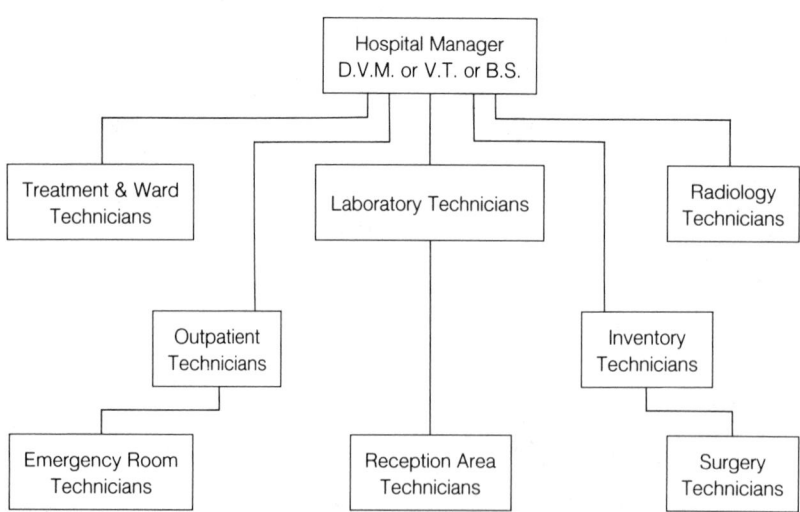

Figure 12-2. Flow chart for technician utilization in a multiperson practice

tasks that technicians must be able to perform. All accredited programs provide 2 years of college-level work. To meet the demands of veterinary practice, the technician must be skilled in handling all domestic species. Each accredited program submits an annual report detailing the number of graduates, job opportunities, number of instructors, and a yearly update on the existing program. Every 5 years a team of educators and members of the CATAT group conducts a site visit for the program to be fully accredited.

With the expanding number of technicians and increased awareness of continuing education, there are many educational opportunities for technicians at the local, state, and national veterinary meetings. Only a few states have mandatory continuing education requirements for recertification of veterinary technicians.

Each practice should provide for continuing education and in-house training for their technicians. Ideally, this should be on a yearly basis. As new skills or techniques evolve, they can be introduced to the technician, and in turn these skills can be used to enhance the quality of the practice.

□ Utilization of the technician

Technicians can be used in a practice to increase the quality of the practice as well as enhancing efficiency and greater productivity. In many practice situations a technician can be added in lieu of another veterinarian.[4] The use of a technician for routine support activities can prevent "burn out" of the veterinarian (Fig. 12-3). In the following section, recommendations for utilization of the technician in various areas of the hospital are discussed.

Reception area

With the increased awareness of the need for effective internal marketing, the role of the technician in the reception area can be vital to the growth and stability of a practice. Table 12-1 outlines a job description for a technician whose primary responsibility is the reception area and outpatient activities. Ideally, this person can interface with clients and help create a caring, considerate personality for the practice (Fig. 12-4). In some cases, clients can relate

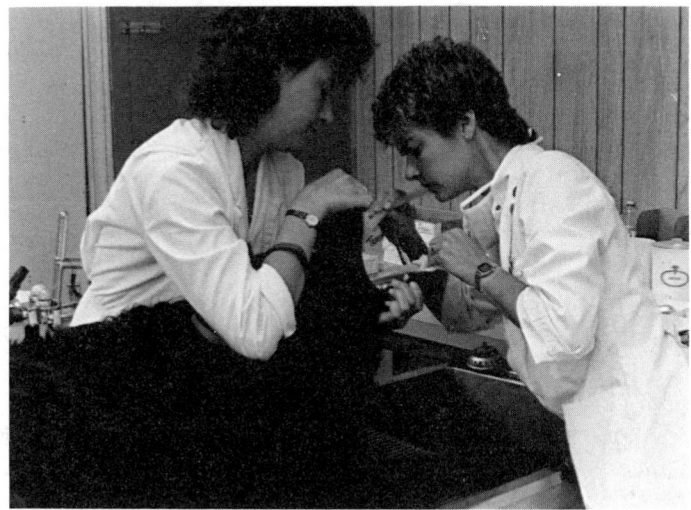

Figure 12-3. Technicians intubating patient before surgery

Table 12-1
Job description — outpatient technician

Ensure clients are handled in an efficient professional manner

Interface clients with doctors, for example, if one doctor is unavailable, to facilitate another doctor in seeing the client

Keep the exam rooms stocked and in neat and tidy order

Ensure the reception area and hospitality center are clean and neat

Answer questions regarding dietary management, parasite control, neutering, and so forth

Counsel clients with regard to outpatient care, home instructions, and medication administration

Help funnel bandage changes and suture removals into the treatment room to keep exam rooms free

Ensure that no one waits in an exam room for more than 3 minutes

Promote sales and activities in the hospitality center. Research and offer new and innovative products for sale in the hospitality center

Interface with all other supervisory technicians to ensure orderly, professional, and timely patient care

Coordinate all releases/inpatient information by maintaining the in-hospital log status sheet, e.g., animal name, doctor, diagnosis, progress report

Collate emergency room (ER) callbacks for ER doctors

Ascertain that all records have home care instructions, and if the doctor is unavailable, explain these to the client

Conduct daily callbacks and progress checks of discharged hospital patients

better and communicate more freely with a technician than the doctor.

In some practices, a reception technician helps market perscription diets and answers questions regarding neutering and behavioral problems and helps determine whether an animal should be presented for examination (Fig. 12-5).

Laboratory

The graduate technician is well versed in routine laboratory procedures. It is common for complete blood counts, culture and susceptibilities, stool analysis, and urinanalysis to be performed in the veterinary hospital. In-house service not only enhances the quality of service the hospital provides but helps speed treatment and diagnosis. In most instances in-house service can have a positive economic impact for the hospital.

With the availability of microsample computerized blood chemistry instrumentation, many large practices can provide in-house biochemical profiling. In several areas of the country a large practice may offer this service to other practitioners in the area. Most veterinarians use reference laboratory services for biochemical profiling, histopathology, and other sophisticated clinical pathology. Table 12-2 illustrates the respective tests for in-house and reference laboratory analysis. This table illustrates suggested areas of division between the laboratories.

Surgical support

Veterinary technicians can contribute considerable expertise and skill in the surgical theater (Fig. 12-6). Depending on the size of the practice, technicians may work exclusively in the surgical area or find themselves involved in this area only briefly each day.

Instrumentation and sterilization

Technicians are thoroughly trained in all aspects of instrument sterilization (Fig. 12-7). They are familiar with the care of most surgical instruments. In most practices that employ technicians, they are solely responsible for the care, setup, sterilization, and maintenance of the surgical instruments, sterilizing devices, and the surgical suite. They should also be responsible for maintaining the operating suite in a clean, aseptic fashion and should frequently monitor the cleanliness with periodic bacterial cultures.

Patient preparation

Preoperative preparation is an important part of any surgical procedure. It is helpful to have a written protocol so that patient preparation can be standardized.

In most instances, the technician does a more thorough job of clipping the surgical site and preparing the surgical area (Fig. 12-8). The veterinarian may become somewhat lax in routine preparation of the surgical patient due to mental distractions from other more pressing cases. The technician may be responsible for patient preparation and positioning as well as setting up the surgical instruments, gowns, and gloves for the surgeon. The technician may then also be responsible for circulating and monitoring anesthesia (Fig. 12-9).

Surgical assistance

The veterinary technician is well trained to provide assistance in the operating room.[5] An experienced, well-trained technician can anticipate the needs of the surgeon. This contrib-

(Text continues on p. 224.)

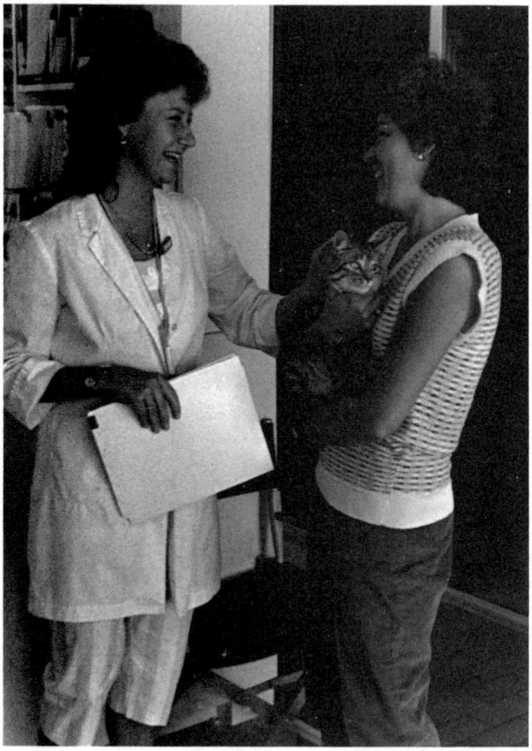

Figure 12-4. Technician offering home care instructions to client

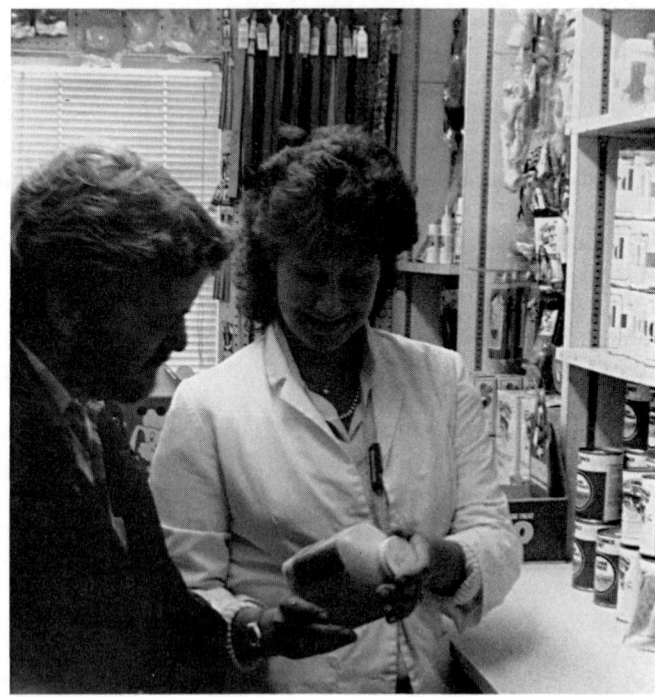

Figure 12-5. *A technician can enhance the profitability of a retail area*

Table 12-2
Suggested in-house tests

Complete blood count	Blood urea nitrogen
Felv	Sodium/potassium
Coagulation panel	Blood glucose
Prothrombin time	Coombs, direct
Partial thromboplastin time	CO_2 — blood gas analysis
Fibrinogen	Creatinine
Whole blood clotting time	Total bilirubin
Platelet count	Bromosulfalein dye excretion
Calcium	Urine analysis
Complete fecal	Knott's test
Brucellosis, slide agglutination	Aerobic/anaerobic cultures
test	Bacterial susceptibility
Fungal cultures	
Biochemical profiling	

Suggested Tests for Reference Laboratory

  Histopathology
  Biochemical profiles
  Special serological tests

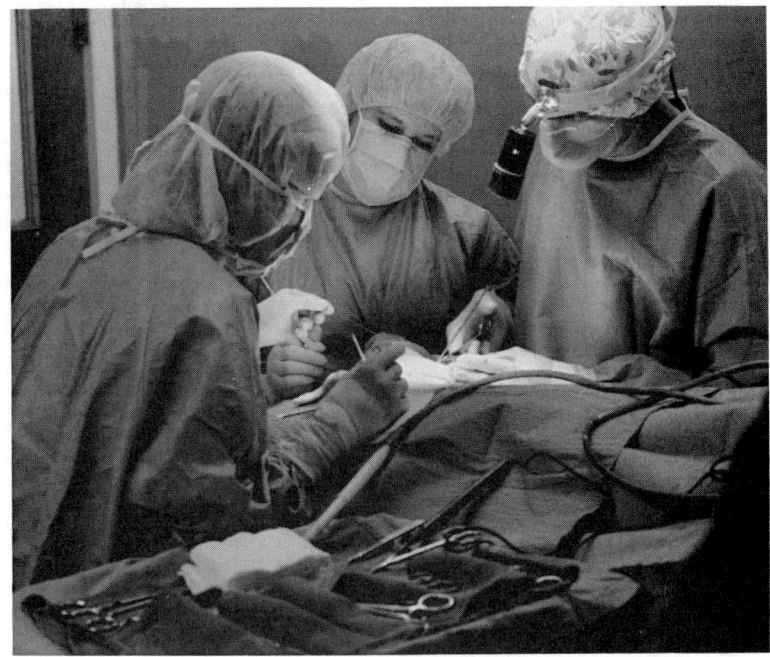

Figure 12-6. Technician assisting during major surgical procedure

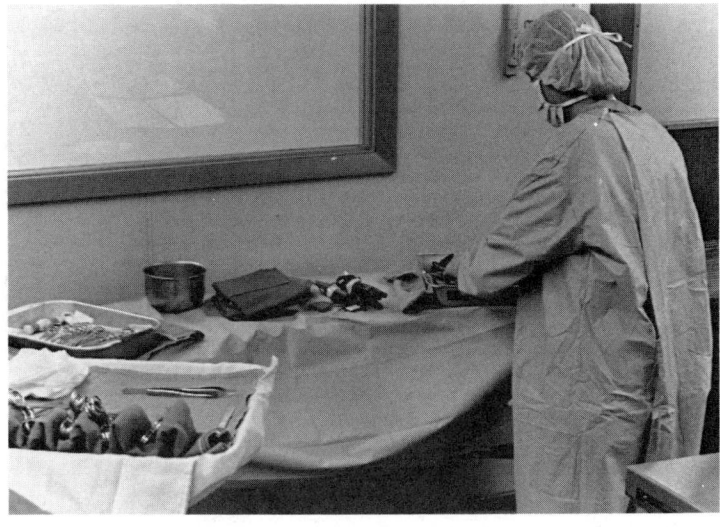

Figure 12-7. Technician setting up instrument table before surgery

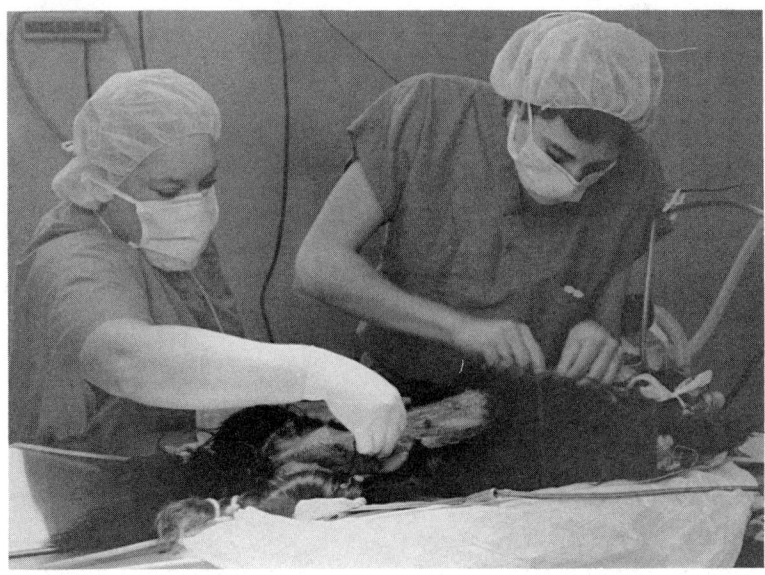

Figure 12-8. Final preparation before surgery

utes to time economy and improves operating efficiency and, in many cases, the quality of the procedure. The surgical assistant handles instruments, applies suction and lavage, applies hemostasis, handles tissues, cuts sutures, and helps manipulate instruments and tissues. Indeed, having a full-time surgical assistant is a luxury few veterinary surgeons experience.

Surgical follow-up

Technicians should be responsible for maintenance of the surgical log and records of drugs and supplies used during surgery. They should be encouraged to examine all postsurgical patients and report any abnormalities such as excessive hemorrhage or discharge,

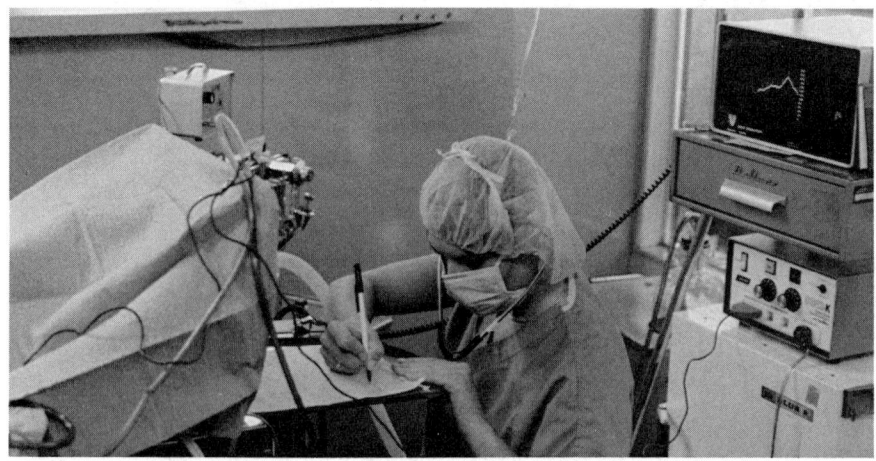

Figure 12-9. Technician monitoring anesthesia

gaping wounds, self-mutilation, and removal of drains or catheters. In many instances, technicians can remove sutures postoperatively. Technicians may also be helpful in performing telephone follow-up checks on all surgical patients.

Instrument preparation

The technician is responsible for cleaning and preparing all surgical instruments. They generally reassemble all surgical packs, arrange for their sterilization, and arrange them in the surgical area so they are readily accessible.

Table 12–3 illustrates a job description for a technician working full-time in the surgical suite.

Anesthesia

In many states, the Veterinary Practice Act defines the role of veterinary technicians with regard to anesthesia administration. Generally, they may administer preanesthetic and in some states anesthetics, but only with the vet-

erinarian physically present in the same room. All veterinary technology programs provide training in anesthesiology. It is curious that human anesthetists with 2 years of training routinely anesthetize thousands of people each day, but in many states veterinary technicians with similar training are prohibited from doing so for animals. In any case, veterinary technicians can make a real anesthesia contribution to their practices, employers and patients.

Technicians should conduct a presurgical evaluation of the patient. Body weight and temperature, pulse, and respiration (TPR) should be measured, drug dosages should be calculated, and general health should be assessed. The technician then may administer the proper preanesthetic drugs and assist or perform anesthesia induction. Intubation of the patient and anesthesia maintenance are important skills that can be developed. Monitoring of the patient by the technician may include TPR, direct or indirect blood pressure determinations, core body temperature, oscil-

Table 12-3
Job description — surgery technician

Cleanse, prepare, and sterilize all surgical packs, equipment
Complete aseptic preparation of OR before surgery and between cases
Position surgery patients on OR table
Perform aseptic skin preparation of the patient
Perform surgical preparation — clipping
Assist in surgery as sterile scrub nurse:
    Prepare sterile backup table and Mayo stand
    Prepare sterile instruments
    Gown/glove surgeon
    Assist surgeon with draping patient
    Assist surgeon by providing retraction of tissues, passing sterile instruments
Assist as nonsterile circulating nurse in OR
    Provide sterile items needed by sterile team
    Log biopsy tissue specimens and ensure delivery to the laboratory
Acquire orthopedic implants, specialty instruments
Prepare daily surgery schedule
Perform general maintenance of surgical equipment
Keep records — surgery report of items used in procedures

loscopic monitoring of cardiac activity, and assessment of the plane of anesthesia. In special procedures, operation of a respirator or collection of arterial blood for blood gas analysis may be necessary. It is important that these findings be charted frequently and recorded in the patient's permanent file. This ensures that accurate, precise anesthetic monitoring is conducted, and should problems arise, appropriate action can be taken and documented as part of the medical record.

Technicians can be very useful during the recovery process. Their presence ensures a quiet and peaceful recovery and allows for timely extubation, relief of pain, and a safe uncomplicated recovery. The era of placing a paddling, incoherent animal back in its cage unattended or allowing a horse to repeatedly bang its head on the floor is gone. The technician should remain with the patient until there is complete recovery.

Upon completion of anesthetic recovery, the technician should record the signalment, dosages, and drugs in the appropriate log books. They may be responsible for maintenance of a controlled substance (e.g., narcotics) log. Specific controlled substance requirements are discussed in Chapter 18.

Radiology

Radiographs are an important part of most diagnostic evaluations; they are used to monitor recovery or progression of disease and to help render a diagnosis. To fulfill these objectives, excellent-quality radiographs are a necessity. This responsibility usually is left to the veterinary technician. Technicians should be responsible for obtaining the radiographs and making sure that they are accurately labeled and that adequate protection against radiation both for themselves and others is provided. In many busy practices, 50 to 100 films are taken each day, and this repetition allows technicians to become very effective.

In addition to routine radiography, the technician can assist with or perform special radiographic diagnostic procedures. Contrast radiography with air, barium sulfate, or other contrast materials can be accomplished. In general, it is helpful to have a written hospital protocol for each special diagnostic procedure. In this way, each person's role is defined so that dosages and intervals of time are standardized. The technician can be helpful in more complex procedures such as myelography or arthrography by assisting the veterinarian.

The technician should be capable of either manual development of radiographs or the use of an automatic processor. Maintenance of developer and fixer integrity and minor troubleshooting on film quality are also helpful. In general, placing the developer or manual tanks on a routine cleaning and maintenance schedule helps ensure long equipment life and excellent film quality. Because radiographs are legally a part of the medical record, they should be carefully stored and filed. We recommend that films be kept at least 5 years. An efficient and simple filing system and log book should be maintained by the technician.

Treatment technician

Technicians can be very helpful in the ward area and the treatment room. Assigning these duties to one or several technicians will ensure that treatment is done on a regular schedule. For example, a regular time should be set up for four-times-daily medication (8 AM, 2 PM, 8 PM, 2 AM) to ensure that all inpatients receive their medication.

Careful monitoring of subjective and objective data can be helpful in both treatment and diagnosis. The veterinarian should be able to rely on the technician to perform these tasks.

In many hospitals veterinary technicians are responsible for supervision of the kennel staff or are involved in the routine maintenance of hospital cleanliness. They should understand the importance of cleanliness of the wards and patient. Learning by example can be very effective; therefore, if the veterinarian demonstrates concern for cleanliness and can show by example his concern for cleanliness, the message will be clear.

It has been demonstrated many times that compassion, touching, and gentle nursing care may alter the course of an otherwise fatal disease (Fig. 12-10). In no other place is this more evident than in the busy medicine and surgery wards of a veterinary hospital. Sick animals separated from their loved ones with no means of communication are subjected to numerous painful and frightening experiences. Bridging this gap and ensuring that the patient is nurtured, fed, nursed, and loved is the veterinary technician. Table 12-4 illustrates a suggested job description for in-hospital treatment technicians. Their technical training ensures that they are capable of inserting intravenous catheters, of safely administering drugs and fluids, and of providing the medical needs of hospitalized patients. It is recognized that the experienced technician may be better qualified than the new graduate in performing

procedures such as urinary and intravenous catheterization.[6]

In large veterinary hospitals and in some institutions, technicians may be solely involved in the care of critically ill patients. In practices where many animals are hospitalized, careful attention to detail and careful monitoring of vital signs can be invaluable. Technicians may also be involved in central venous pressure monitoring, systolic blood pressure monitoring, and electrocardiographic monitoring of critically ill or injured patients (Fig. 12-11).

The technician with primary ward and treatment room responsibilities can often alert the veterinarian to a hospital patient's rapid deterioration or crisis. Many times the veterinarian's time is monopolized by outpatients, surgery, and telephone calls so that he or she gets into the ward only once or twice a day. Animal owners appreciate knowing of an animal's progress, either favorable or unfavorable, as it occurs rather than being informed that "Cindy" was found dead in her stall or cage.

It is helpful to assign one technician the primary responsibility of charting the medical record. The medical record is often the veteri-

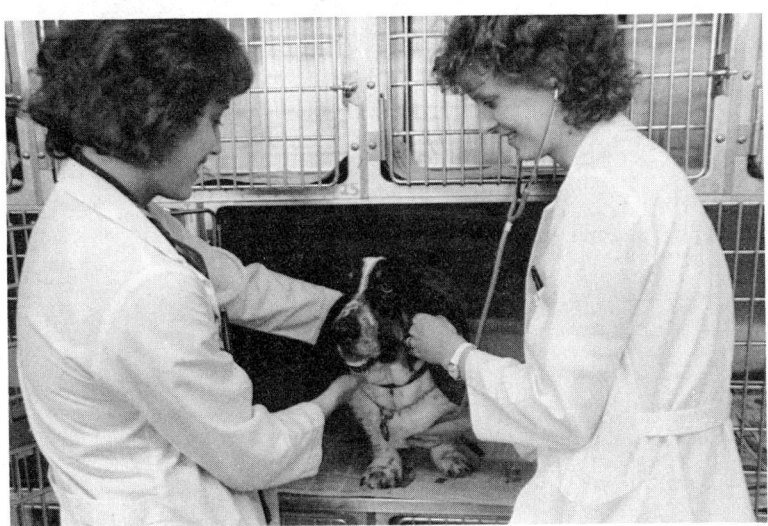

Figure 12-10. Technician providing hospital treatment

Table 12-4
Job description — in-hospital treatment technicians

Nursing Care

Administer fluid therapy
Provide physical therapy
Monitor food/fluid intake and bowel movements (BM)/urine
Manage diets (special diets, nasogastric feeding)
Administer drugs
Groom/bathe/trim nails on animals
Insert intravenous catheter
Provide isolation care

Kennels

Supervise maintenance/basic cleaning and feeding

In-hospital Case Records

Keep record of TPRs, hourly reports; BM/urine
Record weight
Assist with record of charges

Recovery/Intensive Care Monitoring

Monitor oscilloscope hookup
Monitor vital signs
Monitor capillary refill time

Transfusions

Collect/administer whole blood

Wound Management

Prepare and flush superficial lacerations and cuts and provide extended
nursing care of postoperative incisions, drains

Electrocardiograms

Perform and record electrocardiograms

Elementary Bandaging

Minor Procedures — Including Dental Prophylaxis

Bandage Removal and Suture Removal

Pharmacy

Type script, fill medications
Maintain drug stock, vaccines, bandaging material, crash cart
Record controlled substance use

Euthanasia/Disposal

Record outgoing cadavers, ash return, public health hold

Restraint

Perform venipuncture and procedures

Instrument Maintenance

Maintain cold tray, ultrasound, cryosurgical unit, oscilloscope, O_2 and
anesthesia machines

(continued)

Table 12-4
Job description — in-hospital treatment technicians (Continued)

Client Communication/Education
Administer home care as dictated by veterinarian
Provide basic education

Emergency Cases
Assist with resuscitation and emergency care

Injection Anesthesia
Assist with injectable anesthesia maintenance by monitoring vital signs

narian's chief defense in malpractice claims, and it should receive careful attention. Figure 12-12 shows a sample in-hospital record sheet. Places for problem identification, treatment, technician's notes (left column), and doctor's notes (right column) are illustrated. These records become a legal document, and all drugs, treatments, and observations should be recorded. Not only does this foster good pa-

tient care, but it helps the veterinary team avoid mistakes with medications, treatments, and nursing care.

Hospital management

Many technicians have had previous training in the business world. These people can be further trained to blend technical and business

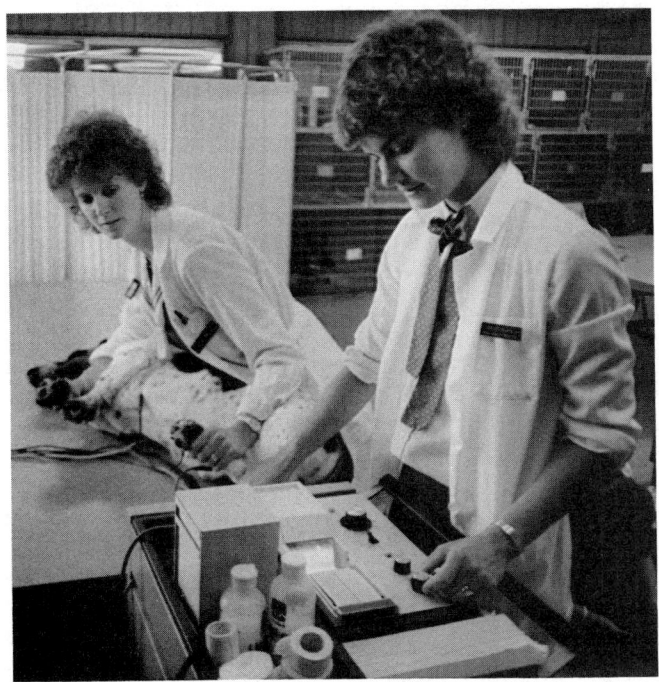

Figure 12-11. Technicians obtaining ECG information

PATIENT DAILY RECORD

PATIENT NAME: _____   DATE _____

PROBLEMS

1.
2.
3.
4.

TREATMENT

1.
2.
3.
4.
5.

COMMENTS

T	P	T	WT.	

Figure 12-12. Patient daily record

skills. In several cases technicians have been trained to perform all of the routine hospital management functions. They can be helpful in personnel management and recruitment as well as be trained to maintain financial and accounting records for the practice. It is advisable to gradually increase their level of responsibility because this position must be built on trust, reliability, and confidentiality.

As the profession is thrust into the computer age, there are many computer vendors eager to train technicians and veterinarians in their use. The technician with technical training in computers can be a real asset in implementing computerization. We recommend that a practice carefully evaluate its needs and have a good manual system in place before computerization. Computerization cannot be expected to solve unresolved problems such as poor record keeping, lack of financial accountability, and omission of data.

An effective reminder and recall system can be invaluable to a practice. Most people appreciate a telephone call or postcard to remind them that their animal is due for its annual vaccinations, physical examination, or dental examination. A technician working in the hospital management area can be very helpful in maintaining the recall system. In some hospitals a technician calls all owners the day after their animal's discharge from the hospital. This very personal service is usually deeply appreciated by the client and can be an excellent practice builder.

Newsletters are becoming an important way to keep in touch with veterinary clientele. A properly written newsletter helps clients understand their animals and their problems. It also lets the client know about the support staff that is available to provide quality animal care. In reviewing a recent newsletter, three of the four articles were written by veterinary technicians. Newsletters, client follow-up phone calls, and reminder cards are all forms of internal marketing that can be done by the techni-

cian. Chapter 6 has additional suggestions concerning professional marketing.

Inventory control

In a busy veterinary hospital it is possible to receive 10 to 12 telephone calls from commercial salespeople and often that many visits each day. Veterinarians are often too busy or unwilling to hear of a vaccine special or be detailed about some new drug. The technician can not only meet and receive information from salespeople but do the ordering as well. In larger practices the information gleaned can be reported to everyone during weekly staff meetings.

With proper records technicians can allow the hospital to benefit from bulk purchases or special sales. By determining the quantity of intravenous fluids the practice used last year or the last 6 months, they might be able to negotiate a bulk price with resultant cost savings. For example,

> Lactated Ringer's solution (LRS) costs $1.52 per liter in quantities of 100 liters.
> LRS costs $1.25 per liter in quantities of greater than 500 liters.
> LRS costs $1.00 per liter in quantities greater than 1000 liters.

The practice used 1200 liters of LRS during the past 12 months. Allowing for growth, an order for 1500 liters of LRS is placed with the stipulation that each quarter, one fourth of the total be shipped and the practice billed as the fluids are shipped. This could result in a $780 saving ($0.52 \times 1500$ liters) to the practice as well as having fluids available when needed. The hospital inventory area would not be crowded with 1500 liters of fluids because the order is being divided into four shipments.

Another area in which technicians can effect costs savings is in the purchase of drugs. With their knowledge of pharmacology, technicians can help take advantage of generic drugs when purchasing for the hospital. Inventory control and management are discussed in Chapter 18.

Emergency room technician

In hospitals providing in-house emergency coverage or in group emergency room situations, the technician can play a vital role. In their capacity they must wear many hats— from receptionist to surgical assistant. It is crucial in emerging medical and surgical problems that the technicians be knowledgeable and energetic, possess initiative, and be able to "think on their feet." They should be able to provide laboratory support, radiology expertise, and a knowledge of anesthesia to work in the emergency arena. Table 12-5 illustrates a job description for an emergency room technician.

Bereavement and pet loss counseling

Understanding the loss and emotional pain one experiences with the illness, loss, or death of an animal is very important. Many times clients express their concerns to the technician. The technician can be very helpful in allowing people to discuss their loss and help them deal with it. A kind word or gentle hug can help overcome their grief. Technicians should receive training to help them deal with and understand death and loss. The Delta Society, dedicated to enhancing the human–animal bond, has excellent resource material and does conduct educational seminars on these subjects. A more complete discussion of patient death and dying is found in Chapter 16.

Table 12-5
Job description—emergency room technician

Reception Area

Greet clients, pull records, obtain history and perform preliminary physicals, answer telephones

Treatment Area

Monitor and administer nightly medications and treatments
Assist veterinarian in minor surgery
Assist in or perform bandaging, catheter placement, monitoring of vital signs

Radiology

Obtain standard radiographs
Assist with special procedures

Laboratory

Perform stat tests as needed

Surgery

Assist or administer anesthesia
Serve as surgical assistant
Monitor anesthesia
Circulate in operating room
Recover surgical patients

Continuing education needs

There are currently 12 states that have continuing education requirements for veterinary technician relicensure. Continuing education for technicians is important because it exposes them to new information and techniques and helps prevent "burnout." The large national veterinary conventions (AVMA, Western Veterinary Conference, Eastern Veterinary Conference, American Animal Hospital Association [AAHA], American Association of Equine Practitioners [AAEP]) all provide excellent continuing education programs for technicians. Veterinarians should underwrite the cost of these endeavors because their practices and patients directly benefit.

National and local technician associations

In 1982 the National Veterinary Technicians Association was formed; however, this association has not yet developed into an effective national organization. Such an organization would allow them to address the problems of state reciprocity, relicensure, certified vs. noncertified technicians, and a host of other problems.

Many local and state organizations sponsor continuing education programs, and the need for education forms the underlying foundation for the technician organization. Again, technicians should be encouraged to join or form these organizations because their increase in knowledge will mean the betterment of the practice and their profession. Strong support must come from the veterinary profession if the local, state, and national groups are to develop.

Legal consideration

Unfortunately there is little uniformity from state to state with regard to licensure, accreditation, or registration. Veterinarians should consult their state's practice act for clarification. It would seem logical that all states recognize the efforts of the AVMA CATAT and only certify, register, or license graduates from accredited programs. By doing this they can ensure that adequately trained professionals will be available.

Liability coverage relates to the individual states' practice act, but in general all agents or employees of the veterinarian fall under his liability blanket. The veterinarian is ultimately liable. The AVMA liability insurance coverage does provide for insurance protection for employees (i.e., technicians hired by the veterinarian and when the technician is acting on behalf of the veterinarian) when the veterinarian and technician are named in the litigation. If the technician is not acting on behalf of the veterinarian and is the only party named in the litigation, the AVMA liability coverage will not prevail. In today's litigious society, all members of the veterinary team should be aware and understand liability protection.

Guidelines for hiring and keeping a veterinary technician

Many times a veterinarian is faced with the decision of whether to hire a technician or instead a new associate veterinarian. In reaching this decision, careful consideration should be given to practice philosophy, expected responsibilities, goals of the practice, and the economics of the decision. In general, the addition of a technician allows veterinarians to expand their capabilities by as much as one half. It also allows for greater control of the practice but does not allow the added flexibility of days off or shared "on-call" duty. Once a decision is made to hire a technician, one should proceed in an orderly fashion for optimal results. A little time spent initially will pay maximum benefits later.

Job description and practice philosophy

A veterinarian should develop a detailed job description and list of duties the technician is expected to perform. It is best to have these duties presented in writing so as to avoid misunderstanding. If you are creating a new position, try to be flexible and imagine yourself having the time necessary to perform all of the required duties. Are the expectations realistic? It is helpful to jot down the practice philosophy. Since the new technician will be an extension of the veterinarian and his philosophy, it is important that both be compatible.

Salary package and benefits

As in any other situation, you usually get what you pay for. Some veterinarians are continuing to expect to hire technicians for $700 to $800 per month and have them work the hours they do with the same dedication and expertise. A fair starting salary will yield great rewards to the practice. If the practice offers such benefits as medical, dental, and eyeglass insurance, continuing education provisions, vacation allowances, credit union participation, buying club privileges, and pension or profit sharing plans, these should be explained to the prospective employee. Realistic expectations and a fair salary and benefit package will yield the greatest return to everyone.

Salary review and raises

It is helpful to decide in advance when salary reviews are to occur and how raises are deter-

mined. Most technicians respond well to merit incentives, and this is an effective way to provide raises. For example, technicians are informed that raises are determined on increased productivity, new ideas or innovations, and acquisition of new skills or responsibility. By informing them initially how raises are determined, they can set their goals accordingly. When there are several employees in a practice, it is helpful to have a formal review with each employee, to document their achievements during the past periods, and to project goals for their future performance.

Regular communication

For people to coexist and work as a team, regular communication is essential. Veterinarians often are too busy to listen and can only give instructions or orders. Veterinary students should receive instruction on personnel management and be taught to develop effective communication skills. By being an active listener you can eliminate many personnel problems (Fig. 12-13).

Hiring the veterinary technician

Once a decision is made to hire a veterinary technician, the veterinarian can contact the state or local veterinary organization, state or local technician organization, and AVMA-accredited technology programs to inquire about available technicians. The local paper or state and national journals may also be helpful.

Schedule enough time for interviewing so that the interview is not rushed or the potential employee kept waiting. The technician can make a tremendous impact on the quality of the practice, so *take adequate time* initially to inform them of performance expectations.

The technician should provide a well-written resume with references that can be con-

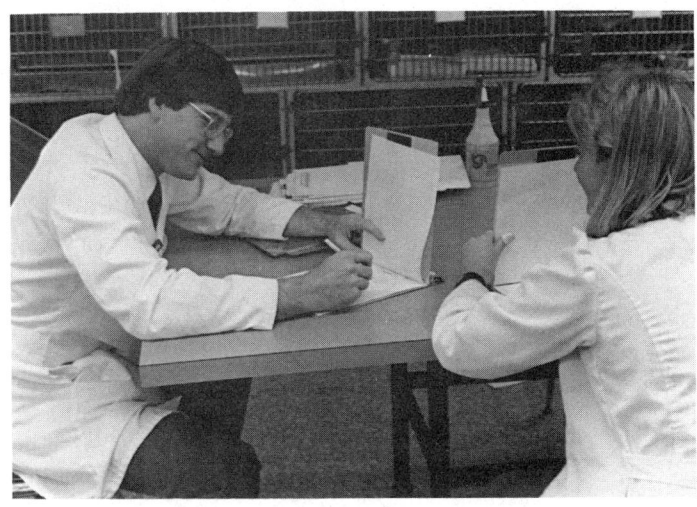

Figure 12-13. *Effective communication between veterinarian and technician is essential in quality patient care*

tacted. We advise contacting all references provided to allow a complete and accurate picture of the candidate.

Many times a prospective technician is invited to work a day in the practice so that both parties can become better acquainted. Once a decision is made to hire an individual, take the time to explain the salary, job description, and benefits that are provided.

In many cases an employment contract can be very helpful. Such a contract can be exercised after a 30- to 90-day trial period. This gives the employer the security of knowing that the employee will be there for the specified time, and the employee has the security of employment for that period. Chapter 3 contains a complete background in personnel management.

Summary

The use of technicians in veterinary practice is continually expanding. These professionals can bring enhanced quality and expertise to a practice. Their presence allows the veterinar-

ians to better perform the tasks for which they were trained, and the result is better patient care. Mutual trust and regular communication and realistic remuneration are prerequisites to a successful veterinarian–technician relationship.

References

1. Wise JK: Survey of accredited animal technology programs in the United States. Survey conducted between March 5, 1982, and April 29, 1982. Vet Tech
2. American Medical Association: Survey Compiled by Department of Scientific Activities, August 27, 1985
3. Lukens RL: Veterinary technician trends: A survey of Purdue graduates. 1982 survey of Purdue university graduates. Vet Tech
4. Reddig W: AHT's: More than pretty faces. Vet Econ 34, 1985
5. Mallard L: The role of the veterinary technician as surgical scrub nurse. Comp Cont Ed Tech 5, 1984
6. Childers HE: Animal technician. Vet Clin North Am 13:661, 1983

Chapter 13

☐

Improving professional effectiveness through time management

Ray L. Russell

The quality of a person's life is directly related to the control he has over the events of daily living. Efficient use of time is necessary in a veterinarian's life to meet the demands of practice, profession, family, and community. Learning to balance the demands for time is essential; otherwise practice life will be a stressful instead of a satisfying experience.

Have you ever wondered why you are able to accomplish more on some days than others? Often the days that are the busiest seem to go better than the slow days. Many times it is more difficult to complete the treatments and surgeries when the schedule is light than when the schedule is overbooked.

The answer is in Parkinson's law, which states: "Work expands to fill the time available for its completion."[1] To illustrate, assume one has 4 hours of surgery, treatments, and appointments but 8 hours to complete the work. It will nearly always take the full 8 hours. Conversely, if one has 8 hours of work and only has 4 hours to do it, a good portion of the work will be accomplished in the time available.

The secret of time management is learning how to use the time available and work on activities with the highest priority. Service is all veterinarians have to sell; therefore, selling services requires time. Bernard Baruch, the late statesman, said, "The person that can master time, can master nearly anything." Practice success is closely linked with the degree to which one can use time and control the events in daily life.

☐
Understanding time

Although it is often said, "Time is money," it would be more accurate to say "Time is life," because life is made up of time. Each person has 24 hours a day, and that is it! You cannot save it, you cannot store it, you can only spend it.

Two very important questions should be asked at the onset: What do you want more time for? and, How much more time do you want? So many people are caught in the activity trap. They are so busy that they do not have time to do the important things. The person desiring more out of a practice and their personal life should be constantly asking the following questions: What is my purpose? How effective am I? What can I do to improve? What have I actually accomplished today? Is this the thing that was the most important for me today?

□ Time management plan

Time management is developing the habits necessary to control the events in daily life. To control these events and improve productivity as a practitioner, it is important to break the subject down into major topics. The following five major topics will help organize your thinking and understanding of the subject a little more clearly: (1) developing a personal philosophy, (2) learning to focus, (3) developing specialized knowledge, (4) increasing energy and alertness; and (5) building a support team.

Understanding these five strategies and putting them into action will help add at least 2 extra hours to each day. The basic principles are the same for a large- or small-animal practice. Although this chapter will refer mostly to hospital practice, the ambulatory clinician can use the same techniques with minor modifications.

Research has demonstrated that using time effectively is the highest priority of hospital managers.[2] Even though the daily goal is to add 2 extra hours to personal effectiveness, it is entirely possible that a greater overall bene-

fit could result. Studies have confirmed that the majority of people operate routinely at less than 50% of their effective level. I have studied the subject over the past 30 years and have frequently observed people doubling their productivity by applying the principles outlined in this chapter.

Developing a personal philosophy

People have varied expectations in life, so it would be foolish to prescribe how a person should use his time. One practitioner may desire to increase income, whereas another may desire to improve the quality or quantity of practice. Still others desire more time off or the ability to control the hours of practice. Stages of practice and circumstances may alter the short- and long-range objectives. Therefore, the first step in initiating a time management program necessitates sufficient time in defining short- and long-range goals. Although most veterinarians may have some plans in mind, according to a study of veterinary managers, very few practitioners have written plans.[2]

The simplest way to make a written plan is to take four blank sheets of paper and list at the top of the first, "My Lifetime Goals"; on the second, "5-Year Goals"; third, "Annual Goals"; and last, "If I Were Bitten by a Rabid Dog and Expected to Be Dead in 3 Months, I Would Want to Accomplish the Following." On each sheet list eight to ten major things to be accomplished within the specific time frame. Subheadings such as practice, financial, physical, intellectual, family, social, spiritual, and so forth may be used to better organize and balance the various goals.

Do this now! Do not worry about doing it perfectly. Just do it! Compare your lifetime goals with the goals written on the sheet when supposing death in 3 months. This is the acid test to see whether your goals are congruent. If your lifetime goals are not similar to what you would do if you had only 3 more months to live, then sufficient thought has not been given to what is important in your life. After completing this first step, plan a 4- to 8-hour block of time for refining and improving the first draft. Even though this may seem like a lot of time, it is imperative to have a clear idea of what you will be spending your time doing.

These written objectives then bring into focus the priorities of life. They should be reviewed every day, and each day's activities should work toward these goals. Lifetime goals are accomplished by daily planning and sticking to the items that have been selected as the highest priorities.

Each year, the yearly goals should be reviewed and rewritten (updated). The lifetime, 5-year, and 3-month goals need only be redone about every 5 years. The secret is in spending sufficient thought in planning and putting into writing these goals. Even though this is a more simplified system than would usually be used in a corporate setting, it is adequate and can work miracles in both practice and personal life.

In addition, take one more sheet of paper and focus specifically on the more detailed practice goals such as What gross income do I want? How can I produce this gross? Am I satisfied with my net income? What specific steps can be taken to increase the net? What practice improvement ideas should be implemented this year? How much time off do I want? Specific goals regarding continuing education, facility improvement, staffing, and so forth should also be included.

What do these goals have to do with time management? The answer is that they are very important because personal philosophy and objectives will determine how time is used. This plan on paper is crucial to improved time utilization. Many people waste valuable time because of unclear objectives and goals. If the goals are not clearly stated and understood, it is difficult to prioritize and reach the specific

objectives. Therefore, clearly defining your own specific practice philosophy and setting goals is essential to planning and organizing your use of time.

Focus

The major problem with achieving goals is the inability to concentrate and focus. This results from the tremendous time demands in today's busy world. People fall into the time trap and become engrossed in activities that do not always lead to their goal. Each person has specific time wasters that rob his ability to concentrate on the most important project at hand.

Time wasters

All people have time wasters that prevent them from being as effective as they might be. To improve your ability to focus and get a job done, it is important to identify your personal time wasters. Some of the most frequent time wasters are telephone interruptions, drop-in visitors (such as pharmaceutical salespeople), failure to delegate, failure to plan, not setting priorities, managing by crisis, attempting to do too much, personal disorganization, failing to say No, indecision, procrastination, leaving tasks unfinished, socializing, poorly trained staff, and failure to communicate clearly. R. Alec MacKenzie in his book *The Time Trap* gives a much more complete explanation that would be helpful to the veterinarian.[3]

Take a sheet of paper and list as many potential time wasters as possible. Prioritize the list by number from the biggest time waster to the smallest. Once these time thieves have been identified, you can work to get rid of them or at least minimize their effect upon your ability to get a job completed.

Priorities

One of the time wasters previously described deserves extra comment because unless you continually work on setting and sticking to priorities your entire schedule will be ruined. Prioritizing needs to be done each morning as the day is planned. It is the most important element in using time wisely. Failure to prioritize will almost always reduce your ability to effectively manage your time. One of the most effective methods of prioritizing time is to make a daily list of the things that must be accomplished. Label each item with A, B, C, or D. The As are the highest priority and must be done. Bs are important but can wait. Make everything else a C or D. Go back again and put a numerical subheading by each letter such as A-1, A-2, B-1, and so forth. One must force oneself to work in the order of highest priorities. The good manager will then hold the Cs and delegate the Ds. Work on the Bs only after completing all of the As.

The 10-second test

One of the most effective techniques for concentrating and more effectively focusing your energy is to apply what I call the *10-second test*. This simply is asking four questions about everything you do. The first question is Why am I doing this? The second is Who else could do it? The third is "Does it need to be done at all? and the fourth is What priority does it deserve? If you develop the habit of automatically asking these four questions, your ability to prioritize will be greatly improved. A much greater awareness of personal activities also results.

Time log

To understand how you use your time and evaluate time wasters, it is necessary to keep a time log for at least 1 week. Two weeks would be better, but usually 1 week will give sufficient information to help formulate a time management plan.

A sample time log is illustrated in Figure 13-1. It can be tailored to fit your daily activities. Fill in the headings and record the time in the left-hand column. Using a stopwatch will help track specific times. Some suggested headings to use are Reading, Telephone, Mail, Management, Clients, Surgery, Interruptions, and Other. Check the appropriate square, or make a note in the box and record the amount of time in the left column. At the end of the day the totals can be made and priorities assigned. The percentage of time can be calculated on a daily basis and summarized at the end of the week.

Another example of a daily time log can be found in Figure 13-2. This log requires filling in the proper headings across the top and then checking the appropriate boxes.

Time analysis

A careful analysis of the time log summaries will reveal how effectively each day's time is being used. It normally is very revealing as to how much time is wasted on the telephone or in nonpractice activities. Remember, veterinarians are trained to practice veterinary medicine and that is where they produce the most income. Technicians can do the support activities that will free the veterinarian to practice medicine. The only way to evaluate how time is being spent is by keeping and analyzing a time log. Even though it may seem like a lot of bother, keeping a log is the only way to evaluate time use effectively. A new daily time log should be made at least once a year.

Once the daily time log has been completed for a 1- to 2-week period, a 2-week time inventory should be completed. An example of a time inventory is found in Figure 13-3. The activities listed on the left of the page should reflect all activity within the period. By reviewing the time expanded in each activity (as documented from the daily time log), priorities can easily be observed. A rank could be assigned to each area (1 to 5) as related to your personal performance in achieving specific priorities. If the rankings in the various areas (PE, study, family, profession, and so forth)

(Text continues on p. 242.)

TIME LOG

Start time: 7:45 am Date: Wednesday 8-23-87

Time	pri	Read	min	pri	Tele.	min	pri	Mail	min	pri	Man.	min	pri	Client	min	pri	Treat.	min	pri	Surg.	min	pri	Inter.	min	pri	Other	min
8:00																						C	Looking for dog	15			
9:30													A	Exams	90												
9:40				B	Judges	10																					
9:56																						B	Drug sales	16			
10:30													A			A	Hosp. treat	34									
10:40																						C	Johns working	10			
11:20																A	✓	40									
11:45																A	Radio. ✓	15									
11:55				B	Jones	8																					
1:30																									A	Rotary	90
2:00																						C	Kennel J. Jones	30			
2:30													A	Khien. CK	30												
2:45													A	Rich. CK	30												
3:00	B	Journal AAHA.	15																								
3:40													A	Exam cumbron	40												
4:00																						C	Cafe drop in	20			
4:45													A	X-ray Wilson	45												
5:05				A	Return calls	20																					
6:10													A	Exams	65												
6:25				A	Tel.calls Jones, samoin	10																					
6:40										A	Ins. app.	15															
6:53							B	Mail	13																		
Total		B – 15			A&B 48			B – 13			A – 15			A –300			A – 99						C/B– 91			A – 90	Tot. 671
% of day		2.2			7			1.9			2.2			44.7			14.9						13.6			13.5	

EXECU-TRENDS®

Figure 13-1. Daily time log

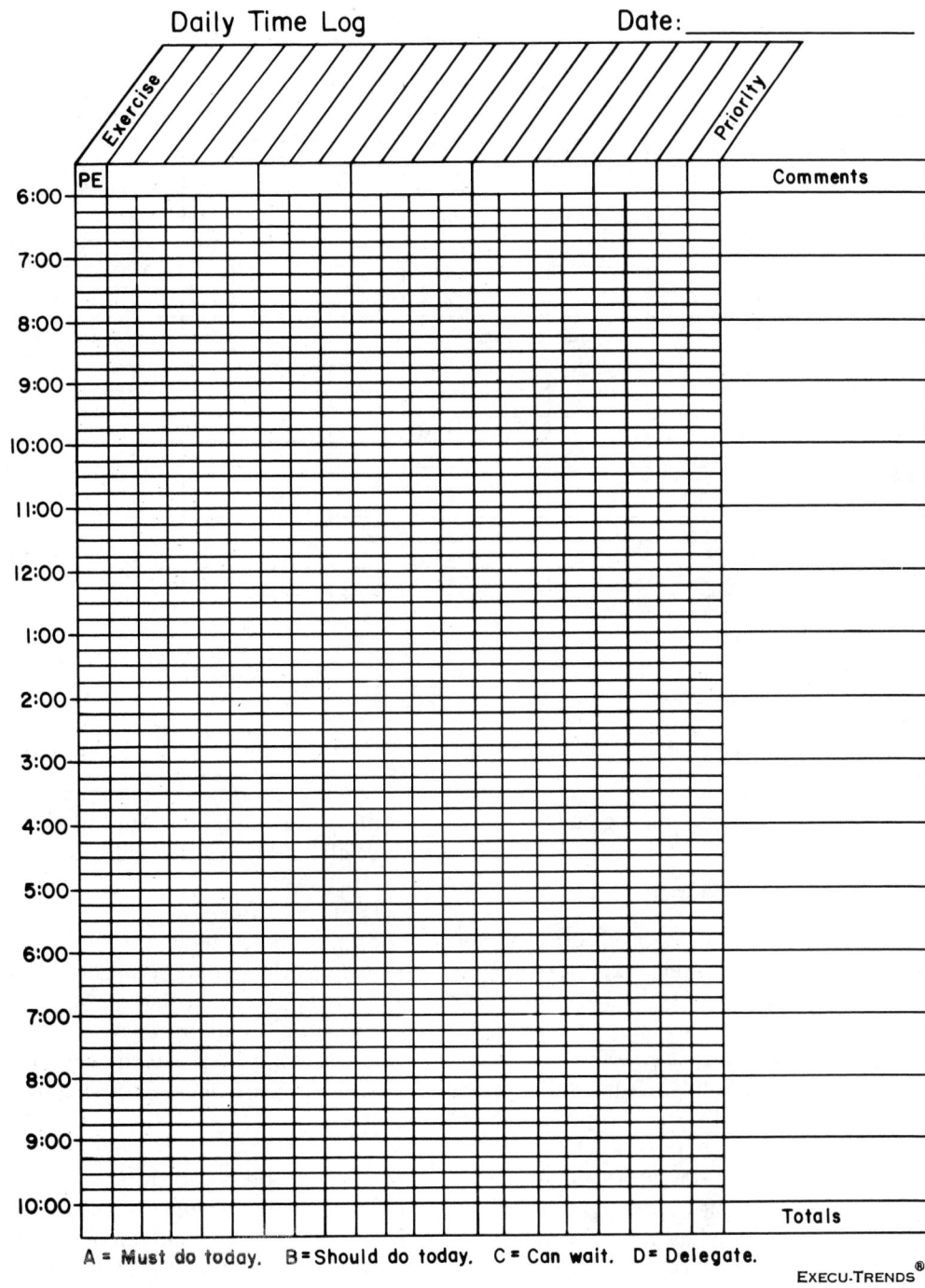

Figure 13-2.   Time log that only requires checking the appropriate box

Two Week Time Inventory

ACTIVITY		SUN	MON	TUE	WED	THU	FRI	SAT	SUN	MON	TUE	WED	THU	FRI	SAT	Tot.	Ave.	Rnk
Exercise	PE																	
Plan & Meditate	Study																	
Church Reading																		
Professional Read.																		
Outside Reading																		
Family Activities	Family																	
Maintenance																		
Family Back-up																		
Clients	Professional																	
Surgery																		
Treatment																		
Back-up / Emerg.																		
Church Assignment	Church																	
Church Meeting																		
School	Comm.																	
Civic																		
Telephone, Business	Tel.																	
Telephone, Personal																		
Other																		
Total Hours																		

Rank: 1 = Excellent   2 = Good   3 = Average   4 = Poor   5 = Rotten

EXECU-TRENDS®

Figure 13-3. Time inventory sheet

are not acceptable, then the daily priorities must be changed to meet the goals.

Specialized knowledge

The easiest way for a person to develop and grow is by acquiring specialized knowledge. Time invested in continuing education is time well spent. The time spent studying this chapter will increase your awareness of how time is spent and thereby help you to use time more wisely. People grow in direct proportion to the specialized knowledge they obtain.

The professional's first priority should be to increase practice knowledge and skills. As professional knowledge and proficiency increase, a higher quality of professional service can be provided in a shorter period of time. This same principle applies to managing the practice or putting to work time management skills. Investing time in education and gaining specialized knowledge is like putting money in the bank.

Let us examine some specific ideas of how specialized knowledge can expand the professional's ability to get a job done. Peters and Waterman point out that the most successful corporations in America have a bias for action.[4] The following are practical ideas of how to act in some routine practice procedures.

Modeling

One of the best ways to learn is to visit the practice of a respected colleague. Observe how he practices, and incorporate his best procedures into your practice. Every practitioner will be superior in one area or another. Take the best idea from each practice, and if it fits your philosophy and is an improvement, incorporate it into the practice. This is referred to as *modeling*. Modeling is what MacDonalds or any other successful franchise does. If one store is very successful and those techniques are duplicated in another location (if the location is equal), the success can be duplicated.

A bias for action

All the knowledge in the world will not help until it is put into action. Whatever is learned must be acted upon or used within a short period of time, or it is usually lost. How many times have veterinarians attended a seminar and learned a new skill only to forget how to do or use the skill because the skill was not evaluated immediately in the practice? One of the finest practitioners in the country always tries everything he learns as soon as possible after returning from a meeting. Over a period of time the new knowledge and newly learned skills can make a big difference in not only the quality of the practice but in the time it takes to accomplish a given procedure.

Time management system

It is important to develop a system for calendaring, setting daily goals, recording important communications, and having telephone numbers and important information at your fingertips. Through the years I have tried many systems, but since 1958, the one that has been the most effective for me has been the Day Timers, Inc., system. In addition, I have a record book to carry management information, financial reports, notes from seminars, and so forth. This combination along with a good filing system will provide the needed organization to improve time management. Several thousand of my associates, friends, and others have also used the system effectively.

Normally in a small-animal practice the receptionist would have the standard size notebook, and the DVM would carry a pocket or junior size depending upon individual preference (Fig. 13-4). The right side is usually used to record notes, telephone conversations, and other important information. Instead of keeping appointments on the right page, record any notes or information that might be needed for reference later. A large-animal practitioner, however, could use the right side very effectively to keep track of appointments, treatments, and time used on each call. The Day Timers was developed for use by attorneys to keep a record of their billable time. It can also be used as a daily time log or diary.

The monthly practice calendar is the most important part of this system (Fig. 13-5). Record every appointment immediately as it is made. Lines can be drawn to accommodate a multidoctor practice. Appointments and practice activity can be scheduled every 5, 15, 30, or 45 minutes. Do not try to keep two calendars for yourself. It does not work! Throw away any second calendars! However, this does not mean that your receptionist should not keep a calendar of your appointments.

In addition to the monthly practice calendar that will be maintained by the receptionist or secretary, a personal business schedule can be maintained by each veterinarian or technician. This personal monthly calendar would have personal and business events outside of the regular practice calendar (Fig. 13-6). Practice appointments should not normally be entered except for large events.

Reading

Most practitioners spend a great deal of time reading. Much of this reading may be irrelevant material or junk mail. Learn to sort out the important material from the trivia. A speed reading class may be taken at a community college or a specialized seminar to increase reading speed. With a little practice, you can greatly increase your reading speed. If the practice has more than one DVM, assign certain professional journals to each and have

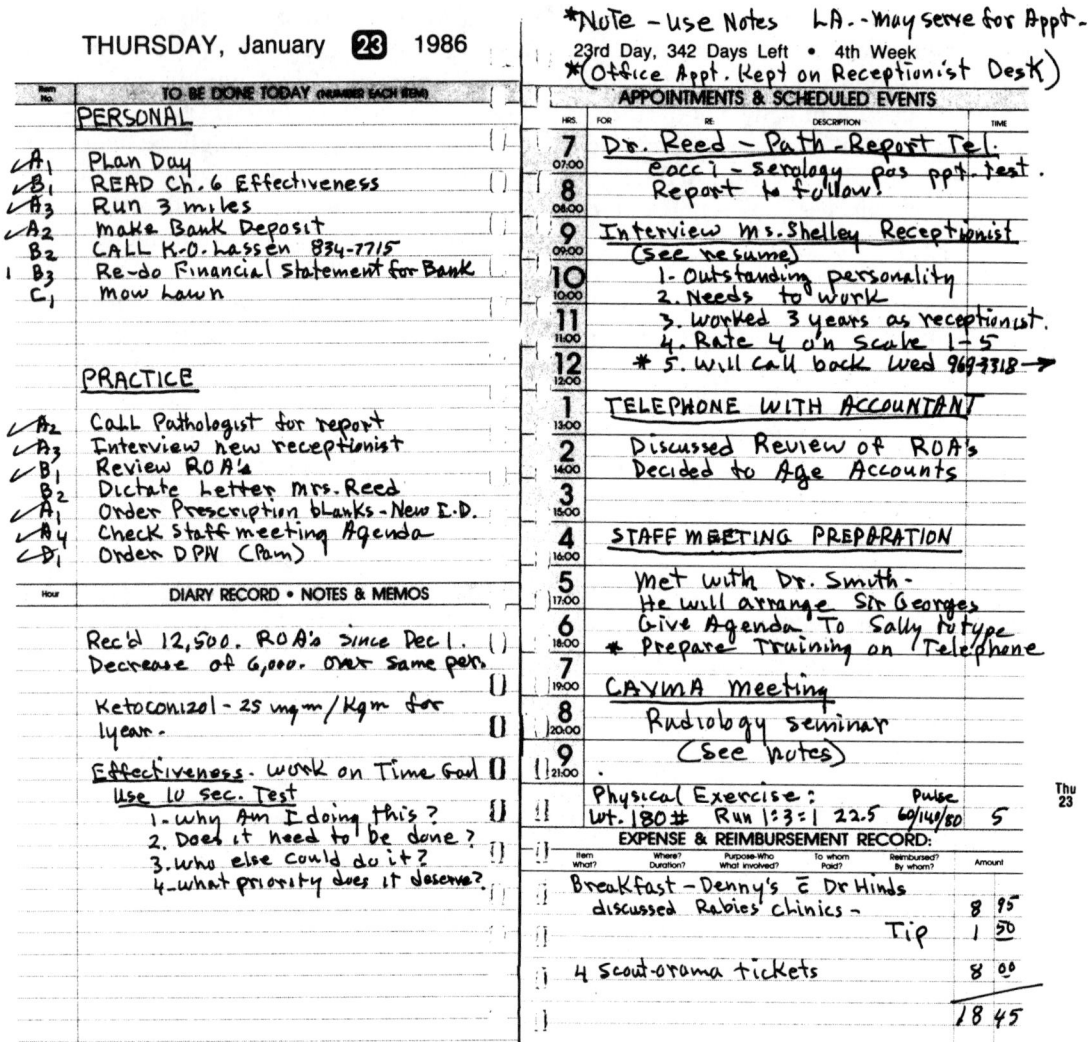

Figure 13-4. Sheets for one day from monthly Day Timers, Inc., publication (Courtesy of Day Timers, Inc, Allentown, PA)

them give an oral report on the important contents at a staff meeting.

Mail

Nearly every practitioner's desk is loaded with mail, journals, and other pieces of paper. This mail could be opened and sorted by the receptionist or secretary. But most often it is opened and read by the DVM. The veterinarian usually lays it on the desk and then comes back to it several times before making a decision for action. This is a waste of time! Learn to handle mail only once. Make a decision as to what action is required the first time the mail is reviewed. Either pitch it in file 13, file it, or take appropriate action so it is not reviewed more

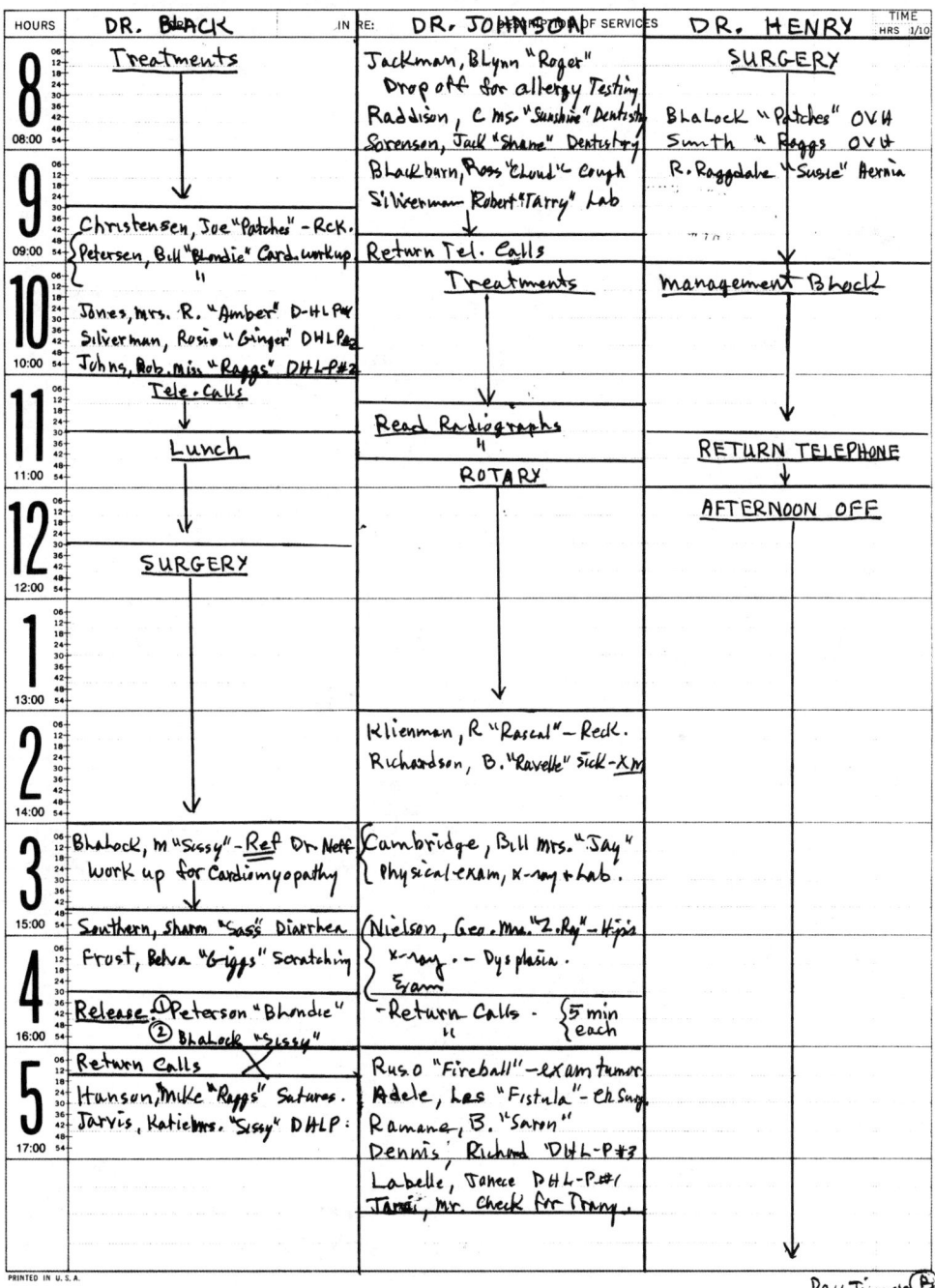

Figure 13-5. Example of appointment scheduling for three-doctor practice using a Day Timers, Inc, Schedule Book (Courtesy of Day Timers, Inc, Allentown, PA)

AUGUST 1987		**NOTES FOR THIS MONTH** ① Use 10 sec. Test before Scheduling! ② Learn to say "Yes" and "No"!				

SUN.	MON.	TUES.	WED.	THURS.	FRI.	SAT.
A.M. Church 10-12	Hold Appt. till noon					Rotary picnic 11:00-5:00
NOON P.M.						
EVE. ③⓪	③①					①
A.M. Church 10-12		Partner mtg 6:30 A "Bobs"			Mesa CR. mtg. 7:00	
NOON P.M.			Rotary 12-2 off ↓	Interview Recept. ↓		Family picnic Hole N' Rock
EVE. ②	③	Staff mtg 7:00pm King's ④	⑤	⑥	⑦	⑧
A.M. Church 10-12				CVMA Seminar 10-4		
NOON P.M.			Rotary 12-2 off ↓	↓	Barbeque 7:00 Bowman's	
EVE. ⑨	⑩	⑪	⑫	⑬	⑭	⑮
A.M. Church 10-12	Dentist 7:30-8:30				mtg.D.C. Wright 7:00 "Bobs"	Vacation Pine Top →
NOON P.M.			Rotary 12-2 off ↓			
EVE. ⑯	⑰	⑱	⑲	⑳	㉑	㉒
A.M. Vacation	Pine Top ——————————————————————————→					Return Home
NOON P.M.						
EVE. ㉓	㉔	㉕	㉖	㉗	㉘	㉙

Figure 13-6. *Monthly Day Timers, Inc, calendar for personal schedule and major business events (Courtesy of Day Timers, Inc, Allentown, PA)*

than once. The best use of the veterinarian's time is to train a secretary to take care of most of the routine correspondence. A simple handwritten note to her either directly on the letter or on a small self-adhering piece of paper is all that is needed. Dictate more complex or longer letters rather than personally writing or typing them. If you insist on doing your own letters, then by all means obtain a word processor!

Desktop management

Clutter and disorganization wastes time. Take the time to go through your desk and throw away or store the things that are seldom used from the immediate work area. Keep only the things that are used frequently in a drawer. A clean, organized desk will save time. The old adage that a clean desk is the sign of an empty mind is false. An organized desk and office will also allow support staff to find materials quickly in periods of your absence.

Telephone

The telephone can be the practitioner's best friend or greatest enemy, depending upon some very basic principles. For example, it can save time if used properly, or be the greatest time waster in practice if used incorrectly. It can build or destroy a practice, depending upon the skill and training of those who answer the telephone.

Every practice should provide 24-hour emergency telephone service. Therefore, an answering service is essential. Many practices use answering machines to good advantage, although some clients object to them. Most practices need to use rotary phones so that incoming calls will roll over on another line when the primary line is busy. Three or four lines is the maximum number one receptionist can handle efficiently. Phones should be checked periodically by the telephone company to see the percentage of busy signals. The telephone company will provide a computerized busy signal study. This will determine when extra lines are needed and be an important factor in determining labor needs for the front office.

If the practice phone system is a few years old, it should be reevaluated because new equipment technology has made many timesaving features available such as intercoms, automatic dialing, call forwarding, and so forth. Many new types of telephone pagers are also available that can be very helpful.

Other timesaving ideas are to set a specific time to make callbacks, avoid telephones in exam rooms, use a speaker phone in surgery for hands-free conversations, answer phones between the second and third rings, screen all calls to conserve the DVM's time, properly identify the practice and receptionist, never keep the caller holding more than 60 seconds without coming back on the line, and use private lines for personal calls and calling out. Additional phone usage information is found in Chapter 2.

The new practitioner has a tendency to talk too long on the telephone. Good communications are important, but economy of words is appreciated by many clients and will help conserve time. The client will develop more confidence in both the veterinarian and practice through thorough but concise conversations. Lengthy explanations often leave the client wondering, "Who is this doctor trying to convince, me or himself?"

Keep a stopwatch or egg timer by the telephone and routinely time conversations. It will be surprising how much time is spent on the telephone. Most conversations can be taken care of in 3 minutes or less. It often helps to make a short outline of the essential things to be covered with the client before placing the call.

Delegation

Many people fail to delegate because they have never learned the specialized knowledge to effectively do it. Begin by asking the questions given earlier in the 10-second test. Then follow these steps: (1) select the right people with the ability to perform the task, (2) make sure they understand specifically what the task entails, (3) let them know that you have confidence in them and their ability to do the task, (4) commit them to do the task, (5) agree on a deadline, (6) let them use their own imagination and creativity to complete the task, (7) tell them to report on their progress, (8) do not do it for them, and (9) reward them when the job is completed.

Delegation is grossly underused in veterinary medicine because veterinarians will not delegate unless they have spent some time in planning. As mentioned earlier, studies show that most veterinarians do not spend much time in making written plans. There is no motivation of employees without delegation, and there is no delegation without planning.

Saying no

Most people end up doing things they do not want to do because they do not know how to say No. Here is a simple four-step formula for saying No: (1) listen, (2) say No, (3) give reasons, and (4) offer alternatives. This formula works amazingly well. Learning when to say Yes and No is one of the most important lessons of life that will save an immense amount of time.

Medical records

Keeping medical records up-to-date every day not only saves time but makes money. A policy should be set that no veterinarian leaves the clinic without every medical record being completely up-to-date. It may take extra time, but it will greatly improve the quality of medicine practiced and will increase income by as much as 30%. Technicians should be used to make entries and keep logs up-to-date. Dictating equipment can also be used to conserve time. Computers that are touch or voice activated will be the standard before long and will save a great deal of time.

Scheduling appointments

Many practitioners use only 15-minute blocks for appointments. It is better to provide for three or four different length appointments. A referral or complete medical workup will take longer than a recheck or vaccination. A better breakdown would be 5-, 15-, and 30-minute appointments. Referrals and initial workups will take more time than is allocated in a 15-minute appointment. Remember to charge more for longer appointments because time is the basis for the fee. Fees for office calls can be made in three types: (1) brief, (2) regular, and (3) extended. The length of the call determines the type.

The typical large-animal appointment is 60 minutes, but this could vary with travel distance and the case. Training of the scheduler is essential to recognize the time that should be allocated for different appointments. Most doctors tend to underestimate the time it takes.

Planning should be done in each individual practice for the times best suited for examinations, treatments, and surgery. A mixed practice requires special considerations. Some practitioners prefer scheduling surgery for early morning, others during midday, whereas some schedule Monday, Wednesday, and Friday. Regardless, times need to be set that will maximize the practitioner's time (see Fig. 13-5). Leaving it to just happen is a poor use of time.

Thirty years ago, appointments did not exist in many veterinary hospitals. Today, most practices are appointment practices. Some clinics are, however, reverting back to a no-appointment status. This is especially true in the multiperson practice that is growing. The wave system is where all clients have one appointment for specific times (i.e., 9:00, 12:00, 4:00, and so forth). Having operated under both systems, I believe the appointment system is much better to maximize the veterinarian's time. However, this is a decision that will depend on the veterinarian's personal philosophy and type of practice.

Regardless of how well a practice plans and is organized, there will be delays on occasion. Good client communications are necessary when a delay is anticipated. Explain the reason for the delay and ask the client whether another time would be better. Provision for emergencies should also be made. The staff should be trained to handle emergency cases immediately. A policy for walk-ins should also be developed. If you are on appointments, it usually works well to advise walk-in clients that clients with appointments will be treated first, but just as soon as there is an opening they will be worked into the schedule. They normally will make an appointment the next time.

Computers and word processors

More practices are turning to the computer to save time and do a better job of marketing, controlling, and organizing the practice. The time is near when nearly every practice will depend on the computer to keep the practice competitive. In fact, it may be difficult to survive in business without a computer. After the initial shock of computerization, it would be difficult to ever go back to the old manual system. Typewriters are obsolete today. This chapter would have taken nearly twice the time to write manually. The word processor makes communicating with the client and the potential market an easy task. Think of the computer as an extension of one's brain, just as machinery is an extension of one's limbs. More information concerning practice computerization can be found in Chapter 5.

Patient workups

Technicians can save the veterinarian a great deal of time by getting basic information, weight, temperature, and major complaints. This is not only time effective but appreciated by most clients. Waiting can be made more enjoyable and educational by using videos or other visual aids. Nail trims, preparation for surgery, radiographs, laboratory samples, and other preparations of the patient can be done by the technician while the veterinarian is taking care of other patients.

Treatments

Under the direction of the veterinarian and in accordance with the individual state's practice act, the technician should be trained to administer medications, insert catheters, take laboratory specimens, and assist in the general nursing care and treatment of the patient. This not only saves a great deal of time but allows the DVM more time to diagnose and manage cases more effectively. This in turn results in better-quality veterinary medicine.

Surgery

Many veterinary surgeons use a technician to scrub on major surgical procedures. An assistant surgeon can greatly speed up surgeries if the veterinarian and technician are working together as a team. Presurgical and postsurgical procedures can also be completed by the technician. Please refer to Chapter 12 for additional information on use of the veterinary technician.

The aforementioned areas are only a partial listing of timesaving ideas. Specialized knowledge can save hours of time every day in practice. The challenge is to be conscious of time and how improved time use can increase practice effectiveness. Constant observation and learning new ideas and techniques will be valuable in one's quest for greater professional effectiveness.

Increasing energy and alertness

Anything that will increase energy and alertness will improve one's ability to concentrate and be more productive. The three main ways to maintain energy and alertness are by *getting adequate sleep, eating properly,* and *exercising.* If any one of these three is ignored for long, general health will decline and result in the loss of energy and effectiveness.

Workaholics

Many veterinarians become workaholics. This has been demonstrated as not an effective use of time. Even though the practice may take long hours, generally there is a way to cut the time spent to a reasonable amount and still get the job done. In my first 5 years of practice, 90-hour weeks were not uncommon. After making and analyzing a time log, a plan was made that decreased my hours by 30 per week, and yet my gross income nearly doubled. Extralong hours are counterproductive and may physically wear out the practitioner.

Stress

Numerous studies have shown that most serious illness is the result of stress. Therefore, it only makes sense to put as much balance into practice life as possible and not neglect diet, rest, and exercise. Evaluate your own life and see what changes can be made to increase energy and alertness. Practice enthusiasm will remain stronger, and a higher-quality medicine will be delivered in a shorter time when physical fitness becomes a priority.

So-called burnout is the result of too much work with not enough diversion. Vacations are a must for the practitioner. Veterinarians owe it to themselves and their clients to get away on occasion. Short vacations and continuing education seminars will do wonders to keep the professional alert, interested, and motivated. It is not how hard you work but how smart you work that makes good sense as far as managing time is concerned. Chapter 17 discusses the recognition and control of practice stress.

Building a support team

One common fault among many veterinarians is that they try to do everything themselves. In today's high-technology society it is foolish not to surround yourself with a complete support team. This team not only includes front office personnel and veterinary technicians but should include a competent accountant, attorney, banker, insurance agent, and management consultant. Each of these specialists can make the practice money if the right person has been selected and they are used properly.

The in-house support team constantly needs building. This means selecting the right people to begin with and then adequately training them to do the job they have been hired to do. Some practices are leasing their entire staff. The leasing company makes their payroll, supplies medical insurance, and sets up a retirement plan. The leasing of employees may be helpful in certain practice situations when highly skilled part-time people are needed. Selection and training of personnel are discussed in Chapter 3.

Team building

Building a support team is an ongoing process. It means sending employees to continuing education seminars and holding in-house training meetings. Staff meetings and coaching/counseling sessions will have a positive benefit in building a united team. A team with high morale is almost always more productive than a staff that has been neglected. Through team building, a highly competent staff can be developed that will produce results. The best time management possible is an efficient, well-trained staff. After all, management is getting things done through others.

In today's market, there is an adequate supply of veterinarians available for employment. Finding and hiring the right one is much more time effective than making a mistake and going through frequent professional staff changes. Our practice constantly had a flow of potential veterinarians from the internship program operated with students from various veterinary colleges. Maintaining a challenging environment for professional growth will allow the practice to hire the best of these interns after graduation. This wise use of resources is one of the most time-effective methods of screening potential professional employees for the practice. It not only saves training time but allows all practice employees to know the skills and qualities of every new professional staff member.

Synergy

As one builds a strong practice team, a synergism starts to result that greatly increases productivity. Each team member can make a contribution that produces greater results than any one member could achieve alone. The combined use of outside specialists may be the extra edge needed to improve the practice. Referring specific cases to a specialist can be very time efficient to both the client and referring veterinarian. The referral system is discussed in Chapter 20. The resulting synergism makes sense in getting the most out of everyones' time.

□
Summary

Good management dictates self-management. When practitioners have control over their time and lives, chances are excellent that outstanding results will be achieved. An assessment of one's effectiveness as well as an audit of the practice may reveal some important problems that can be remedied by instituting a time management program. Breaking time management down into five specific parts will allow a better understanding of how to build a meaningful time management program. The five important areas are (1) developing a philosophy, (2) focusing, (3) obtaining specialized knowledge, (4) maintaining energy and alertness, and (5) building a support team.

There it is, a very simplified course on time management. This chapter would normally take a 1- or 2-day workshop to properly teach the techniques to change time effectiveness and life. It will do little good just to read this chapter. It will require personal involvement and practice of the suggestions to change old long-standing habits. Just having the information will not work unless it is put into action! Good luck as you reach for an excellent way to professional effectiveness.

□
References

1. Parkinson CN: Parkinson's Law. Boston, Houghton Mifflin, 1957
2. Russell RL: Evaluation of Management Practices of Veterinary Hospital Managers. Masters' thesis, University of Phoenix, 1983
3. Mackenzie AR: The Time Trap. New York, Amacom, 1972
4. Peters TJ, Waterman RH: In search of Excellence. New York, Harper & Row, 1981

□
Suggested reading

Drucker PF: The Effective Executive. New York, Harper & Row, 1967

Lakein A: How to Get Control of Your Time and Your Life. New York, Peter H. Wyden, 1973

McKay JT: The Management of Time. Englewood Cliffs, NJ, Prentice-Hall, 1958

Moskovwitz R: How to Organize Your Work and Your Life. Garden City, NY, Doubleday & Co, 1981

Odiorne GS: Effectiveness. Minneapolis, DirAction Press, 1967

Winston S: The Organized Executive. New York, WW Norton, 1983

Chapter 14

□

The practice manager

Donald R. Dooley

The concept of having an outside manager or someone other than the veterinarian or veterinarians who own the practice manage has been around for years. The proliferation of veterinary emergency clinics since the early 1970s has provided an opportunity to demonstrate the concept in action. This demonstration has shown the concept will work.

Many veterinary practices are large enough business enterprises to justify professional, outside management, but the nature of practice ownership has been in the way. Because the majority of veterinary emergency clinics are owned by groups of veterinarians who do not work in the clinic and really want little if anything to do with the management, it has become possible to use outside management.

The reason outside management has not worked well in the past and is not apt to work well in most practices is due to the on-site existence of the owner or owners. The on-site owner is almost always the reason why the practice is not as profitable as it should be. Two good reasons for having an outside manager are relieving the owner of all of the routine, mundane nonveterinary chores of running a practice and making the practice more profitable.

Those who like the concept of an outside manager very often think outside managers will make their practice more profitable because they will be able to reduce the practice's expenses and increase the profits. This may be possible to a small degree on a short-term basis, but the real potential for increasing profits is in increasing production. Very little reduction of expenses is possible in most practices. Profits are the difference between income and expenses, and in nearly all practices, the lack of profitability is due to the lack of production rather than an excess of expenses.

Thus, if a manager is to be effective, he must have the authority to control the productivity of the veterinarians on the staff, including the productivity of the owner or owners. This means that for the manager to be able to perform he must have the authority to deal with the individual staff veterinarian's productivity, whether the staff veterinarian is an employee or owner. Not only does the manager need to be able to demand a specified level of production from the individual veterinarians, he must have the authority to remove and replace veterinarians who do not meet those demands. If this authority is not given (it is unlikely the owner, who is usually the problem, will give authority to remove himself), it is obvious that the manager does not have the ability to change the practice productivity.

This is why a concept that looks so good in theory has not been successful in more practices. In far too many cases where it has been tried, it quickly became evident that the manager was nothing more than a junior executive with a good deal of responsibility and no authority to perform. All that is achieved in such cases is a great deal of frustration on the part of both owner and manager. In some practices the manager has become an errand person for the owner with a title of manager. There is nothing wrong with this situation if everybody is happy and the position pays adequately.

Now let us set this rather negative viewpoint aside and look at what a manager can and should be doing in a practice where true management is possible. Again, this is a practice where the manager has full authority to manage the practice and every staff member in it. The manager may still be responsible to an owner or owners for broad practice philosophy and policy guidance but has full authority to implement both policy and philosophy.

The responsibilities of a practice manager,

listed in order of importance, are (1) practice income production; (2) personnel management; (3) purchasing; (4) maintenance; (5) bookkeeping, accounting, and legal; (6) banking; and (7) miscellaneous.

To keep the practice's income near its potential, the manager must (1) hire the right veterinarians, (2) let them know what is expected, (3) monitor their progress, (4) coach them when needed, (5) reward them for good performance, and (6) remove them if necessary.

□
The professional staff

Hiring the right veterinarian is the most difficult part of practice management. Most veterinarians have good medical and surgical skills, and some have the ability to produce income. Finding a veterinarian with both is extremely difficult. Good medical skills are a product of good training and the right attitude. Income production is the result of having the right attitude. There is no conflict or compromise between quality medicine and high income production because quality medicine is the basis of high income production. Poor-quality medicine is dishonest and should never be tolerated. Overcharging for poor-quality medicine is not only dishonest but in the long run destroys the practice.

Fortunately most veterinarians have a great deal more medical ability than they ever use. The quality of medicine they allow themselves to practice is far below what they are capable of were it not for their attitude toward veterinary medicine and their clients. To practice quality medicine a veterinarian must have a strong belief in the value of veterinary medicine to society and the individual client and the client's desire and ability to pay for quality veterinary medicine.

The ability to use quality veterinary medicine to produce an acceptable level of income depends on the veterinarian's self-image and attitude toward his ability to practice quality veterinary medicine. It takes a positive self-image to be able to demand and get the best from life, and without it people will be willing to settle for an income far below their potential. If a staff veterinarian is willing to settle for a low personal income, he will never be concerned about increasing the practice's income.

The veterinarian needed to staff a profitable practice is a veterinarian with good medical skills and attitudes that will allow him to practice quality medicine and produce income. Both veterinary schools and continuing veterinary education provide the ability, but it will be up to the manager to find and enhance the desire for productivity and income.

Unfortunately there is no easy way to find productive individuals. Interviews with several veterinarians will be required to find the right combination of skill and attitude. Some are easy to weed out simply by observing their grooming, posture, and dress. Others will eliminate themselves during the interview. However, the only way to tell how a veterinarian practices and produces income is to put him to work. For this reason, it is not as important whom you hire as it is whom you retain. Make sure the veterinarian you hire understands that he is being hired for a 90-day probationary period followed by semiannual reviews.

Professional expectations

Informing the veterinarian hired of what is expected of him is very important. You cannot achieve specific performance if you keep the expectations secret. The practice manager must first make an income projection for the whole practice before projecting individual income requirements.

To make an income projection for the whole practice, start with the past year's income. If last year's net income was less than desired,

adjust for that in this year's income projection. Adjust for any anticipated additional expenses (adding more staff, equipment purchases, or repairs); then add an inflation factor to last year's expenses. To complete the income projection for the new year add a margin of profit to this adjusted gross figure.

Break down the total practice income projection into individual projections. The first step is to remove income that does not come directly from veterinarians (boarding, grooming, pet food sales, and so forth). The remainder is then divided among the total number of staff veterinarians either equally or based on past performance.

A further breakdown of the individual projected practice gross could be on a monthly or daily basis. The monthly projection is made by dividing each monthly total for the previous year by the total for the year. Then multiply the projected total by the monthly percentages. To determine a daily average simply divide the monthly projection by the number of working days in the month or, for the individual veterinarian's projection, by the number of days the veterinarian is scheduled to work.

A very helpful income figure is the average charge per client or, in the case of a large-animal practice, the average income per hour worked. This average fee is necessary to make sure any increase was not from just seeing more clients or working more hours. There should be an increase in the average charge per client or per hour every year. If there is not, the individual veterinarian or the practice is doing less per client or being less efficient each hour. Use past records of client numbers to make this projection. If the staff veterinarians have not been accounting for their hours in the past, do some estimating and then start documenting the hours worked.

Discuss specific income projections thoroughly with each veterinarian on the staff to make sure they fully understand their income production. Document in writing specific income items that will be credited toward their projected goal. They also need to know how the figures are compiled and have access to any income figures they need to verify the accuracy of your figures. In other words, they must know they will be treated fairly and accurately.

Income monitoring and reporting

Monitoring and reporting income progress are very important tasks of the practice manager. These data can be extracted from the bookkeeping system by hand from the daily receipts or compiled by an electronic cash register or the daily report from a computer. A weekly report is best because most veterinary practices seem to cycle on a weekly basis (cases start Monday and are usually completed by Sunday). Reports should show the total production for the period, average daily production for the period, number of clients seen or hours worked for the period, and average production per client or hour. The report should provide figures for the current reporting period, month to date, and year to date (Fig. 14-1).

Obviously if the practice has several veterinarians, an electronic cash register or computer would help put this information together. If computer equipment is used, make sure the proper software program is available. Most programs are designed to provide a breakdown of individual procedures performed but not the average charge per client. Tabulating the number of individual procedures performed is of general interest but has little to do with the productivity of the practice. Make sure the program provides useful information for managing the practice (see Chapter 5 for additional information on computers).

In addition to written reports made available to individual veterinarians regarding their individual production and practice production, some practices use graphs and charts prominently displayed to keep everyone informed on the progress of the individual's and the practice's production. Graphs in the form of "thermometers," commonly used by fund raising organizations, make a good visual display of production on a daily, weekly, or monthly basis. Some practitioners feel this makes the hospital or clinic seem like a sales office. They fail to see that the hospital or clinic *is* a sales office and the manager is responsible for the sale of veterinary medicine to the practice's clients.

Coaching the veterinarian

Coaching veterinarians in the sale of veterinary services to the practice's clients has been the subject of several books and is too broad a subject to be covered in this chapter.[1-3] For the purpose of this chapter, the manager must devote a large part of his time to coaching the staff veterinarians on good, honest sales techniques. It can be an uphill battle at times. Some veterinarians mistakenly think professional sales have no place in a veterinary hospital. These veterinarians will usually be "failures" and must be sorted out and moved on as soon as possible.

Selling in a veterinary hospital is needed to allow the practice's clients to know what veterinary medicine has to offer them. Because veterinarians are not taught professional sales as a part of their training and most of them do not have prior sales experience, it becomes the manager's job to train and coach them. The success or failure of a practice manager will depend a great deal on his ability to train and coach the staff veterinarians in professional sales skills.

Rewarding performance

Rewarding outstanding performance and positive behavior is the best way to encourage it. Veterinarians must be rewarded for performing as requested. Historically we have discouraged productivity in veterinary practices by

End-of-Month Report

	AUG	SEPT	YTD
Total Charges	$50,302.00	$59,299.00	$597,281.50
Total Collected	47,607.00	60,353.24	591,275.84
Special Deposits			
Stock Purchase	0.00	0.00	2,000.00
WC Refund	0.00	0.00	3,616.00
Tax Refund	0.00	0.00	534.73
Drug Co. Refund	0.00	0.00	573.95
Other	25.00	0.00	25.00
Total Deposits	47,632.00	60,353.34	598,025.52
Total Checks	43,288.73	51,582.82	556,124.68
Equip. Purchase	0.00	0.00	1,293.40
Net Gain/Loss	4,343.27	8,770.52	43,194.24
Net Gain/Loss (%)	9.1	14.5	7.2
Reg. Bank Balance	21,883.46	25,894.51	37,312.91
Trans. to Savings	0.00	0.00	20,000.00
Trans. from Savings	0.00	0.00	20,000.00
Dividends Paid	0.00	0.00	40,000.00
Stock Buyback	0.00	0.00	2,000.00
Computed End. Bal.	26,226.73	34,665.03	34,665.03
Adjustments (Peter)	−332.22	0.00	(2,548.72)
Regular Clients	377	497	4,982
PHS Cases	42	29	475
PHS Wildlife	40	37	321
Blood Donors	6	0	44
Total Cases	465	563	5,822
Dr. A	143	152	1,624
Dr. B Cases Seen	78	168	1,369
Dr. C	76	161	1,462
Relief Drs	80	16	527
Total Regular Cases	377	497	4,982
Dr. A	$130.88	$139.12	$126.27
Dr. B Charge per Case	117.24	140.12	129.70
Dr. C	111.41	107.01	100.23
Relief Drs	104.44	93.44	98.67
Total Regular Cases	118.52	127.59	116.65
Dr. A	$18,716.00	$21,146.00	$205,066.00
Dr. B Gross	9,145.00	23,540.00	177,566.00
Dr. C	8,467.00	17,229.00	146,532.00
Relief Drs	8,355.00	1,495.00	51,997.00
Total Regular Cases	44,683.00	63,410.00	581,161.00

Figure 14-1.   End-of-month report

paying veterinarians for breathing steady and staying healthy instead of producing income. It has been customary to base salaries on the number of years of service rather than on production. This encourages veterinarians to take it easy, keep stress to a minimum, and live long and nonproductive lives.

If you want a specific behavior, then it must be rewarded. To encourage veterinarians to be productive, base their reward (salaries) on their production; the more they produce, the more they earn. A sales worksheet to monitor the productivity of each veterinarian is found in Figure 14-2. This is the same income commission basis that sales organizations have successfully used for years. Some veterinarians paid on a commission basis will pressure their clients and become unprofessional to increase their salaries. This is not an indictment of the system but means that an unprofessional individual was exposed by the system of salary determination and should be terminated.

The percentage of income production paid is usually between 20% and 25% depending on the profitability of the practice and fringe benefits paid. Assuming the practice's profitability can afford 25%, the next consideration is the fringe benefits. If no fringe benefits are paid, a straight 25% may be appropriate. If, however, insurance, professional dues, continuing edu-

cation, vacations, and sick leave are to be paid, the percentage may need to be reduced to 20%. If a profit-sharing or pension plan contribution is to be made, an even lower percentage may be appropriate.

When establishing the payment percentage, it is important to determine the exact income base. For example, will pet food sales or prescription refills be included? What about the division of income for cases where two or more veterinarians are involved? In this latter case it should be the veterinarian who sold the procedure who gets credit. After all it is not difficult to hire someone to perform the medical procedure, the difficulty is hiring someone who can sell the procedure. Keep in mind that you will get the behavior you reward, so be careful what you reward.

There are other ways of paying veterinarians. One may pay a salary plus bonus and base

Doctor Sales Worksheet

SALES-BY-DOCTOR WORKSHEET, For the month of: _____, 19_____

	This Month	Same Month Last Year	+ or − (%)	This Year to Date	Last Year to Date	+ or − (%)
Dr. _____						
Gross Income:	$_____	$_____	____%	$_____	$_____	____%
Number of Clients Seen:	_____	_____	____%	_____	_____	____%
Average Charge per Client:	$_____	$_____	____%	$_____	$_____	____%
Dr. _____						
Gross Income:	$_____	$_____	____%	$_____	$_____	____%
Number of Clients Seen:	_____	_____	____%	_____	_____	____%
Average Charge per Client:	$_____	$_____	____%	$_____	$_____	____%
Dr. _____						
Gross Income:	$_____	$_____	____%	$_____	$_____	____%
Number of Clients Seen:	_____	_____	____%	_____	_____	____%
Average Charge per Client:	$_____	$_____	____%	$_____	$_____	____%
Dr. _____						
Gross Income:	$_____	$_____	____%	$_____	$_____	____%
Number of Clients Seen:	_____	_____	____%	_____	_____	____%
Average Charge per Client:	$_____	$_____	____%	$_____	$_____	____%
Dr. _____						
Gross Income:	$_____	$_____	____%	$_____	$_____	____%
Number of Clients Seen:	_____	_____	____%	_____	_____	____%
Average Charge per Client:	$_____	$_____	____%	$_____	$_____	____%

Figure 14-2. Doctor sales worksheet

the bonus on a portion of the gross or net income. For example, payment may be based on a salary plus a percentage of the increase in gross income. This means a percentage will be paid of the increase in the practice's gross income for the current month compared with the same month last year. Keep in mind that humans have short attention spans; the reward has to be kept as close to the behavior as possible for it to be effective. Most bonusing should be done on a monthly basis. No one can get very excited in January about something they are going to be rewarded for in December.

Terminating a staff veterinarian

Removing a staff veterinarian is never a pleasant task, but if the desired profitability is to be maintained, it may be absolutely necessary. Of course, there are other reasons to remove staff veterinarians in addition to low income production. They may not be able to get along with the rest of the staff or the practice's clients. Regardless of the methods used in selecting staff veterinarians and coaching and rewarding their behavior, there will be individuals who simply do not fit into the practice and practice philosophy for one reason or another.

This does not mean there is anything wrong with them or with the practice. It simply means they or the practice are in the wrong place at the wrong time. Since it is easier to remove one person than to completely change a practice and its philosophy, the individual must go. The purpose of your action is to simply remove the veterinarian from your practice, not to destroy him. If possible send them away with their egos intact. Do not hesitate to give them a good recommendation in another situation. Just because they did not work out well in one situation does not mean they would not be fantastic in another practice.

Again, removing a veterinarian is an unpleasant task, but do not put it off. Terminating a staff member will not be easier later and will not become easier regardless of how many times it is done. If dismissals become easy, the manager needs to reevaluate his own feelings and job effectiveness.

This has been a brief overview of managing the veterinary staff of a veterinary practice to achieve efficient income production. Obviously it is more complex than would be indicated here, but this overview will provide some guidelines to be used. In addition to salary incentives there are other things the veterinary staff will need to achieve their potential productivity.

□
Personnel management

One important ingredient a veterinarian needs to practice quality medicine and produce income for the practice is a quality support staff. This makes personnel management a very important aspect of practice management. Good personnel management consists of several parts: (1) attracting good employees, (2) selecting good employees, (3) training, (4) scheduling, and (5) retaining and releasing them when indicated. A complete description of personnel management is found in Chapter 3.

Employee attraction

Be careful how ads are worded when advertising for employees. Do not be too restrictive; some very excellent employees started without the right education or experience. There are times when it is best not to mention that the business is a veterinary practice. An ad for a receptionist might read: "Receptionist wanted for small business, must be able to type, use calculator, and answer the telephone. Call (your phone number)." Not mentioning that the business is a veterinary hospital might spare your practice from receiving applications from an army of "pet petters."

Employee selection

Selecting the right employee for the position requires that homework be done before talking to the applicants. Different positions require different skills and personalities. The receptionist position is a sales position and requires a person who is people oriented. There are good receptionists in veterinary practices who don't care for pets. They do a good job for the practice because they like people and deal very well with the practice's clients.

A veterinary technician position requires certain knowledge and abilities but also requires that the employee like animals. The technician should be a meticulous person who is careful about details. Obtaining high-quality radiographs and accurate results on laboratory tests requires attention to detail. A veterinary technician must like animals and medicine and must be meticulous in details. This is almost the opposite of the good receptionist who is people oriented and cannot be bothered with details.

Training

On-the-job training is a very important part of personnel management. Even if the new employee comes with training and experience, specific practice techniques will warrant a training program. When training is left to chance, it can become a major cause of poor job performance.

Take the time necessary to prepare a list of needed skills for each position in the practice. After the new employee has been hired (or as part of the employment interview), have the employee review the list and demonstrate those skills already mastered. After the employee has demonstrated his proficiency, a training program should be set up for the remainder of the needed skills.

Training should not be done in a haphazard manner; it must be organized. First of all set aside time to do it, preferably outside the normal working hours. It is helpful if this training can be done before the employee officially starts work. Training sessions should be limited from one-half hour to 1 hour. Do not try to do it all at once and exhaust the employee; the results will be poor. Start by explaining what is to be accomplished; then demonstrate the skill. Ask the employee to do the procedure and repeat it until it is right. Encourage the employee to ask questions.

Part of a training program should be retesting quarterly or semiannually to make sure bad habits have not taken over. Proficiency retesting is a part of every good quality assurance program. Just because someone demonstrated the ability to do something right 6 months ago is no assurance they are still doing it correctly.

Scheduling

The scheduling of employees has a strong influence on the quality of medicine a veterinarian will practice. A veterinarian will practice a higher quality of medicine when assisted by a veterinary technician who can take good radiographs and do accurate laboratory work. The manager must provide the veterinarian with the best possible employees if high-quality medicine is to be practiced. Poor-quality medicine affects the practice's income in a negative way.

Study each staff position to determine the optimum utilization times of the day for each employee. Each practice is different in its scheduling of clients, so each practice will have different staffing needs.

Key employees must have the assistance they may need. An excellent veterinary technician without an assistant to hold animals will be inefficient. To have an expensive employee standing around waiting for a veterinarian to become available to hold an animal is the ultimate in poor personnel use. For the receptionist to be an effective salesperson, she needs to be at the counter greeting and dealing with clients, not running around the hospital taking animals back and forth and getting pet food for clients. She may need a gofer to run errands. A gofer may not be needed all day, but there will be periods of peak activity. A good receptionist is too valuable to use refiling records and other clerical work, especially in a hospital large enough to have a practice manager.

Retaining staff

Retaining a staff once it is put together is an ongoing concern. The author believes all practices can be divided into two groups: (1) practices that have current personnel problems and (2) practices that are about to have problems. Single people get married (never to a person who will stay in the area), and the married reproduce or become single again. As their lives change, so does the staff. It is a numbers game: the larger the staff, the shorter the periods when the staff stays together operating smoothly.

Although turnover is costly, it is also normal. Perhaps the only thing worse than turnover is what would have to be done to keep it from happening. Even though turnover is costly, it also has its benefits. New employees often bring new enthusiasm and new ideas with them when they join the staff. Also, employees tend to age like wine: some get better with age, but some turn to vinegar. To retain employees as long as possible, communication, competitive salary, and personal respect must be present.

Employee communication should be both written and verbal. Personnel policies should be written out so there are no misunderstandings. Policies should address pay periods, overtime pay, sick leave and holiday pay, paid vacations, uniform allowances, health insurance, employee discounts for veterinary services and supplies, and so forth.

Caution should be exercised with verbal communication. The message that is actually delivered is not as important as the interpretation by the listener of what was said. If it is important, follow important verbal information with a written confirmation.

Verbal communications handled in the form of a staff meeting should be done carefully. Staff meetings held on a routine scheduled basis such as every other Tuesday noon are dull, boring, and nonproductive. Just because it is Tuesday noon again is not a reason to have a staff meeting. Only have staff meetings when there is a reason. This can be determined by having a sheet of paper on the bulletin board for employees to use to request a staff meeting.

Before a staff meeting is held, the agenda for the meeting should be published on the bulletin board. Staff meetings without an agenda tend to wander out of control. Attendees at staff meetings should understand that management is more interested in solutions than in problems and that no solution is too ridiculous to be considered.

Every staff meeting should have a chairperson and a secretary. Neither of these people should be in management. The position of chairperson should rotate among the staff to give everyone some experience in managing a group discussion. The secretary takes minutes, types them up, and distributes them to every staff member as soon after the meeting as possible. The minutes are necessary to document discussions and decisions.

Personal respect may be the most important reason why employees stay in a practice. Some work is a bit degrading at times and can have an adverse affect on an employee's self-esteem. If self-respect is shown to all employees, they will maintain a healthy self-esteem from which all will benefit. A survey of veterinary technicians who have left practice found that a perceived lack of respect from their employers was the reason most often given for leaving practice.

Respect is demonstrated by listening and actively soliciting suggestions and comments. Ask if there is anything that could be done to make their work easier or more productive. The people doing a job have the best ideas for improving the performance of that job. Not all the suggested ideas need be implemented, but it does not cost anything to listen respectfully and thank the person. When new ideas appear not to have negative reactions, they should be used on a trial basis.

Demonstrate respect by always speaking in a professional manner and tone with all people, but especially with employees. Never criticize an employee in public, and try never to praise them in private.

A great and inexpensive way to show respect for an employee is by giving them their own business cards. This is only for those with some authority as office manager, head receptionist, head technician, chief ward attendant, laboratory technician, and so forth. The only thing that makes employees feel better than giving them their own cards is to ask for one to give to a client.

Salary and incentives

The right amount to pay varies from community to community and even from practice to practice within the same community. The right salary to pay is the amount required to keep good employees and keep them working.

Salaries and performance should be evaluated at least twice per year. This does not mean raises are given twice a year. Each employee should have the opportunity to discuss their job performance and how it relates to their income.

In addition to individual salaries, consideration may be given to incentives for support staff to help achieve and maintain income production. Receptionists control the number of clients seen. The way they handle the telephones has a great bearing on whether the practice will see the caller. If more clients need to be seen, the receptionist needs an incentive to put forth the extra effort. Veterinarians and practice managers love to see new clients, but to a receptionist a new client is only extra work that will not be encouraged on a very busy day. Extra work is only enjoyable when it produces extra income, so pay the receptionist for new clients. Some practices have the clients pay this extra amount. Charge the client a record setup fee, and give a percentage to the receptionist. Clients do not object to a $3 or $5 initial visit or record setup fee, and the receptionist suddenly discovers the joy of seeing new clients.

Technicians do a much better job of recording charges for work done on hospitalized animals than do veterinarians. They especially remember everything done if they are getting a small percentage (1% or 2%) of the increase in this month's income compared with the same month last year.

Do not include all support staff in the incentive program. Only those who are in a position to make a difference should be rewarded. The additional advantage of rewarding only those with some authority is that it gives those below them something to work toward. If the one receiving the incentive leaves, another staff member will want to move up and take on the extra responsibility.

Releasing an employee

Letting an employee go or letting go of an employee can be a great morale booster for the rest of the staff. Long before management knows an employee is not pulling his weight on the staff, the rest of the staff knows it. Keeping a nonproductive staff member on the staff has a very negative effect on the staff. When employees see a fellow staff member getting by with things, they wonder why they should work so hard. By contrast, when they see a person being let go for poor performance and they are retained, it sends the message that performance is important.

Having to let an employee go after you have invested a great deal of time and effort in him is the most unpleasant thing a manager has to do. No matter how many times it is done, be assured it will never get easier. There really is no good way to do it other than to be as kind and considerate of the other person as possible. One should be direct, specific, and concise.

The opposite of having to let an employee go (a nice way of saying you fired them) is letting go of an employee. One of the most exciting things a manager can experience is the wonderful experience of having an employee outgrow the practice. To bring employees into a practice, train them, and watch them grow until they leave the practice and go to bigger and better things is one of the most rewarding things a manager can do. It is almost the same as raising a child and seeing him turn out well. This should be the goal of the manager for every employee on the staff.

A nice agreement to have with employees is a promise to help them achieve their career goals, and in return, the employee agrees to help hire and train their replacement when they leave. The author is pleased to state that every employee he has helped to grow and go on to better things has honored his side of the agreement. This will keep the turnover in personnel from adversely affecting the practice.

In addition to a good support staff, the staff veterinarians need a few other things to be able to consistently practice quality veterinary medicine. Next to a good support staff in importance is an adequate supply of quality drugs and supplies and adequate equipment. This is where the practice manager puts on the hat of a purchasing agent.

☐
Purchasing

Being a good purchasing agent is a balancing act. It is a matter of being adequately stocked without being overstocked. A purchasing agent tries to buy at the best price without spending more time and money than could possibly be saved by shopping. The purchasing agent has to take service into consideration as well as price. The purchasing agent's work can be broken down into three major jobs: (1) maintaining inventory records, (2) doing the actual purchasing, and (3) evaluating equipment needs.

Inventory records

Maintaining inventory records starts with deciding what information is wanted so that the appropriate information will be fed into the record system. The organizational format of the inventory system will be somewhat dependent upon the information being monitored. To keep the inventory turning over as often as possible and yet maintain an adequate supply, the following information will be needed: (1) product name and description, (2) suppliers' names and phone numbers, (3) date and amount received, (4) reorder level, and (5) price (Fig. 14-3). The price listing has nothing to do with maintaining the inventory but can be used for comparison purposes when making the next purchase.

Make sure the product name and description are complete because many names are similar and most drugs come in several strengths, formulations, and sizes. Where necessary some items such as suture materials should also include catalog numbers.

Suppliers' names can be kept on a single

CARD NO._____
DESCRIPTION   PART NO._____

SERIAL NOS. OR MODELS ON WHICH USED				MAXIMUM		LIST PRICE			AISLE	
				MINIMUM		COST PRICE			SECTION	
				CLASS		SOURCE			BIN	

SALES RECORD — BIN CHECKS

YEAR	JAN.	FEB.	MAR.	APR.	MAY	JUNE	JULY	AUG.	SEPT.	OCT.	NOV.	DEC.	ANNUAL	DATE	COUNT	DATE	COUNT
19																	
19																	
19																	

PURCHASE RECORD — STOCK RECORD

DATE	ORDER NO.	QUANTITY	√	INVOICE NO.	REC'D	√	BACK ORDER	REC'D	DATE	SOLD	BALANCE	REC'D	DATE	SOLD	BALANCE	REC'D	DATE	SOLD	BALANCE

AIGNER FORM NO. 25-247   PRINTED IN USA

Figure 14-3.   Inventory card

page or card for quick reference. Then, rather than writing the full name with each item you can just use a code name or number (Fig. 14-4).

When an order is received, it should be checked against the packing slip that accompanies the order. When the billing invoice that goes with the order arrives in the mail, it should be matched with the packing slip. The invoice is then checked against the packing slip to make sure everything charged was received. The invoice can then be recorded in the inventory records. The date the shipment was received and the amount of the item received will allow a determination of the product usage.

The reorder level of each item is determined by checking the past usage, the best quantity to buy to get a good price in keeping with the usage, and the length of time it takes for delivery. The reorder level is the minimum quantity of an item that will trigger a new order for that item.

Another important item to record from the invoice is the price of the item. This is necessary to quickly determine the cost of any item. If the price goes up, an adjustment in the dispensing price of that item should be made. If it is not a dispensing item but one consumed in the hospital or clinic, the increase should be placed on a list of items that have increased during that month and given to employees who use the product. For example, the staff veterinarians need to know when the price of bandage materials increases so they can increase the fee for bandaging.

There are a number of ways to record inventory information. The most popular seems to be the inventory card file. After trying several systems, however, the author's preference is inventory sheets in a loose-leaf binder (Fig. 14-5). It is easier to thumb through a loose-leaf

SUPPLIER NAMES

Name_____

Address_____   Average delivery time:_____

Phone_____

Name_____

Address_____   Average delivery time:_____

Phone_____

Name_____

Address_____   Average delivery time:_____

Phone_____

Name_____

Address_____   Average delivery time:_____

Phone_____

Name_____

Address_____   Average delivery time:_____

Phone_____

Name_____

Address_____   Average delivery time:_____

Phone_____

Name_____

Address_____   Average delivery time:_____

Phone_____

Name_____

Address_____   Average delivery time:_____

Phone_____

Figure 14-4.   List of supplier names

binder and make notations than to take individual cards out of a file, make a notation, and then refile them. Either system is available in most office supply stores.

We have now entered the computer age so that inventory control can be done with a computer. The computer may be neater and even a bit faster than working by hand. One must be careful not to spend too much time and money on employees entering information that has little value into the computer. For example, some computer programs encourage the entry of usage of drugs and supplies as well as the purchases. This can be extremely time-consuming and provides no more information needed for purchasing than just recording the amounts purchased. The level of usage is the important factor in guiding purchasing. Please refer to Chapter 3 for information on computers in practice.

Drug and supply purchases

The actual purchasing can be done quickly and effortlessly by being prepared, calling the correct supplier, and ordering from a written order list. Being prepared is very important, especially if the order is being placed by telephone. Being prepared means knowing the name of the item, the strength, style, length, size, and amount of the item needed before dialing the telephone. Do not be in a position of playing guessing games. Know which supplier should be called for specific items, and group them on your call list accordingly.

The reason for using a purchase order form or an order list is to document your order in case questions arise before receipt of the order. The purchase order will also serve to record any special prices that were quoted when the order was placed. The purchase order can be used to time the shipment from placement to receipt.

Be careful about becoming overly excited about shopping for better prices while order-

ing. The competition among suppliers is very strong, and their margins are too small for very big differences in prices. Sometimes the apparent real bargain is offset by the short dating on the item. It is better to build a relationship with a supplier who provides good service and will give breaks when possible. The author knows from the experience of being a salesman calling on veterinarians that few companies or their representatives do favors for the shoppers.

Equipment purchase

Evaluating equipment purchases is one of the more complex duties of the purchasing agent. The question is most often not what the equipment costs but what is it costing the practice to not have the equipment. For example, an x-ray processor may cost between $4,000 and $8,000, so the most-often asked question is, How many radiographs does the practice have to take to justify purchasing a processor? The question is irrelevant because once the processor is purchased the usage of radiographs will increase enough to justify the expenditure.

It is the practice manager's duty to monitor the work being done by the veterinarians and make sure they are not hampered in their attempts to practice quality medicine by a lack of needed equipment. Equipment should not be purchased just because the veterinarians think it would be fun to have. Equipment should only be purchased when the practice is unable to practice quality veterinary medicine without the item.

When purchasing a piece of equipment, the integrity of the supplier is important. Equipment will break down or wear out. If it does either sooner than it should, the quality of the supplier will determine repair or replacement satisfaction. When income is being lost because the practice has a useless piece of equipment, it is little consolation that a few

(Text continues on p. 268.)

MINIMUM	DESCRIPTION	COST	SUPPLIER	JAN.	FEB.	MARCH

©1971 Medical Management Publishing Co.

Figure 14-5. *Inventory sheet*

APRIL	MAY	JUNE	JULY	AUG.	SEPT.	OCT.	NOV.	DEC.	TOTAL

Figure 14-5. Inventory Sheet (Continued)

hundred dollars was saved when it was purchased. The ability and desire to provide a repair loaner can be more important than the brand name of the equipment or any small savings made when purchasing the equipment. Before purchasing a major piece of equipment ask for the name of practices that have bought the same equipment from the supplier from which you are considering making your purchase, and then call the references and see whether they are satisfied with the after-sale service.

The author does not wish to infer that price is not important, but there is an overemphasis on price in the market, and there is a need to stress the importance of quality and service. Additional price can be passed on to the client, but the cost of running out of a needed item due to poor delivery service or being without a piece of needed equipment is borne by the practice. Please refer to Chapter 18 for specific information on inventory and equipment control.

□
Maintenance

Maintenance is a close relative of purchasing. At times parts or equipment will have to be purchased to maintain the building and equipment in good conditon. Maintenance can be divided into two types: (1) preventive maintenance and (2) repair maintenance.

Preventive maintenance is done on a regular, scheduled basis before there is a breakdown calling for repair work. Examples of scheduled preventive maintenance are

1. X-ray processor—should be serviced at least once each month, more often if necessary depending on usage
2. Anesthetic vaporizers—need to be cleaned and recalibrated at least once per year or more often depending on usage
3. Laboratory equipment—may need reca-

librating on a regular basis as recommended by the manufacturer
4. Microscope—should be cleaned and adjusted annually
5. Fire extinguishers—should be checked and recharged as necessary at least once each year
6. Roof—a roofing company should inspect and do minor patching annually, preferably just before the beginning of the wet season
7. Heating/air-conditioning units—should be inspected and serviced as necessary on a quarterly basis
8. Professional floor and cleaning service — should be done on a weekly or biweekly basis, with the floors being completely stripped and rewaxed at least once or twice each year
9. Landscaping service—should visit at least monthly

There may be other things that should be on the list, depending on your building and how it is equipped. It is the responsibility of the practice manager to make sure these inspections and services are performed. The most efficient way to maintain equipment is to arrange annual contracts with service providers. A calendar is marked when the service is to be performed and checked to make sure it was done rather than having to remember to find someone to do the work each time. Good preventive service will greatly reduce the cost of breakdowns and equipment being unavailable for a long period of time.

Repair work should be anticipated. All owners and managers hope equipment will not break down, but a plan should be in place when it eventually happens. For every piece of equipment in the practice a log should be kept of the name and phone number of the company who will perform repair service. When buying equipment attention needs to be directed to repairs as well as the availability of loaner equipment during repairs. Some equipment must be sent back to the manufacturer, a process that may take weeks or months, and a loaner will be needed to replace the equipment while it is out of the practice.

In addition to the equipment in the practice, there is the building that houses the practice. A plumber familiar with the building is needed so that everything is not new when you call him in an emergency. Another important repair person is the electrician, again preferably someone who has some familiarity with the building. For the minor things like leaky faucets and temperamental light switches, a handyman will fill the bill. Local senior citizen agencies are a good place to look for a retired contractor who would like a little part-time work or a construction worker who would like to do a little part-time work.

You should compile a maintenance book with all the names and numbers of service and repair people needed to keep the building and equipment in "like new" condition. Also, in this book record the names of companies from whom you would buy replacements because sometimes the repair will consist of replacing a piece of equipment.

Good maintenance is important because it affects the quality of medicine practiced. Veterinarians tend to not use equipment that is unreliable, and they definitely cannot use it if it is broken or unavailable. Also a poorly maintained building has a negative affect on staff morale and projects a poor image for clients.

□
Records

The practice manager will spend a major portion of time with bookkeeping, accounting, and legal work. Because much of this work has to do with income production, an accurate reporting system must be established to provide information necessary to analyze and monitor the practice's progress and make the necessary decisions. In addition to the need for information the income from the client must get to the bank without going astray. Occasionally information will be required about a case for the state Veterinary Board of Examiners or an attorney, so a good medical record system is necessary to provide accurate, reliable information.

Whether taking over an existing system or setting up a new one, a thorough and complete check of the system should be completed. Understand, of course, that every system is a compromise and no system is going to provide everything. If it did, it would be too time-consuming to be practical. When setting up the hospital's book and record keeping systems, keep in mind that the purpose of the practice is to provide veterinary services to the animal-owning public, not to do paper work. In addition to making sure the system provides the safeguards and information needed, make sure it is not providing the employees with too much useless "busy work." There are three types of information commonly derived from bookkeeping systems: (1) "Oh wow, that is fantastic!" information, which is usually useless; (2) interesting information that is useless; and (3) useful information.

For years veterinary hospitals have spent hours and hours of their bookkeeper's time compiling totals of different procedures performed or different department percentages. It is, of course, interesting to note how much less surgery was done this year than was done last year, or whether more or fewer radiographs were taken, but this is basically useless information. After years of asking veterinarians whether they have ever made a management decision or made any changes in their style of practice based on these numbers, I have determined that this is not only useless information but that it is also extremely costly. With the proliferation of computers in veterinary practices, useless information is now being compiled at a rate never dreamed of in the past.

This is not to say that all the information coming out of a computer is useless, but the time has come to stop compiling information no one understands or wants. The practice manager must make sure the information gathering is efficient and purposeful.

The major needs of the practice bookkeeping system are as follows:

1. Provide the client with a written estimate of work to be done.
2. Provide the client with an itemized breakdown of charges.
3. Record the charges for services performed.
4. Record the number of clients seen.
5. Record the number of financial transactions.
6. Record the money collected.
7. Provide for recording and collecting charges not paid at the time service was performed (accounts receivable).
8. Provide controls to make sure all monies collected are recorded.
9. Break down the income into categories needed to pay veterinarians who are working on a percentage basis and provide the manager with information needed to be able to manage the practice efficiently.
10. Provide the accountant with accurate numbers needed to prepare financial statements and compile tax forms.
11. Provide needed information to pay employees and properly record payroll information for employees and the accountant.

Because the aforementioned information will be compiled differently in most practices (because some will have "handwritten" systems, others will have electronic cash registers, and still others will have computers), the discussion here will be limited to the purpose for each item.

Fee estimate

The written fee estimate is a very important part of client communications. Verbal estimates are worth less than the breath it takes to give one. Only the written fee estimate given a client has value. The written estimate should be in duplicate so that the client can have a copy and the practice can keep one (Fig. 14-6). Veterinarians may claim they cannot estimate accurately because of the variables in medicine, but this is not true. They can anticipate what they intend to do and then add 10% to 20% to cover unforeseen problems. The total estimate can then be given as a range rather than a specific fixed amount.

To help veterinarians learn to estimate accurately, make sure when the charges are figured that everything done is included. If the charges exceed the estimate, simply have the client pay the estimated amount and then provide the veterinarian with both the estimate and the charges so that the next time a similar case is presented he will be able to give a more accurate estimate. By doing this the estimates will become accurate within a month or two. If the veterinarian is allowed to shave the charges to fit the estimate, the estimates will never be accurate and always too low.

Charge slip

The service items listed on the charge slip are the ultimate financial purpose of having a veterinary practice. All practice income comes to the practice through the charge slip (Fig. 14-7). Unfortunately not everything done in a veterinary practice finds its way to the charge slip. Approximately $40,000 worth of work done by each veterinarian every year somehow never reaches the final client bill. There are many psychological reasons for this, but sometimes it is the charge slip itself that is to blame.

For example, in many practices if an animal

DR._____ OWNER_____ PET_____ ADMIT DATE_____

ESTIMATE		
OUTPATIENT SERVICES	____	OFFICE VISIT
	____	RE-CHECK
	____	HEALTH CERTIFICATE
	____	OTHER
	____	D.H.L.P. - PARVO
	____	F.V.R.C.P.
	____	RABIES
	____	
	____	TREATMENT
	____	NAIL TRIM
	____	INJECTIONS
	____	PRESCRIPTION DIETS
	____	MEDICATION
	____	
	____	
	____	
	____	SALES TAX
	____	COMPLETE BLOOD COUNT
DIAGNOSTIC SERVICES	____	BLOOD CHEMISTRY
	____	URINE ANALYSIS
	____	CYTOLOGY/HISTOPATHOLOGY
	____	CULTURE/SENSITIVITY
	____	HEARTWORM TEST
	____	COLLECTION COST
	____	RADIOLOGY/DIAG. FILMS
	____	BARIUM
	____	ELECTRO CARDIOLOGY
	____	CONSULTATION
	____	ANESTHESIA/SEDATION
	____	TRANQUILIZATION
INPATIENT SERVICES	____	SURGERY
	____	DENTISTRY
	____	EXTRACTIONS
	____	OXYGEN THERAPY
	____	HOSPITALIZATION
	____	INTENSIVE CARE
	____	DAY CARE
	____	BOARD
	____	IN HOSPITAL MEDICATION
	____	INJECTION
	____	
	____	
	____	FLUID THERAPY
	____	I.V. CATHETERIZATION
	____	URINARY CATHETERIZATION
	____	BLOOD TRANSFUSION
	____	CAST/BANDAGE
	____	SPLINT
	____	
	____	
	____	EUTHANASIA/DISPOSAL

CASTRO VALLEY VETERINARY HOSPITAL
2517 CASTRO VALLEY BLVD. ● CASTRO VALLEY, CA. 94546
PHONE (415) 582-3656

Office Hours:

Monday - Friday
Hospital hours: 8-12:00, 2-6:00
Doctors hours: By appointment

Veterinary service is provided during nighttime hours as necessary in the judgement of the veterinarian in charge. Continuous presence of qualified personnel may not be provided. Critical cases are transferred by owner to the Alameda County Emergency Pet Clinic. 352-6080

Calling Hours:

You may call regarding your pets condition between the hours of 10 - 12:00, & 2 - 6:00.

Telephone Calling Procedures:

Since the doctors will be seeing patients or doing surgery during office hours, they may not be available to speak to you at the time of your call. The receptionist will take your telephone number and your call will be returned as soon as possible. Should you need to speak to the doctor personally, the receptionist will make you an appointment.

Fees:

The doctor, or a member of the doctors staff, will discuss all charges with you before any work is done; should you have any questions please do not hesitate to ask them. The doctors will not exceed the given estimate without again checking with you (should it be necessary to do so.) We feel it is important for you to know what the charges will be.

Payment:

Is to be made when the service is performed or when you pick your pet up. If you wish to charge, we do accept bank cards. If you have any questions, please check with the receptionist ahead of time.

Prescription Refills:

All prescription refills require the doctors approval, so when possible please call before you drop by to pick-up a refill, so that your file may be pulled and the prescription ready for you when you arrive. Should you be unable to call, please keep in mind there will be a short wait at the hospital.

Emergencies:

Other than during office hours, please call; (415) 352-6080

I am the owner of the above pet or am acting as an agent for the owner and accept full financial responsibility. The doctor has explained the medical condition of my pet, the proposed regimen of treatment or surgery and possible complications. I authorize the doctor to proceed as discussed.

OWNER/AGENT_____

INSTRUCTIONS:

TOTAL CHARGES	
DEPOSIT	
BALANCE DUE	
TOTAL PAYMENT	

FEE SHEET No. 12205

Figure 14-6. Fee estimate form

CASTRO VALLEY VETERINARY HOSPITAL

2517 CASTRO VALLEY BLVD. ● CASTRO VALLEY, CA 94546
PHONE (415) 582-3656

DR. _____ OWNER _____ PET _____ ADMIT DATE _____

ESTIMATE		DATES	COSTS	COSTS	COSTS	COSTS	COSTS	TOTAL
OUTPATIENT SERVICES	____	OFFICE VISIT						
	____	RE-CHECK						
	____	HEALTH CERTIFICATE						
	____	OTHER						
	____	D.H.L.P. - PARVO						
	____	F.V.R.C.P.						
	____	RABIES						
	____							
	____	TREATMENT						
	____	NAIL TRIM						
	____	INJECTIONS						
	____	PRESCRIPTION DIETS						
	____	MEDICATION						
	____							
	____							
	____							
	____	SALES TAX						
	____	COMPLETE BLOOD COUNT						
DIAGNOSTIC SERVICES	____	BLOOD CHEMISTRY						
	____	URINE ANALYSIS						
	____	CYTOLOGY/HISTOPATHOLOGY						
	____	CULTURE/SENSITIVITY						
	____	HEARTWORM TEST						
	____	COLLECTION COST						
	____	RADIOLOGY/DIAG. FILMS						
	____	BARIUM						
	____	ELECTRO CARDIOLOGY						
	____	CONSULTATION						
	____	ANESTHESIA/SEDATION						
	____	TRANQUILIZATION						
INPATIENT SERVICES	____	SURGERY						
	____	DENTISTRY						
	____	EXTRACTIONS						
	____	OXYGEN THERAPY						
	____	HOSPITALIZATION						
	____	INTENSIVE CARE						
	____	DAY CARE						
	____	BOARD						
	____	IN HOSPITAL MEDICATION						
	____	INJECTION						
	____							
	____							
	____							
	____	FLUID THERAPY						
	____	I.V. CATHETERIZATION						
	____	URINARY CATHETERIZATION						
	____	BLOOD TRANSFUSION						
	____	CAST/BANDAGE						
	____	SPLINT						
	____							
	____							
	____	EUTHANASIA/DISPOSAL						

I am the owner of the above pet or am acting as an agent for the owner and accept full financial responsibility. The doctor has explained the medical condition of my pet, the proposed regimen of treatment or surgery and possible complications. I authorize the doctor to proceed as discussed.

OWNER/AGENT _____

INSTRUCTIONS:

TOTAL CHARGES	
DEPOSIT	
BALANCE DUE	
TOTAL PAYMENT	

FEE SHEET   No. 12205

Figure 14-7.   Charge slip

is hospitalized for 4 or 5 days, there is no charge slip to record the day-by-day charges. The daily charges are either recorded in the medical record and, we hope, transferred to the charge slip when the animal is discharged, or the veterinarian records the charges from memory on the day of discharge. The charge slip should allow the charges to be recorded on the day they are performed or, better yet, at the time the procedure is performed.

The charge slip must be easy to use and have the necessary categories. Because veterinarians are hesitant to charge for many things they do, the charge slip must accommodate all practice activities to allow all services to be recorded. Keep in mind, however, that being too complex is just as bad as being too brief.

The charge slip should have two or three copies, depending on the requirements of the accounting system. Make sure the client has a copy of the itemized charges, not just a cash receipt. The reason for additional copies will be covered when discussing financial controls.

Financial accountability

Recording the charges from the charge slip on some type of daily income record is the next step. In addition to the charge slip the practice needs some way of summarizing the day's financial activity. It is necessary to record the daily charges as well as the total cash received. One purpose of this is to develop an accounts receivable control. Monitoring the accounts receivable requires comparisons between the charges and the amount collected.

Other reasons for recording both charges and cash received are to monitor the average charge per client visit, the gross income per hour for the practice, and the individual gross income per veterinarian. The daily charges relate to the clients seen during the same time period. Money collected could come from a prior time period (paid on account), so the money collected on a given day may not relate to just the client seen that day.

Recording the number of clients seen is necessary for a number of reasons. For example, it is necessary to know the number of clients being seen to determine the proper staffing of the hospital. A practice with three veterinarians each seeing 500 clients per month is probably not able to provide quality service and will not reach their income potential. Hiring a fourth veterinarian would correct the imbalance problem. However, a practice with four veterinarians each seeing only 200 clients would be better off with three veterinarians.

The number of clients being seen is also needed to monitor what is happening to your practice. To know the health of the practice, the gross income must be compared with the client numbers. Is the practice seeing more or fewer clients during the time periods under comparison? Without an accurate client count any comparisons and evaluations are just guesses and probably very inaccurate.

Of course, the number of clients seen is needed to be able to figure the average charge per client for each veterinarian and for the whole practice. This is very important in multiveterinarian practices because unfortunately all veterinarians are not created equal. Two practitioners from the same class in veterinary school who are practicing the same quality of medicine and using the same fee schedule may have a difference in their average charges of 50% or more. One veterinarian may be charging double what the other charges while working in the same practice. The practice manager has the responsibility for the income of the practice and, therefore, must know what each individual veterinarian is charging. When large average charge differences develop between two veterinarians, the manager must bring specific examples to the attention of those involved for resolution.

The number of financial transactions is another important figure to help monitor a practice. The ratio of financial transactions compared with clients seen can be very helpful information. Unless there are major changes such as changes in merchandising pet foods, grooming, or boarding in the practice, the ratio of clients to transactions should stay approximately the same. When this ratio changes, it can indicate a change in practice style by the staff veterinarians.

It is not unusual for a veterinarian after a number of years in a practice to treat more and more cases over the telephone or to authorize medication refills without examining an animal that should have been seen. An increase in the number of transactions compared with the number of clients seen without another plausible explanation is an indication that this is happening.

Keeping track of the money between the client and the bank is, of course, very important. On the daily financial summary sheet next to the charges should be a column for the money actually received. There should also be breakdowns of how the money was received and whether it was in the form of cash, check, or bank card. This is necessary for verification of the deposit.

It is extremely important to keep accurate financial records. There are no good reasons for the money not balancing to the penny at the end of each day. Deposits must balance against the total money received. The cash taken in and the cash in the deposit must be exactly the same. If employees are allowed to cash checks from the cash drawer, their checks and the cash taken out must be recorded on the daily summary. It is better to use a petty cash fund, but if payments are made from the cash drawer, every cent taken must be recorded.

If the manager is not demanding about the accuracy of the cash drawer, no one else will be. Sloppy cash drawers invite people to steal. The manager should be fanatically meticulous about the handling of the practice's cash and demand the same of others. The potential problem of missing cash can be reduced or eliminated through tight accounting and control of the cash drawer.

Accounts receivable also need to be regularly monitored. Be sure to review the bookkeeping system by looking for system leaks and checking to see that safeguards are being used properly. One of the common leaks in many systems is the failure of the amount charged to be posted to the accounts receivable. If the client is allowed to charge and the account is posted at a later time, there is always a danger of the record being refiled or getting lost without the charge ever being posted to an accounts receivable card. Most good systems have safeguards to keep this from happening, but many times shortcuts are taken that circumvent the safeguards. Clients will not pay if they are not billed, and they will not be billed if the charges never get posted to the accounts receivable.

Another potential leak is in the receipt of money after the client has been billed. As money is received, it must be recorded not only in the daily financial summary but also on the accounts receivable card. A very common form of embezzlement is to receive a check on account and not record it, throw away the accounts receivable card, take the same amount of cash out of a deposit, and put the check in. This is another reason to check the cash amount as well as the total deposit amount daily.

It will be up to the manager to establish accounts receivable policies. Some important questions will be who is allowed to charge, the minimum limits allowable, when and how often the client will be billed, when to use telephone calls for nonpaying clients, and when to turn bad accounts over to a collection agency or take them to small claims court.

It is also the responsibility of the manager to decide how to handle both insufficient funds and stop-payment checks. However bad checks are handled, the important point to keep in mind is the quicker the action, the better the chances of full recovery.

Record controls

Record keeping controls are a must even if only one completely trustworthy employee is handling the money. Embezzlers have two traits in common with most honest people: they are very likable and they are very hard workers. Most commercially available record keeping systems, whether handwritten, cash registers, or computers, have built-in safeguards. The problem is that the systems tend to get modified as they are used or the control measures are not used by management.

The basis of the controls in most systems is the sequential numbering of the charge slips and money receipts. If these numbers are used as intended, it will not be impossible to steal, but it will be very difficult. There is no completely secure system, but by making sure numbered charge slips and receipts are used, the majority of the problems will be eliminated.

To make the record numbers mean something to the employees a fanatic attitude must be established about missing records, whether it be a charge slip, receipt, or any other form that has a number. Going a little bit crazy every time one is missing will ensure that these records or forms are not thrown away or otherwise misused. Spending 2 days tearing the hospital apart looking for a missing form will impress the staff with the concern for accuracy and honesty. This means the manager cannot dare to be casual in the use of records or forms either. Set an example of accuracy and honesty, and it will usually be followed.

Most of the financial management information needed can be derived from the daily financial summary. Do not be willing to accept the information provided by the system, but decide instead what information is needed to manage the practice, and insist that the system provide that information. Make sure the information provided is on a continual, long-term basis. If specific information is needed only occasionally, do not set up a system that provides the information on a continual ongoing basis.

When using production information, *how* the income is produced is of little value, it is *who* produced it that really matters. Unfortunately most systems are not people or human oriented, they are oriented more toward things and procedures, and this information is more interesting than useful. If the practice is considering computerizing or in any way changing the financial system, decide what *you* want from the system, write it down, and then insist the salesperson provide that from the system. The practice should have the information reported that is important, not the information the software salesperson thinks should be reported.

In addition to the practice manager, the accountant is the other person who will be using the bookkeeping system. The bookkeeping system will be providing the accountant with information needed for paying sales taxes and filing tax forms. The information provided will also be used for the income portion of the financial statements, so the accountant should have input into what information the system should regularly provide.

Payroll is another part of the bookkeeping system. When setting up a payroll system it is advisable to consult with the practice's accountant. Tax laws keep changing, and not adhering to the changes can be very costly, so keep in close touch with an up-to-date accountant. The payroll informaton necessary varies but includes employee information concerning deductions, payroll information to complete W-2 and W-4 forms, time card information, and so forth. There is certain information the employer is required to provide employees and specific records that must be kept.

Work out with the accountant who has the responsibility for providing the necessary information for paying payroll taxes on time. Decide who will keep employee records, and make the information available to employees when requested from the employer.

Even accountants who work full-time in the tax and accounting areas have trouble keeping up with regulation changes, so the practice manager should not try. The cost of mistakes is too great to take chances.

Medical records

Medical records have more to do with the medicine practiced than with the management of the practice, but there are some things about the medical record that are of concern. As the practice's manager there are a number of things about the medical record to be aware of such as (1) the size, shape, and form; (2) usefulness to relief or new staff veterinarians; (3) usefulness in answering complaints; and (4) the efficiency of use.

The size, shape, and form of the records are important considerations because they all affect storage space. If laboratory reports and other additional forms are kept with the medical record, large folders will be necessary. The major problem is that they take considerable room, and some hospitals simply do not have room for these files. The manager will have to evaluate the practice's record needs, veterinarian's wants, and space available and then choose the best compromise.

The usefulness of the records to relief or new staff veterinarians is very important. The records are really a veterinarian's memory of past treatments. They also provide others access to the attending veterinarian's memory. Without good records a relief veterinarian or staff veterinarian may be completely starting over with an ongoing case.

The Problem-Oriented Veterinary Medical Record (POVMR) used in most veterinary schools and many research and training facilities would be ideal. Unfortunately, this record system is not practical in most private practices. However, modifications of the POVMR can be used and should be considered.

It is necessary to provide the relief or new veterinarian with a quick reference to the patient's past health history. For this purpose a record system should keep the vaccination history together on one page. Past treatments should be organized to quickly show diagnosis, treatment or surgery, and follow-up. To make this a quick reference, the diagnosis should be underlined, written in a different color ink, highlighted with a highlighter pen, or printed if the rest of the record is written. The purpose is to make it catch the reader's eye quickly.

The same differentiation should be used for treatment or surgery, especially the names of the medications used. In other words, any veterinarian should be able to pick up the medical record and quickly determine what the veterinarian writing the record was treating or at least thought he was treating, what medication was used for treatment, or what surgery was performed and the outcome.

The usefulness of the records in answering complaints is similar but slightly different. Staff veterinarians should be admonished to write their records as if they were writing them to an attorney because they might be. Again, they should be complete with a diagnosis, treatment or surgery, and follow-up. Unfortunately, an amazing number of treatments and surgeries are completed without any diagnosis being recorded. The practice manager should call the state's Board of Examiners in Veterinary Medicine's executive secretary to ask what things are most commonly omitted from the record. Steps should be taken to make sure those items are present in the practice's records.

If the doctor gives the client a very grave prognosis, it should be recorded. If the client elects treatment even if the animal has almost no chance of recovery, the veterinarian should note the grave prognosis in the record and have the client initial it. The same is true of any suggested diagnostic testing or treatment the client refuses. It should be written in the record that the veterinarian suggested the procedure but the client declined and the client should initial that statement. Properly written records are a defense against complaints without additional explanations being necessary.

Of course, if the record is to be read by others, it should be legible and copyable. If the veterinarian cannot write legibly, perhaps he should learn to type or have someone else do the writing. When using different color pens, make sure the color can be copied.

Efficient records are those that make it possible to spend less time on paperwork than on medicine. Keep in mind the purpose of the practice is to help clients with their animals' medical problems, not to write records. Consider using stamps or preprinted forms for things that are written often. Using stamps instead of additional pieces of paper for laboratory reports and euthanasia releases can save filing excessive amounts of paper. By keeping surgical releases and euthanasia releases simple enough to fit on a reasonable size stamp, they can be stamped on the back of a record sheet rather than adding a separate slip of paper.

Be careful about the excessive use of initials and abbreviations. Some practitioners get carried away with using initials and abbreviations in an attempt to save time. A year later even the attending veterinarian cannot guess what the initials meant, so it would be impossible for anyone else to decode what was written.

Financial status reports

The third type of record you will need to be concerned with is the practice's financial status record. These are the reports prepared by the accountant. The most common reports are the profit-and-loss (P/L) statement, the balance sheet, and various tax forms. The practice manager should always keep close track of the finances of the practice. To do the necessary monitoring, the manager should keep and understand the following records: (1) monthly P/L statement and balance sheet; (2) copies of all tax forms, filed and paid; (3) the manager's P/L statement of the operational income and expenses; and (4) cash flow records.

P/L statement and balance sheet

The P/L statement and balance sheet are compiled by the accountant from the income and expense information provided by the manager. The additional expense to have these reports done monthly is minimal over quarterly reports, so monthly reports should be requested. In addition to the column of figures for the current month there should be a column of figures showing year-to-date. If possible it is nice to also show the year-to-date figures for the same period of the previous year on the same page to make comparisons (Fig. 14-8).

The balance sheet reports the financial condition as of the date at the top of the sheet, and the P/L statement reports what activity took place in the practice during the period covered by the statement. The manager must be able to evaluate both reports because they describe the health of the practice and provide early warning of problems. This will be discussed in greater detail when describing the manager's P/L statement.

Tax forms and payments

Copies of all tax forms and payments must be kept for a given period of time that your accountant can explain, but before you file them, read them. Try to understand what they are about, and when you do not understand them, ask your accountant. It is always a good idea to

Veterinary Emergency Clinic, Inc., 154
Profit and Loss Statement
Five-Month Period Ending August 31, 1986
For Internal Use Only

Sales & Revenues

551 Professional Services	$44,897	$48,979	100.00%	$243,961	$271,907	100.00%
552 Tax Paid Drugs Sold	2,048			4,564		
559 Interest Earned				257		
Total Sales & Revenue	$46,945	$48,979	100.00%	$248,782	$271,907	100.00%

Cost of Sales

661 Cost of Drugs	$9,295	$6,896	14.08%	$35,938	$31,771	11.68%
662 Cost of Taxable Items	120			120		
663 Hospital Supplies	369			369		
664 Outside Lab Expense	69	86	0.18	69	324	0.12
665 Other Costs	604	813	1.66	3,302	3,415	1.26
666 Surgical Supplies	86			86		
667 X-Ray Supplies	299	775	1.54	299	960	0.35
668 Laboratory Supplies	94			94		
Total Cost and Sales	$10,936	$8,570	17.46%	$40,277	$36,470	13.41%
711 Professional Wages	$18,562	$23,492	47.96%	$91,129	$98,763	36.32%
722 Lay Wages	11,173	11,411	23.30	59,630	56,856	20.91
770 Professional Sub Contr.	700			2,050		
771 Administrative Expense		700	1.43	4,077	4,250	1.56
773 Laundry & Uniform	152			533		
774 Promotion				39		
775 Bldg. Loan Interest	3,504	3,415	6.97	3,504	17,141	6.30
780 Depreciation Reserve	2,137	1,210	2.47	11,294	6,050	2.23
781 Dues and Subscriptions	142			172	41	0.02
782 Insurance	849	2,780	5.68	6,088	9,350	3.44
783 Interest & Bank Charges	97			10,430		
784 Miscellaneous	50			64		
785 Office Expenses	338	585	1.20	2,246	2,959	1.09
786 Supplies Maintenance					293	0.11
787 Accounting & Legal	270	280	0.57	1,635	1,690	0.62
788 Rent	45			186	270	0.10
789 Repair and Maintenance	569	578	1.18	3,220	2,854	1.05
790 State Franchise Tax				1,000		
791 Employment Taxes	1,010	1,007	2.06	8,887	8,281	3.05
792 Property Taxes	397			1,184	1,548	0.57
793 Tax Other & Licenses				30	30	0.01
794 Telephone	642	617	1.26	2,883	3,108	1.14
796 Utilities	405	464	0.95	1,802	2,112	0.78
798 Staff Meetings					1,270	0.47
Total Operating Expenses	$41,042	$46,539	95.03%	$212,083	$216,866	79.77%
Net Profit or Loss	$ 5,033—	$ 6,130—	12.49%	$ 3,578—	$ 18,571	6.82%

Figure 14-8.   Profit and sales statement

get your taxes done early enough so you can take your time and look the forms over before you mail the payment or the form to the tax agency. Most accountants are accurate, but they are human and can occasionally use a wrong number. If the taxes are much different than you expected, do not hestiate to question them.

Manager's P/L statements

The manager's P/L statement of operational expenses is important to keep. Remember that the accountant is primarily a tax preparer, not a business manager. The accountant's function is to prove to the tax agencies that the practice is bankrupt and does not owe taxes. If the accountant does the job well, the result can be a distorted and depressing picture of the practice's finances. Creative accountants can show a practice having a loss when in truth the practice is having a very good year.

The manager should take the accountant's P/L statement and extract items such as depreciation, interest (income and expense), and any other expenses not directly related to the operation of the practice. One needs to know what is happening in the practice financially by using actual income and expense figures from the practice. Also when compiling these figures, for simplicity divide them into six categories (Fig. 14-9). This will provide a quick reference for comparing with other years. These categories are

1. Professional staff—all income or costs related to the veterinarians whether they are employees or owners
2. Support staff expense—all of the salary, tax, and fringe benefit costs associated with the support staff
3. Supplies—all medical supplies, drugs, office and janitorial supplies
4. Outside services—outside laboratory service, animal disposal, consulting services, accounting and legal costs

5. Housing costs—all costs associated with housing the practice such as utilities, maintenance, rent, insurance, and so forth
6. General overhead—anything that does not fit one of the aforementioned categories such as lawn care

There are a few things to keep in mind when using this statement in evaluating the practice's financial condition. To simplify the evaluation process start by expressing each expense as a percentage of the practice's income. Keep in mind that when the expenses are expressed as a percentage of the income that percentage resulted from two numbers, not one. In other words, if the expense is a higher percentage of the income than should be, it is more apt to be the income that is too low rather than the expense being too high. Also it is easier to adjust the percentage by raising the income than it is to lower the expense.

Of the six items listed one should really not be considered an expense. The professional staff costs are really a part of the net income of the practice. One goal of the practice manager is to increase this amount both as a percentage and in actual dollars each year. The other expenses should go up in dollar amounts each year but should remain level or drop when expressed as a percentage of the income. When all costs and expenses move together in one direction, it is the income that is fluctuating. If one of the costs or expenses is changing at a rate much different from the other costs and expenses, the problem is with that individual cost or expense.

Do not be concerned about comparisons with national or area averages or any other practice, the only valid comparison is with your own practice's past performance. Signs of a healthy practice are when client count and income have increased enough to raise the percentage of net (or professional) income

Manager's Profit and Loss Sheet

MANAGER'S PROFIT AND LOSS EVALUATION: Date: _____

_____ Year to Date Figures

Income:

  Charges: $ _____

_____ Clients or Transactions: _____

               Average Charge: $ _____

  Amount Deposited: (minus returned checks) $ _____

Operating Expenses:

  Support Staff: $_____   _____%*

  Supplies $_____   _____

  Outside Services: $_____   _____

  Housing Costs: $_____   _____

  General Overhead:$_____   _____

  Professional Staff: $_____   _____

    Total Operating Expenses: $ _____

Operating Profit:**   _____$ $ _____

1. Support Staff: all of the salary, tax, and fringe benefits associated with the support staff. 16% to 20%
2. Supplies: all medical supplies, drugs, office and janitorial supplies. 10% to 15%
3. Outside Services: outside laboratory, animal disposal, consulting services, accounting and legal. 5% to 6%
4. Housing Costs: all costs associated with housing the practice such as utilities, maintenance, rent insurance, etc. 10%
5. General Overhead: anything that doesn't fit one of the above categories. 9%
6. Professional Staff: all income or costs related to the veterinarians whether employees or owners. (See operating profit note below.)

* Percentage of amount deposited. Divide expense by the amount deposited.

**Add operating profit to professional staff expense to determine the professional income of the practice. The goal for the practice should be a professional income of 40% to 50%. This is the most significant figure of all because it is the reason for practicing in the first place.

Figure 14-9. Manager's profit and loss sheet

while the percentage of expense has decreased.

Cash flow records

Cash flow records are the basics of the practice's finances. They are simply the practice's checking and savings account balances at the beginning of the month, plus the amount deposited during the month, minus the checks written, the bills left to pay, and the payroll to be met. A good measurement of the cash flow is to measure it in days. How many days do the bills have to wait before being paid? Assuming a 30-day average month, if the bills left to be paid at the end of the month (including payroll) are equal to the amount of income generated during the month, the practice is 30 days behind. If the bills are 50% of the amount available to pay them, the practice is 15 days behind.

The goal, of course, is to be able to pay the bills as they arrive and have a small cash reserve at the end of the month. The manager cannot afford to rely solely on other financial reports but must know the cash position at all times.

Banking

Banking is another part of the practice manager's job description. It is important to have a strong relationship between the practice and the practice's bank. The bank is not just a place to store money, but rather it is people renting money to other people and exchanging money as directed. The practice manager should know and be recognized by the bank officers where business is conducted. Personalize the transactions by being acquainted with the banker, and make sure they know something about the practice. Some day the practice may need a short-term loan, and it will be too late to make the banker's acquaintance.

Establish a line of credit with the bank before it is needed. Make sure that if a check is accidentally written for more than the account balance the bank will not return the check, especially if it is a tax check.

The banker should be known well enough that when a loan is needed for an equipment purchase or remodeling the best possible terms will be offered. Loan terms are not etched in stone as bankers would like to have us believe. At times, banks have little money to loan, and acceptable terms can be difficult to obtain. At other times they have excess money and are anxious to provide excellent terms. Most bankers like to suggest that we need them more than they need us, which, of course, is untrue.

Another item that can be negotiated with the banker is the credit card discount. The author has practices with credit card discount rates of 1.25 to 2 percentage points lower than the amount paid by other practices in the same area. Discount rate negotiations are not always successful, but it costs nothing to try.

Miscellaneous duties of the manager

The practice manager will also have other responsibilities that are not quite as well defined as those already discussed. For example, the manager should take full responsibility for cleanliness of the facility and aspire to a reputation for managing the cleanest practice in the country. My definition of cleanliness in a veterinary practice is a practice where no dust can be found on plant leaves, picture frames, door casings, or window sills; no hairballs or dead flies under the x-ray machine or surgery table; and no hair or lint around the casters of any equipment with wheels. When you get these items completely taken care of, the rest of the hospital will usually be clean. The manager should be careful not to do any of the cleaning, or the staff will just stand back and watch. Make them do it and be a beast about cleaning until they keep the hospital as clean as wanted rather than having to deal with the manager.

Part of being clean is being odor free. Since the manager is in and out of the practice more than the rest of the staff, he should be aware of unpleasant odors. When the manager comes in from outside and experiences an unpleasant odor, it should be traced down and eliminated rather than accepted as a part of veterinary medicine. Fecal examinations should be done under an exhaust fan and should not permeate the whole room.

The practice manager also has the responsibility to provide positive leadership. If the staff manager does not have a positive attitude, what hope can there be for the rest of the staff?

The veterinary profession already suffers from more negativity than it can deal with successfully. If the manager cannot be positive about the future of veterinary medicine and the practice, then another career choice should be made.

Providing the practice with a library of inspirational books and tapes that have helped the manager maintain a positive perspective on life and work is another important function. The manager must provide the practice with positive leadership and be a positive influence on the practice personnel. One way to do that is to be adaptable. The staff should never see the manager upset or out of control. When the manager is unflappable no matter what management disaster occurs, the staff will be amazed and will be confident in the manager's leadership ability.

☐
Choosing a practice manager

If you are a practice owner and are wondering whether you need a practice manager as described in this chapter, there are a few questions you need to ask yourself:

1. Will I be out of the practice, and will I stay out? If you are not currently working in the practice and do not plan to work in it or if you are planning to retire but would like to keep your practice as an investment, you probably could use a practice manager.
2. If I am continuing in the practice, could I let the manager fire my favorite technician or veterinarian without getting involved? If the answer is yes, then you are a rare individual and ready for a practice manager. If you cannot, you are not ready for a manager as described in this chapter. A midlevel executive might fill the bill by allowing the owner some management decisions.
3. Is my practice large enough for a manager? Practice size has nothing to do with it because the practice manager could be a part-time employee if the practice is a small one. A former, successful, retired business manager would make a great part-time manager for a small practice.

When the practice owner is convinced the practice can use a practice manager, how is the right person selected? College degrees or knowledge of veterinary medicine (there is nothing wrong with degrees or knowledge of veterinary medicine) should not become absolute prerequisites for the position. What is needed is a person with management skills. The successful candidate should be someone who has demonstrated management ability in his last position. Maturity is an extremely important characteristic. Do not confuse age and maturity; age does not ensure maturity, nor does youth preclude maturity. Because the manager will also be the leader of the staff, he must demonstrate at least the same or more maturity than the most mature person on the staff.

The manager must respect the veterinarians on the staff and the owner, even if the owner is not working in the practice. The manager must not be overwhelmed by or be in awe of any member of the veterinary staff. The manager cannot manage something or someone he is afraid of or does not respect. The manager must consider himself at least equal to the senior member of the staff. The manager must be neither belligerent and overbearing nor timid and reticent. Self-confidence and self-discipline are two very necessary qualities a successful practice manager must possess.

Admittedly the necessary traits to be a good practice manager are found in few individuals, but they are not impossible to find. Good practice managers are rare, but so is a practice that will tolerate a good practice manager.

Because most practices are still owned by a veterinarian or veterinarians who work in the practice, true practice management will probably be a rare position for the foreseeable future. Many practices have tried to turn part of the management over to a practice manager and have finally given up because of the frustrations caused by the conflicts inherent in such a situation. Before giving up on the idea completely, however, consider the possibility of a partial step in the direction of a practice manager.

The owner of the practice can retain the final responsibility and authority for the management of the practice and yet be rid of all of the routine management duties and devote more time to practicing medicine. The process by which this is done is called *delegation*. The duties of the practice manager as listed in this chapter, except for final decisions at the highest level, can be done by other staff members, people already on the payroll. They can be done by the following people:

1. Practice income production: chief of staff—the practice owner, senior veterinarian, or any veterinarian who volunteers for the position who has the respect of the rest of the staff veterinarians
2. Personnel management
   a. Senior receptionist
   b. Senior technician
   c. Sharing the duty and taking care of their respective departments
3. Purchasing
   a. Senior technician
   b. One of the other technicians
   c. Office supplies by one of the receptionists
   d. Janitorial supplies by the person who does the cleaning
4. Maintenance
   a. Maintenance person or handyman
   b. Technician with general equipment repair knowledge
5. Bookkeeping, accounting, and legal
   a. Bookkeeper hired specifically for bookkeeping duties
   b. Office manager (the person above with a different title)
   c. Senior receptionist who is also the office manager, credit manager, bill payer, or whatever title currently being used
6. Banking
   a. Practice owner
   b. Practice owner and the office manager/bookkeeper
7. Cleaning: whoever the owner puts in charge
8. Providing leadership: owner of the practice by demonstrating leadership in delegating duties to other responsible staff members

Delegating is as simple as letting go. Most veterinarians are hesitant to delegate responsibility and authority to their employees because they tend to underrate their employees. Keep in mind that all employees are only using a small percentage of their capabilities, so they are capable of taking on much more responsibility than their current assignments. The only thing holding them back is that they cannot have the responsibility until it is given to them.

Once the decision of employee delegation has been made by the practice owner, do not forget that the employees must have the authority to perform the responsibility assigned to them. An employee responsible for keeping the floor clean must have the authority to purchase a mop when necessary. A monetary limit could be set on any or all areas to allow the owner more control over expenditures. For example, the maintenance manager can have anything repaired without the owner's permission as long as the repairs are under $75. When the repair is in excess of the predetermined limit, then the repair estimate and the cost of a new replacement must be presented to the owner for the final decision.

Veterinarians should either hire a manager or delegate the management duties and concentrate on practicing medicine. After all, if veterinarians had wanted to be business managers, they would have gone to school to get a masters in business administration rather than a doctorate of veterinary medicine.

References

1. Girrard J: How to Sell Yourself. New York, Warner Books, 1984
2. Johnson S, Wilson L: One Minute Salesperson. New York, William Morrow & Co, 1984
3. Mandino O: The Greatest Salesman in the World. New York, Bantam Books, 1985

Chapter 15
□
Practice and the law

Harold W. Hannah

Why should a veterinarian be concerned about the law? Apart from concerns as a citizen, some activities as a professional person are affected by provisions in the Veterinary Medical Practice Act of the state. Therefore, the veterinarian should be familiar with the state's practice act. Veterinarians have a contractual relation with clients and, therefore, should have some familiarity with their rights and duties under such a contract. From that contractual relationship, if it is an unhappy one, may spring a malpractice action. Therefore, one should have some notions about how such actions might be discouraged, about reactions when a suit arises, and about cooperation with the insurer in defending such an action or making a settlement.

Familiarity with the state practice act and taking the right steps to defend a malpractice action represent only some of the areas of the law about which a veterinarian should be concerned. The veterinarian hires both lay and technical personnel and may be liable to them or for their injuries to clients or other persons. Practitioners maintain premises to which members of the public are invited. They may render emergency service, be incorporated, practice in a partnership, practice in a location that disturbs the neighbors—for these and other reasons, veterinarians need to be concerned about the law. It is the purpose of this chapter to discuss some of these issues in a way that will be helpful to the practicing veterinarian.

□
Selecting an attorney

A veterinarian is most likely to need an attorney for the following purposes: to defend in a malpractice action, to recover fees, or to handle certain business matters that arise in practice.

Since the veterinarian's insurer will come to his or her defense in a malpractice action, it will provide the legal services for defense. Though one might make suggestions to the insurer about the lawyers to be involved, the insurer has the right to select the attorneys.

With respect to legal matters for which an insurer does not come to the rescue, and there are many, the veterinarian must choose from the legal profession an attorney to represent him. Many veterinarians know the legal profession in their community and have some judgment about whom they would like to employ. In fact they may have established relations with an attorney who has handled such problems for them as leasing or purchasing property, collecting fees, incorporating, establishing a partnership, interpreting employment contracts, or advising on legislative or administrative pronouncements that affect their practice.

For veterinarians who have not established a relationship with a competent attorney, selecting the right one may not be easy. Here are some suggestions:

- Discuss the needs with other members of the profession, bankers, or business friends who have used legal services, and get their suggestions.
- Contact the secretary of the county or city bar association to see whether it has a referral service. If so, describe the specific needs and get recommendations from that service.
- If a local referral service is not available, the state bar association may operate one. Contact it for suggestions.
- If none of the aforementioned is possible or feasible, select the most appropriate law firm or attorney from the telephone directory yellow pages, arrange an appoint-

ment, discuss the specific needs, and form an opinion about the attorney's ability to handle the legal business. If one has doubts about the attorney chosen, ask to be referred to another attorney. Most attorneys will willingly suggest another lawyer if the matters brought to them are outside their area of expertise.

Just as a client can terminate the services of a veterinarian at any time without liability for payment of services rendered, so can a veterinarian terminate the client–lawyer relationship and seek other legal counsel. However, the sooner this decision can be made, the better, especially if litigation is involved. If the attorney has spent many hours preparing for a trial, including perhaps the filing of a complaint, and the client withdraws at this stage and employs another attorney, the client's costs will materially increase.

Attorneys (like veterinarians) are also subject to malpractice actions and to proceedings for revocation or suspension of license. If a veterinarian should be so unfortunate as to employ an attorney who grossly mismanages his business or fails to file important documents on time, to observe applicable statutes of limitation, or to perform other acts that are important in securing a client's rights, the veterinarian may consider a malpractice action against the attorney; one may also inform the state authority that disciplines attorneys and register a complaint. Legislation and Supreme Court rules generally provide for the establishment of an attorney licensing and disciplinary commission or similar body to hear complaints about attorneys and decide what action, if any, should be taken.

☐
The standard of skill and care

More than a century ago the Supreme Court of New Hampshire said:

The professional man contracts that he will use reasonable and ordinary care and diligence in the exertion of his skill and the application of his knowledge to accomplish the purpose for which he is employed. He does not undertake for extra-ordinary skill. The general rule is well settled, as in other cases in contracts supposed to be mutually beneficial to the parties, that the contractor for services to be performed for another agrees to exert such care and diligence in his employment as men of common care and common prudence usually exert in their own business of a similar kind (*Leighton v. Sargent* 27 N.H. 460 [1883]).

In a suit against the United States for alleged negligent certification of cattle for interstate shipment, the Court said:

The nearest analogy that occurs to us is the duty of one who undertakes a matter requiring expertness to bring reasonable skill and knowledge to his task according to the then state of the art and to execute it with ordinary care that involves no guarantee of the results. Such is the duty of a medical practitioner on man or beast (*U.S. v. Russell & Tucker,* 95 F2nd 684 [1938]).

Veterinarians are not held to a standard of perfection; they are held to the standard of other practitioners generally. The "locality rule," one that held that the standard of skill and care of a professional person should be measured against practitioners in their locality, once generally accepted, is no longer the prevailing rule.

Mistakes in diagnosis do not automatically spell liability. Here again, the courts will measure the veterinarian's diagnostic skill and procedures used against those used by other veterinarians in similar circumstances. If they pass the test, liability should not be imposed.

The specialty practitioner

What about the specialist? Is there a different standard? Court decisions indicate that there is. If the veterinarian is board certified in a specialty or claims to possess special skills, a disgruntled client would have the right to introduce expert testimony in an attempt to prove that the veterinarian's knowledge and skill were not equal to those of other veterinarians practicing the same specialty.

A veterinarian who is not a specialist but who undertakes a procedure involving a specialist's knowledge and skill may be liable to a client for an unsatisfactory result if the client is able to show that the veterinarian undertook a procedure beyond his skill and knowledge. A veterinarian confronted with such a case (such as cataract surgery) should get the client's consent to refer the animal to a specialist or, if this is not feasible, get a specific waiver from the client before proceeding. Another possibility when a referral is not feasible and the veterinarian does not wish to undertake the case is to explain the situation frankly to the client and suggest other clinics to which the client might take the animal. In large-animal practice, referrals might be made to a state diagnostic laboratory.

If a veterinarian agrees to service the animals of a client over a period of time, there are many points that should be discussed, agreed upon, and preferably stated in writing. Such a practice contract should, as a minimum, cover the following points: (1) the length of the contract agreement; (2) the minimum number of visits the veterinarian will make; (3) a statement about the services that will be rendered; (4) the rate, method of determining, and times for payment of fees; and (5) duties of the client—assistance, having animals confined, and making other arrangements to facilitate the veterinarian's work when visiting the premises.

A herd contract by its very nature imposes duties on the veterinarian that do not exist in the ordinary veterinarian-client relationship. Because of this the possibilities for negligence claims are expanded. Also, there may be more situations in which a conflict of interest could arise — when there are dealings between the contract client and other clients of the veterinarian involving, for example, the examination of animals and issuance of health certificates. A herd contract can be advantageous to both the livestock owner and the veterinarian, and it is not so fraught with potential legal problems as to discourage its use.

Promising a cure

It is not wise from either a legal or practical standpoint for a veterinarian to promise a result. Veterinarians and other professionals may now state many things in general advertising (as long as they are not false, misleading, or deceptive). Statements made to or expectations aroused in a client that amount to a promise on the part of the veterinarian that a particular result will follow are another matter. It is not only unethical (as provided in the American Veterinary Medical Association's *Principles of Veterinary Medical Ethics*) to guarantee a cure, it is dangerous legally. Cases in human medicine have held that when such a promise can be proved the practitioner is liable for a bad result regardless of the degree of skill and care involved in treatment of the patient.

Additional treatment

Important in the veterinarian-client relationship is the understanding by the client of the services the veterinarian intends to render. If an animal is left for a specific purpose, treatment for other purposes is *not* implied, and before proceeding further the veterinarian should obtain the consent of the client.

Though the admission form may contain a general consent for the veterinarian to make any treatment that seems necessary and may also include an exculpatory clause excusing the veterinarian from liability, these provisions are of little protective value in case the veterinarian is sued and the client can prove that he was not advised and informed about additional treatment or surgery. It is well established in any situation where a change in treatment or surgery not contemplated is undertaken that the client is entitled to be informed so that a judgment can be made about additional treatment or surgery. This has additional importance in veterinary medicine because there may be a fee limit beyond which the owner would not wish to go in the treatment of an animal. Billing for unrequested treatment stands high among the complaints made against veterinarians by their clients. Thus, it behooves veterinarians to explain the proposed treatment or surgery so the client can make a decision based on adequate information.

Besides obtaining informed consent for treatment or surgery, there are other activities for which a veterinarian should have written authorization. This applies especially to euthanasia, disposal of the animal's body, and necropsy. The body of the animal belongs to its owner, and there should be a clear understanding between owner and veterinarian about what the veterinarian is permitted to do if the animal dies while in the hospital. Euthanasia may be traumatic for the client or for members of the client's family (please refer to Chapter 16). Hence a written authorization signed by the party who has authority either as owner or agent is desirable.

Unless the veterinarian knows the client's family or has dealt with the members previously, he should be cautious about doing anything based on authorization by a minor. This is especially true when euthanasia is requested. If there is any doubt about the authority of a minor, or for that matter any other agent of the owner, to request either treatment, surgery, or euthanasia, the owner should be contacted. Situations may arise in which it is impossible to contact the owner before the veterinarian must make a decision. If during surgery an unexpected complication arises or another diseased organ is discovered and an immediate decision is necessary, the veterinarian will be protected if in performing the additional procedures testimony introduced would convince the judge or jury that most other veterinarian would have reached the same conclusion.

In emergency situations that do not involve the veterinarian's client but where the veterinarian may be present, for example, at the scene of an accident involving animals, and euthanasia or treatment was performed on an injured animal, the veterinarian may be protected as a matter of common law. Some states, however, have adopted legislation like that in Illinois that provides that

> A veterinarian who on his own initiative or other than at the request of the owner gives emergency treatment to a sick or injured animal at the scene of an accident shall not be liable in damages to the owner of such animal in the absence of gross negligence. If the veterinarian performs euthanasia on the animal, there is a presumption that it was a humane act necessary to relieve it from pain and suffering (Ill. Rev. Stat. ch. 111 par. 7018).

The medical record

Of vital importance to veterinarians if they are sued for malpractice is timely and adequate documentation of treatment and the recording and preservation of adequate medical records. Additional information on malpractice may be found in Chapter 8. Records should be made promptly and be complete and accurate—

something that may not be easy for a busy large-animal practitioner away from the clinic for long periods of time. Even a busy large-animal practitioner, however, should consider that part of the job is making field notes or other memoranda that can be put into acceptable record form as soon as they are returned to the clinic. Timeliness is important—the longer the time gap between the rendering of service and the making of records, the more suspect the records become, not only for legal purposes but for medical purposes.

When litigation arises and the veterinarian's records are requested, whether or not the veterinarian himself is involved in the litigation, authenticated copies of the records should be made available. Records can be subpoenaed by the requesting party, so they should be made available without additional legal action.

There may be some question about the confidentiality of veterinary medical records. There is some legal authority for holding that because veterinary records concern property and not people they are not confidential. Nevertheless, there are veterinary medical records disclosure of which could be harmful to the client. Thus, in a proper case it would be pertinent to raise this issue and argue for confidentiality.

Views differ on the length of time veterinary records should be retained. It can be said for certain that they should be kept for as long as there is any reasonable likelihood they will be needed in litigation. Because most records do not fall into this category, other considerations apply.

Will the medical record be useful for scientific purposes, historical review of the practice, or for a purchaser of the practice? These additional uses may require that records be held for longer periods of time. Microfilm offers an opportunity for keeping records in a minimum of space, thus permitting their retention.

Other business records of the veterinarian, those having to do with the purchase and sale of real and personal property and the employment of personnel, may be kept for shorter periods depending on statutes of limitation in the particular state. Ten years is a usual time for enforcement of written agreements. However, the records of agreements that are not likely to give rise to controversy may be disposed of in less than 10 years. At any rate, it would be good business and afford legal protection if the veterinarian established a timing system for practice files, a system devised in the light of any state laws or regulations that may be applicable and in the light of practical business advice.

Client responsibility

Questions are frequently raised about the veterinarian's duty to accept a client, especially if there is doubt about the client's ability to pay. The American Veterinary Medical Association's *Principles of Veterinary Medical Ethics* states, "Veterinarians may choose whom they will serve." This means they do not have to establish a veterinarian–client relationship unless they choose to do so. Because no reason is required for refusal to accept a client, refusal for the inability to pay would not violate the code of ethics. Court decisions have followed a similar line with respect to medical practitioners by saying that a physician is not required to accept a patient even under circumstances that would imply a moral obligation for him to do so. Once a client is accepted, however, there is a duty to continue service as long as it is needed or until such time as the client can find another veterinarian after a statement by the attending veterinarian that he intends to discontinue service to the client. It should be noted that "client" has two connotations: in the eyes of the veterinarian it in-

cludes people who customarily come to him for service whether or not he is currently engaged in treating their animals. There is also a legal connotation, namely, that a person is a client of the veterinarian only as the result of a contract to treat an animal or animals, and when that treatment ends in one way or another, the contract ends, and there is no longer, legally speaking, a veterinarian–client relationship.

There are situations under which a veterinarian may be under a continuous duty to respond. This will exist if one is a contract veterinarian or a public veterinarian (with respect to public responsibilities) or is party to an agreement under which 24-hour emergency service is rendered. Questions sometimes arise about how far the veterinarian should go in rendering emergency service — should it go beyond first aid without the consent of the owner of the animal? The answer is no. The veterinarian cannot create a client relationship against the will of the animal owner.

When does a contractual relationship between a veterinarian and client terminate? There are two obvious answers: when the animal dies and when the client tells the veterinarian that services are no longer required. But what is the veterinarian's duty as far as continuing service once treatment of an animal has commenced? There is a duty to continue service, to provide needed post-operative care, to inform the client about aftercare when the animal returns home, in other words, to continue professional services until the animal either expires or until all of the services contemplated and reasonably implied have been rendered. To escape responsibility to a client when the animal requires further care, the veterinarian must notify the client of the intention to terminate services and give the client time to find another veterinarian, during which time necessary services will continue to be rendered for the benefit of the animal.

Payment of fees

What security does or should a veterinarian have for payment of fees? In times of economic stress, particularly in the agricultural community, veterinarians become concerned about their priority among other creditors. It can be argued that because the veterinarians' services may preserve animals or their value for the benefit of other creditors their claim should come first. Some state legislatures have been motivated by this argument and have enacted veterinary lien laws that give them priority over all other creditors. Other states that have not enacted a veterinarian' lien law may nevertheless have laws that would permit a veterinarian to assert a prior claim.

Among these laws are the *agisters lien* (a lien for one who keeps, yards, feeds, and cares for the animals of another) and *statutory liens* for service and storage of personal property. Agisters liens are of no help to a large-animal practitioner because they normally depend on possession, and they may be of little help to the small-animal practitioner because the value of the animal retained in possession for payment of the fee may be so small as to afford no recompense if it has to be sold under foreclosure provisions of the agisters lien law. If an owner's sentimental attachment to the animal is great enough, retaining possession by the veterinarian under an agisters lien or other law that would permit the retention might induce payment.

There is another possibility for the large-animal practitioner or the racehorse veterinarian who treats many animals of high value, and that is to file a security agreement under the Uniform Commercial Code. This would give the veterinarian priority over other creditors who were junior in time of filing. Preservation of an amicable relationship with clients might, however, dictate that the veterinarian not follow this route.

The most useful law for the veterinarian would be one giving him a statutory lien not dependent on possession but preserved by filing. One could then decide in each case whether it is worth the time and expense to enforce the lien.

□
Work contracts and restrictive covenants

What agreements are important when a veterinarian hires another veterinarian? Although there are pros and cons about the desirability of a written contract, controversies that have arisen and litigation that has grown out of these controversies suggest that a written contract is desirable. Among other things, such a work contract should provide for the following:

The beginning and ending date of the contract with provisions on renewal

The method for determining payment of the employed veterinarian—whether a straight salary, a percentage of the income, or some combination of these

A provision on vacations, sick leaves, and leave to attend continuing veterinary medical education programs

Duties regarding emergency service if this is involved

Retirement and insurance benefits

A requirement that professional liability insurance be carried and by whom it shall be paid

Provisions on the use of practice vehicles and expenses connected with their use

Provisions on buying into the practice and becoming a partner if this is contemplated

A covenant not to compete if the employee will sign an agreement containing such a covenant.

There are other considerations, and some of the ones mentioned beg for further breakdown. It is advisable that the employing veterinarian's attorney be asked to draft an employment contract after consultation and after both parties have agreed generally on what they would like to see in the contract. Figure 15-1 illustrates a contract of employment.

A *restrictive covenant* is a provision in an employment contract, a partnership agreement, or a bill of sale that the party leaving or selling the practice will not compete with the covenantee for a stated period of time and in a described area. American courts are divided in their opinions about the enforceability of such covenants. Some hold that if the time is reasonable (2 or 3 years, for example) and the restricted area is not too large the covenant

Contract of Employment

This agreement is made this _____ day of _____ 19_____ between _____ (hereinafter called employer) and _____ (hereinafter called employee).

The term of employment shall be for 1 year from the _____ day of _____ 19_____, to the _____ day of _____ 19_____, and from year to year thereafter unless either party gives the other written notice of termination not less than _____ days before the expiration date of the yearly contract.

It is agreed as follows:

1. Employee shall be paid an annual salary of _____, payable monthly on the first of each month. (Note: other salary arrangements including a percentage of income may be agreed upon.)

2. Employee shall be allowed _____ days annually for vacation and sick leave.

3. Employee shall be allowed _____ days annually for attending continuing education programs.

4. Employee shall carry malpractice insurance satisfactory to employer to be paid for by employer.

5. Employer and employee shall agree on a retirement program for employee, the cost to be shared equally by employer and employee.

6. Employer shall carry Workers Compensation Insurance covering employee.

7. Employee shall perform emergency service equal to that performed by employer and other employees. (Note: other arrangements may be made—payment in the nature of overtime, for example.)

8. Alternate. Employer shall provide to employee a practice vehicle and shall pay for operating expense.

8. Alternate. Employee shall provide a practice vehicle, and employer shall reimburse employee for the use at the rate of _____ cents a mile.

9. After _____ years of employment, employee may, for a price agreed upon by employer and employee, buy into the practice and become a partner, at which time this contract will terminate.

10. Employee shall not while employed by employer practice veterinary medicine for remuneration outside of his employment.

11. If employee terminates the employment, he/she shall not practice veterinary medicine within a radius of _____ miles of employer's clinic (or in the city/county of _____) for 2 years after such termination.

Signed this _____ day of _____, 19_____.

_____
Employer

_____
Employee

Figure 15-1. *Contract of employment*

will be enforced. Other states have concluded that such covenants are against public policy and will not enforce them regardless of how reasonable their provisions might be. Therefore, it behooves one who has been asked to sign such a covenant to obtain legal advice about the enforceability in the particular state. The relation of the covenantor and the covenantee has something to do with enforceability. Courts are more willing to enforce a covenant by the seller of a veterinary practice than they are one made by a junior partner or an employee.

Whether an employee or someone being taken into a partnership should sign a restrictive covenant is not an easy question to answer. It depends on a number of factors — the likelihood that the covenantor will wish to remain in practice in the area, the income outlook in the practice that they join, and the apparent validity of such covenants in the state where they will practice. Another item to be checked is whether in the particular state there is legislation or a rule or regulation that either nullifies or conditions the effectiveness of such covenants.

□
Malpractice — causes

Malpractice can be simply defined as professional negligence. *Black's Law Dictionary* says it is "professional misconduct or unreasonable lack of skill" and further that it is the "failure of one rendering professional services to exercise that degree of skill and learning commonly applied under all the circumstances by the average prudent, reputable member of the profession with the result of injury, loss or damage to the recipient of those services or to those entitled to rely upon them."*

* Black H: *Black's Law Dictionary, 5th ed*, p 864. St. Paul, MN, West Publishing Company, 1979.

To determine whether a veterinarian has been negligent or at fault, treatment of the animal must be compared with the treatment that a majority of veterinarians would have used. Ordinarily expert testimony is required to make a finding in this regard.

What can a veterinarian do to reduce the likelihood that a malpractice action will be filed? The most important protection obviously is the practice of good veterinary medicine. This will not only reduce the likelihood of a suit being filed but will be the best defense if suit is filed. Practicing "good veterinary medicine" implies many things — among them that the veterinarian

Participated in continuing education programs to "keep up"

Had adequate equipment for diagnosis and treatment

Selected lay employees with care and exercised a reasonable amount of surveillance over their activities

Obtained informed consent from clients when treatment or surgery not originally contemplated were deemed necessary

Maintained a friendly and communicative attitude towards clients

Used discretion in permitting clients to assist

Promised no cures or specific results

Adhered to current rules and regulations in the use of controlled substances

Determined the agency authority when a person other than the owner requested services — this is especially important if euthanasia or surgery is requested.

Although many court cases involving specific alleged shortcomings of veterinarians could be cited, most complaints are settled by the veterinarian's insurer. Many are dismissed because an investigation shows the veterinarian was not at fault and the client's complaint stemmed either from a disappointing result or irritation at the veterinarian's manner in dealing with the client. Chapter 8 contains additional information concerning the subject of malpractice.

□
Professional corporations and partnerships

The traditional organizational structure for two or more professional persons who wish to practice together has been the partnership. But with the relaxation of legal rules that prohibited the incorporation of professional persons and the enactment of special incorporation laws for them, many practitioners are now incorporated.

A primary consideration in deciding whether to go the partnership or corporation route is an economic one. Which will net the highest return for the practitioner after all costs, tax liabilities, and other financial obligations are met? But apart from the economic consideration, which should be explored thoroughly before making a decision, there are some important legal differences between a partnership and a corporation that should be taken into account.

Legal nature of the entity

A corporation is regarded as a legal person and in many ways is dealt with as such. Except in a very restricted sense and with respect to some transactions, a partnership is not a legal person. A corporation, for example, makes an income tax return; a partnership does not. A corporation may be perpetual; a partnership will not be unless there are specific provisions in the partnership agreement on taking in new partners, thus keeping the entity alive.

Applicable laws

There are state laws defining a partnership and containing provisions on organization, func-

tioning, and dissolution. Most states are party to the Uniform Partnership Act. Special incorporation laws exist for professional persons. These are titled either professional corporation acts or professional association acts. These laws specify how professional people can incorporate and the conditions that apply to the corporation and its members. Legal services should be employed in organizing either a partnership or a professional association. It is especially important to have legal help in organizing a corporation.

Tort liability — malpractice

A well-established principle of law states that partners are "agents of the partnership and of each other." This means that if a partner whose negligence in carrying on any of the partnership business, professional or otherwise, results in legal action, the other partners and the partnership itself can be included as defendants. If there is a judgment and the assets of the partner or the partnership are not sufficient to satisfy it, assets of the other partners may be taken to satisfy the claim. A corporation, on the other hand, insulates the assets of the nonnegligent members. The negligent veterinarian and the corporation itself can be sued.

Veterinarian-client relationship

Professional association laws provide that the fact of incorporation does not affect the relationship that exists between a veterinarian member of the corporation and a client. A malpractice action can thus be maintained against the veterinarian exactly as though he were a sole practitioner. If two or more veterinarian members of the professional association were involved in treating an animal, a determination would have to be made with respect to the standard of skill and care of each unless a "vicarious liability" argument can be made.

In the field of medicine under what has become to be known as "the captain of the ship" doctrine, anyone assisting a surgeon who is performing an operation, whether the assistants be laypersons or other professionals, can through negligence make the surgeon liable, the theory being that in such closely controlled situations there is a "concert of action" and in effect all are acting as one. Arguments have been made that in a medical corporation an exception should be made to the insulation theory and all members should be subject to liability as in a partnership. It is possible that the courts in a particular state might adopt this theory. It is something about which members of professional associations should be concerned and informed.

Worker's compensation insurance

As employees of a professional corporation or professional association, veterinarians can be covered by worker's compensation insurance. Partners cannot be covered because they are regarded as the employers and not as employees. But some states have made an exception and say they can be covered.

Life insurance and retirement plans

A corporation can offer advantages in the purchase of life insurance by contributing a tax-free portion of the premium, and it may offer opportunities for retirement plans that do not exist in a partnership. In view of the change in laws and the establishment of procedures under which individual retirement accounts can be created tax free, this whole area should be explored thoroughly with a tax expert and an attorney familiar with professional associations before concluding that the corporation would offer significant advantages.

Membership in a professional association

Laws permitting professional people to incorporate uniformly require that only professional people licensed to practice in the state may become members and only a single profession can practice under the aegis of a corporation established under a professional incorporation or association law.

Contracts made by professional corporations or partnerships

A professional corporation, being a legal entity, may purchase and sell real and personal property necessary for the rendering of its professional service. Also, in furtherance of its professional functions, it may make investments, lease property, and execute mortgages or other security agreements. Its business is conducted in the name of the corporation, with appropriate officers signing documents. A state "assumed-name law" may apply, which means that the names of the members would have to be registered with a county recorder or similar officer showing who in fact are the responsible persons. This same law applies to partnerships unless the partnership name indicates who the parties are.

For most purposes, any partner can enter into agreements and make binding contracts, regardless of any agreement that may exist among the partners themselves. Any party dealing with the partnership and having knowledge that a partner does not have authority to sign a particular kind of agreement, would not, however, be protected. Also, the Uniform Partnership Act lists several transactions that are binding only if all the partners sign. Among these are (1) making an assignment of partnership property to secure an obligation, (2) disposing of the goodwill of the business, (3) making any agreement that would make it impossible to carry on the ordinary business of the partnership, (4) confessing a judgment, (5) submitting a partnership claim to arbitration, and (6) transferring the partnership real estate unless agreed to by all of the partners.

Dissolution of a professional corporation

Articles of incorporation or bylaws may contain a provision on dissolution of the corporation. If so, then it can be dissolved when the conditions arise that fulfill the intent of such a provision. If there is no provision and the professional incorporation act does not cover this phase of corporate activity, the general business corporation act of the state may apply. Because the dissolution of a corporation involves many considerations, especially with respect to distribution of property, funds, and receivables, both legal and accounting help are implied.

Perpetuating the partnership — dissolution

A cardinal principle of partnership law is that when a partner dies or leaves the partnership there is a dissolution. This means that partnership assets must be appraised and, in the case of a deceased partner, distribution made to the heirs and devisees. Since a division of partnership assets in the case of either a departing or deceased partner is likely to leave the remaining partner or partners in an undesirable economic position, there should be a written partnership agreement covering this contingency. The basic provision in the agreement should be one that permits the remaining partner or partners to buy out the leaving or deceased partner and that provides that the partners will carry insurance to make this possible. The partnership may be dissolved for other reasons: by bankruptcy or expulsion of a partner or by the express will of a partner. At any rate, a buy – sell agreement, backed by insurance, is strongly recommended. Information on how to buy and sell a practice is found in Chapter 7, and insurance protection is discussed in Chapter 10.

Determining the value of a deceased partner's interest may present difficulties. A written partnership agreement containing some guidelines can be helpful. Besides a division of physical assets, consideration must be given to goodwill, accounts receivable, and unbilled work along with the disposition of files and pending liability claims.

The desirability of a written partnership agreement is illustrated by *Osborne v. Workman,* 621 SW2d 478, a case decided by the Arkansas Supreme Court in 1981. There the partnership agreement provided for continuation of the partnership and that a withdrawing partner would not be entitled to any share of accounts receivable. The Court upheld these provisions over the objection of the withdrawing partner and said that they were not against public policy.

In those situations where a partnership is not to be continued, either because of an event that results in dissolution or because the partners mutually agree to terminate it, a winding-up process is involved. Except to the extent that this is covered in the partnership agreement, certain provisions of the Uniform Partnership Act will apply. These have to do mainly with the determination of values, division of tangible and intangible property, and responsibility for partnership obligations. Unless the winding-up process is straightforward and the partners are in agreement, both legal and tax assistance are implied. An example of a partnership agreement is found in Figure 15-2.

☐
Premises liability

There is more than one reason for having a well-ordered and attractive veterinary clinic.

Partnership Agreement

1. Creation of partnership

   This agreement is entered into on this _____ of _____, 19_____, between
   _____ and _____ to create a partnership for the practice of
   veterinary medicine in the state of _____, in which state the above signatories are licensed to
   practice.

2. Name

   The name of this partnership shall be _____.

3. Duration — insurance

   This partnership shall continue until dissolved by mutual agreement of the partners. It is agreed that life insurance
   payable to the partnership shall be carried on the life of each partner in amounts agreed upon with premiums payable from
   partnership assets. The proceeds of such insurance shall be used to pay the deceased partner's representative the fair
   value of the deceased partner's interest in the partnership, the balance if any to remain with the partnership.

4. Contributions to the partnership

   The beginning assets of the partnership shall consist of the equipment, supplies, and cash contributions from the
   respective partners as shown below. (List partners and their contributions.)

5. Profit and loss

   The partners shall share equally in net profits and shall bear losses in equal amounts. (If the partners are not to share
   equally, their respective shares should be specified)

6. Account procedures and payments to partners

   Monies received by the partners as a result of partnership activity shall be deposited in a partnership account in the
   custody of a bank agreed upon by the partners. Monthly payments from this account shall be made to each partner in an
   amount to be agreed upon by the partners. Bills for materials, supplies, and other obligations of the partnership shall be
   paid from this account. Standard accounting procedures for partnerships shall be used. Books shall be available for
   inspection by partners at all times. At the close of each calendar year there shall be an annual audit by an independent
   public auditor.

7. Professional responsibility of partners

   Unless otherwise agreed upon, partners shall spend an equal amount of time in the conduct of the partnership business.
   Partners shall not, for remuneration of any kind, practice veterinary medicine outside the partnership. However, partners are
   permitted to retain honoraria and royalties from any writings they may do.

8. Vacation, sick leave, continuing education

   Partners shall each be entitled to _____ weeks vacation per year and _____ days sick leave per year.
   Also, partners shall be entitled to _____ days per year for attending professional meetings and professional
   education programs.

9. Records

   Veterinary medical records shall be the property of the partnership and shall be made available to persons outside the
   partnership under policies established by agreement of all the partners.

10. Professional liability insurance — other insurance

    The partnership and each partner shall be covered by adequate professional liability insurance, the premiums to be paid
    from partnership assets. Accident and health insurance and contributions to retirement plans for the partners shall be
    obtained as agreed upon by the partners, premiums and contributions to be paid from partnership assets.

11. Disabled partners

    If a partner is unable to perform his professional duties for a period in excess of sick leave and vacation time, the share
    of income for such partner shall be reduced proportionately under a formula to be agreed upon by the partners. If the
    disability continues for more than _____ weeks and the partner is still unable to perform professional duties, the
    partner's interest in the partnership shall be terminated and an accounting made.

Figure 15-2.   Partnership agreement

(Continued)

12. Withdrawal of a partner

A partner may withdraw by giving written notice of not less than _____ days to the other partners. An accounting shall be made and there shall be paid to the withdrawing partner a pro rata share of fees due at the time of withdrawal and the amount of the withdrawing partner's credit balance in the account. Withdrawal of a partner shall not terminate the partnership if two or more partners remain.

13. New partners

New partners may be admitted to the partnership upon agreement of all the partners and under terms and conditions agreeable to all parties.

14. Expulsion

A partner may be expelled by agreement of the other partners if the partnership agreement has been materially violated or if grounds exist for suspension or revocation of the partner's license. An expelled partner shall be entitled to an accounting and payment from partnership funds as provided for a withdrawing partner.

15. Dissolution

A partnership may be dissolved by agreement of a majority of the partners. Clients shall be notified of dissolution of the partnership. Assets shall be distributed as provided for sharing of partnership profits.

16. Covenant against competition

If a partner withdraws from the partnership, he shall not engage in the practice of veterinary medicine for a period of _____ years within _____ miles of the partnership practice site. This provision does not apply if the partnership is dissolved.

17. Arbitration

The partners agree that if they cannot resolve an issue they shall, before resorting to litigation, submit the issue to arbitration. The opposing parties shall each select one arbitrator, and the two arbitrators thus selected shall name a third. Arbitration shall be conducted and an arbitration decision made in accordance with the laws of the state of _____ on arbitration.

Signed this _____ day of _____ month, 19_____.

_____
Partner

_____
Partner

_____
Partner

Figure 15-2.   Partnership agreement   (Continued)

Besides making a good impression on clients and visitors, the likelihood of a suit by those who claim injury because of the condition of the premises will be reduced. After making certain that adequate and appropriate premises liability insurance is in place, the veterinarian can reduce this potential by

1. Making certain that sidewalks and steps are in good repair and do not present a hazard because of their design

2. Getting rid of ice and snow in parking areas, and on sidewalks and steps as soon and as often as possible (failure to do this has been the basis for a number of lawsuits)

3. Making certain that the entrance is well

lighted so that steps and changes in the level of the floor can be seen

4. Having seats in the waiting room arranged so that people waiting with pets will not have to be so close that their pets can bite each other
5. Having a courteous sign or reminder that clients should closely restrain their pets until they have been taken in for examination
6. Assuming custody of animals as soon as possible so that they will not have to be restrained for long periods of time in the waiting room
7. Informing the receptionist that if an unruly or vicious pet is brought in she should immediately inform the veterinarian or a technician so that custody can be transferred
8. Maintaining a waiting room with floors, furniture, and a placement of furniture that afford a maximum of safety (lawsuits have arisen from slick floors)

A veterinarian, by inviting members of the public to use his services, owes such people a duty of reasonable care to prevent injury while they are on the premises. It is akin to the duty to provide a safe workplace for employees, and similar principles will be evoked by the courts in determining whether liability should be decreed. Some of the things that have led to lawsuits are the absence of a handrail on steps leading to an entrance, foreign matter or slick substances on steps or floors, and the absence of lighting.

It should be pointed out that the veterinarian is not automatically liable just because someone is injured on the practice premises. There must be proof the veterinarian was at fault, and even if this is proved, there are at least two effective defenses. The first line of defense is that the injured party was also negligent, thus contributing to his own injury. The second defense is that the injured party was

snooping, that is, entering portions of the veterinarian's premises he had no right to enter and thus, in the eyes of the law, becoming a trespasser.

□
Liability for acts of and to employees—using technicians and other lay help

The principle that holds that an employer can be held liable for the negligent acts of employees performed in the course of duty is referred to as *respondeat superior,* or sometimes *vicarious liability,* this latter term recognizing that the employer can be held liable though not at fault. Besides hiring competent lay personnel and giving them proper instructions, what defenses can a veterinarian make if sued because of an alleged injury caused by an employee? Here are some examples:

1. Deny that the plaintiff or the plaintiff's animal was injured or the injury is as great as claimed. Before a defendant can be held liable, the burden is on the plaintiff to prove there was injury.
2. Although there may be injury, deny that the employee was negligent in causing it. It might have been unavoidable with no fault involved.
3. Claim that the plaintiff was also negligent, thereby contributing to his own injury. In some jurisdictions this is a complete defense; in others, it is a partial defense (states that adhere to the comparative negligence doctrine).
4. Claim that the employee's actions were not the proximate cause of the injury. The employee might very well have been negligent in some respect, but unless that negligence is the cause of the injury for which the complaint is filed, there is no liability—at least not through that route.

5. Claim that the employee was not in the course of his duty at the time the injury occurred. There are some close cases on this point—growing out of situations where the employee is either going to or returning from work or deviates temporarily from the employment to do something on his own behalf.

Because many of the activities of lay employees are not concerned directly with the professional activities of the veterinarian, an insurance policy or a rider on the policy that covers liability for such things as permitting an animal to escape or injuring third parties while using a vehicle should be purchased and kept current.

As employees of the veterinarian, technicians and other lay help are entitled to a safe place to work and to working conditions that will reduce to a reasonable minimum the likelihood they will be injured while carrying on their duties. Much of the protection that a veterinarian can provide in this regard comes from selecting competent employees, instructing them properly, making certain of their skills and abilities, stressing in detail safe procedures and work habits, and reviewing at intervals situations that arise in the practice from which an injury might be foreseeable. Specific points on personnel management may be found in Chapter 2.

In many states veterinarians are required by law to maintain worker's compensation insurance on employees. In states where this is not mandatory, veterinarians could nevertheless elect to be covered by the plan. Under the plan the veterinarian is liable for any injury that occurs to an employee (with a few exceptions that do not often arise) if the injury is received in the course of employment. Worker's compensation acts, however, and the rules developed under them limit the amounts that can be recovered for particular kinds of injuries. They also prohibit the bringing of a civil suit outside the workman's compensation act. If the veterinarian is not covered by workman's compensation, he should by all means carry employer's liability insurance. A large amount of insurance should be carried because there is no limit generally on the size of the claim an employee might make because ultimately this will be determined by a jury and the court and not under the statutory provisions of a workman's compensation act.

☐
Assistance from clients

When a client assists, one or more concerns may arise, each of which has legal implications: (1) the client may be injured, (2) the veterinarian may be injured, and (3) the animal may suffer because of improper handling and restraint.

The author knows of at least two cat cases that have reached the courts. In these cases the owner claimed damages from the veterinarian for bites and scratches received from the cat. In an Australian case the veterinarian was held liable for the client's injuries; in a Wisconsin trial court case the judgment was for the veterinarian.

In another case involving injury to an owner's agent when he was restraining a horse, the veterinarian's insurer settled for a large amount. In that case the veterinarian's assistant was giving the animal an injection.

Situations vary, and in case of injury to an owner the facts in each incident become important. The following are some things about which the veterinarian should be assured before examination or treatment by questioning the owner if need be:

1. What is the age, experience, physical ability, and temperament of the owner? An inexperienced youngster holding his pony is one thing, and the experienced employee of a racing stable restraining a horse is another.

2. What is the temperament and current physical condition of the animal? Is it mean, does it have some medical problem that would make it abnormally sensitive?
3. Has the owner held the animal before?
4. Has the veterinarian treated this animal before?
5. What conditions surround the animal at the time of treatment? Is it in an excited, confined herd, or is it in the quiet of the veterinarian's examining room or clinic?
6. What is to be done to the animal — injections, oral medication, treatment of a wound?

If the veterinarian is injured while the owner is controlling the animal, the right to recover damages from the owner will be difficult to establish, but it is possible. First, however, it must be ascertained that the owner was negligent and the veterinarian was not negligent, and it is an unexpected occurrence that would induce the court to say the risk was not one that a veterinarian normally assumes. In a Missouri appellate court case a veterinarian called at the premises of the owner of a large Airedale. The owner negligently dropped the leash, and the dog attacked the veterinarian who at the time was not watching the dog but was reaching for some item in his medical bag. The court allowed recovery for the veterinarian's injury and said it was not the kind of risk veterinarians assume.

Injury to the animal resulting from the way the owner handled or restrained it would not be compensable if the veterinarian were not at fault and if the circumstances were such that it was reasonable to permit the owner to hold the animal.

□
The common law nuisance theory

There is a time-honored legal maxim that states in effect that one should so use his property as not to deny others the beneficial enjoyment of their property. A use that violates this precept may amount to a nuisance giving the injured person a right to seek damages or to enjoin the nuisance.

What activities of a veterinarian may create a nuisance? An obvious one is keeping animals, especially dogs, on the veterinary premises under conditions that permit noise, odor, and even unsightliness to interfere with neighbors' enjoyment of their property.

Cats and dogs in residential areas have occasioned a fair number of lawsuits, with the plaintiff generally winning. What defenses might a veterinarian make if sued under the common law nuisance theory? Here are some:

1. My clinic was here first. This argument is sometimes called the "coming to" theory. In some circumstances it can be an effective defense, but in an urban environment where progress means the expansion of the city and the building of more residences, it will soon cease to be a good defense.
2. My clinic is not a nuisance in fact — the plaintiff is overly sensitive. This can be a good defense if the facts bear out the statement. The plaintiff must show there are noises, odors, or other undesirable features that allegedly exist. Furthermore, the plaintiff must show that persons of ordinary sensibilities would be affected in the way they have been affected.
3. My clinic is in compliance with all zoning and permit requirements. This is not a good defense if a nuisance has in fact been created. But there should be compliance in this regard, or else complaining parties will have another basis for complaint.
4. Give me time and I can eliminate the noise (smell or other features). The courts, although they may be convinced that an injunction should be granted, will

nevertheless accept evidence from a defendant that the undesirable feature can be eliminated given a reasonable period of time. If the veterinarian promises to close animal runs, keep animals inside more of the time, or improve sanitary standards — this might induce a court to delay the issuance of an injunction during the time granted to make the required changes.

☐
The steps in a malpractice suit

Malpractice suits are civil actions. Criminal law is not involved. A malpractice suit is one in which a veterinarian's client sues for damages under a claim that his animal has been harmed or has died, as the case may be, due to the veterinarian's professional negligence (failure to meet the standard of skill and care of other veterinarians). Figure 15-3 illustrates in a general way the steps involved once a client decides to commence legal action against a veterinarian.

☐
Defenses in a malpractice action

When a veterinarian is sued in a malpractice action, his attorney should consider every possible defense and explore in detail those that seem appropriate. What are defenses that a court will recognize? Listed here are those that courts will heed:

1. There was in fact no damage, or all of the damages claimed did not occur. This is relevant in every malpractice action. The plaintiff must make a case to show there was damage.
2. The defendant veterinarian's actions were not the cause of the injury. In malpractice actions the theory of proximate cause is important. This means that although the plaintiff may have been injured and there might have been negligence this is not the cause of the injury.
3. The veterinarian was not negligent. This of course goes to the heart of the case once it has been established that damage did result. Through testimony, expert and otherwise, the defending veterinarian's attorney will try to show that the standard of skill and care was met.
4. There was contributory negligence. If the client is negligent in aftercare of the animal or in following instructions given by the veterinarian and it can be proved that this is a contributing cause to an undesirable result, it may constitute either a complete or partial defense depending upon whether the state in which the action arises has adopted the comparative negligence theory. In states that have adopted the theory, the negligence of the plaintiff is only a partial defense and must be compared in degree with that of the defendant.
5. The statute of limitations has run out. Every state has laws barring both contract and tort actions after the expiration of a period of time established by statute. Though these statutes vary from state to state, a usual period for a tort action is 2 years. Though some states have reduced this period to 1 year in medical malpractice actions, veterinarians would not benefit unless the statute specifically includes veterinary medicine. The statute ordinarily commences to run at the time the client discovers an injury that is claimed to have resulted from the veterinarian's treatment. This is a question of fact that the court must determine. A plaintiff's client will try to show that the injury was not discovered until late enough to keep the right alive under the statute. The defending veterinarian, on the other hand, will try to show that the

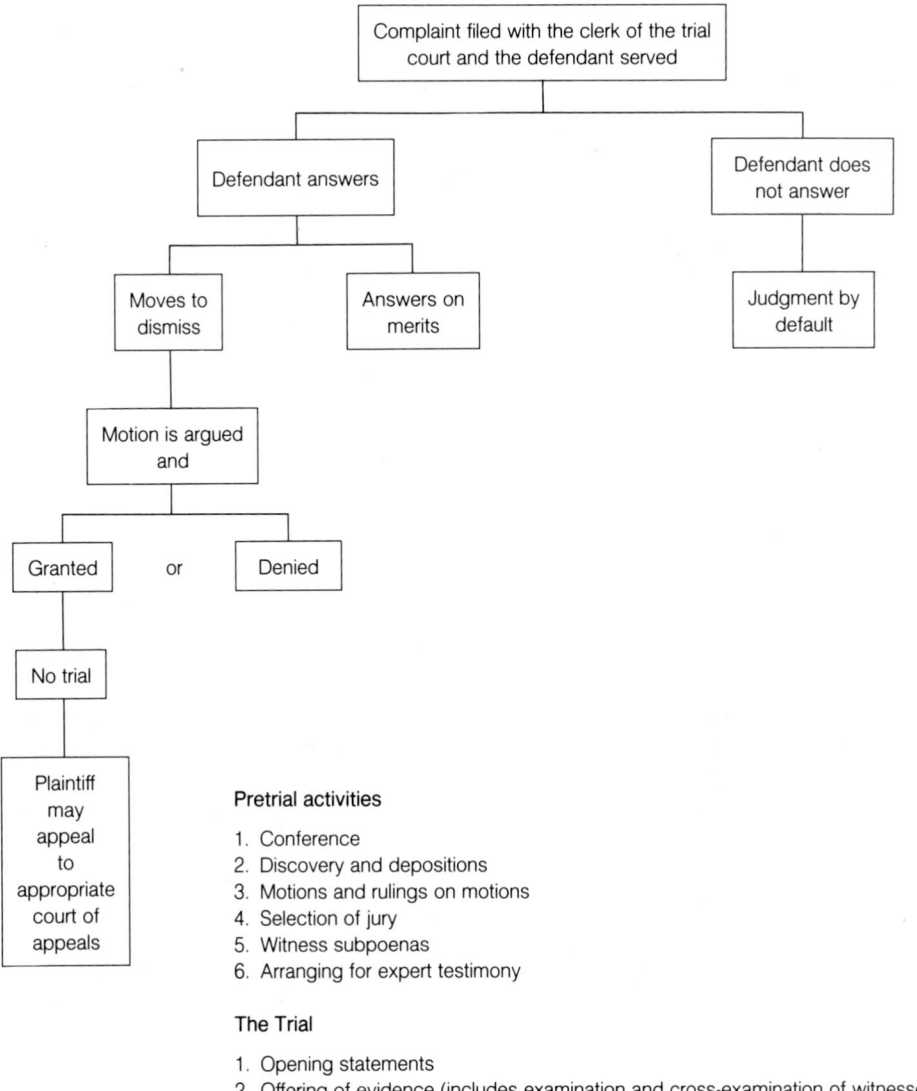

Pretrial activities

1. Conference
2. Discovery and depositions
3. Motions and rulings on motions
4. Selection of jury
5. Witness subpoenas
6. Arranging for expert testimony

The Trial

1. Opening statements
2. Offering of evidence (includes examination and cross-examination of witnesses)
3. Closing arguments — summation
4. Instructions to jury
5. Verdict of the jury
6. Judgment of the court

Appeal or request for rehearing

Either party may appeal an adverse ruling or request a rehearing within the time allowed by court rule.

Figure 15-3.   Steps in a civil action

injury was or should have been discovered earlier and thus the statutory period for filing suit has expired.

Many things can be suggested to veterinarians for avoiding malpractice actions. Out of such a list that might be compiled, two things stand out as more important than all of the others: practicing good veterinary medicine (this has many connotations including continuing education) and establishing a friendly and communicative relationship with clients. Detailed malpractice information is found in Chapter 8.

☐
Punitive damages—mental anguish

Punitive damages are those that may be awarded when it can be proved that the defendant acted in malice or was grossly negligent. They are damages in addition to compensatory damages. Two assumptions support the principle of allowing punitive damages: the plaintiff has been injured, albeit intangibly, beyond the injury for which compensatory damages are allowable, and by awarding punitive damages the defendant will be deterred in the future from acting recklessly, maliciously, or in a grossly negligent manner. In support of this latter objective, many courts will not allow the defendant's insurance to pay for such damages, the theory being that to allow such would simply encourage a defendant to be malicious or grossly negligent while knowing that liability insurance would cover an award for such.

Damages for mental anguish or pain and suffering are on a somewhat different footing. These feelings may exist in a client regardless of the negligence of the veterinarian simply because of the attachment owners oftentimes have for a companion animal. Most courts are reluctant in allowing such damages, but awards have been made in cases involving injury to or the death of animals.

Some states have adopted a statutory prohibition against the recovery of punitive damages in medical malpractice cases. One such law provides that "in all cases, whether in tort, contract or otherwise, in which the plaintiff seeks damages by reason of legal, medical, hospital or other healing art malpractice, no punitive, exemplary, vindictive or aggravated damages shall be allowed" (Ill. Rev. Stat. 1985 ch. 110, par. 2-1115). Whether this language includes veterinarians is questionable, though it might be argued that the phrase "or other healing art malpractice" would include them. Thus if a veterinarian is sued and there is a claim for punitive damages, both statutory provisions and common law holdings in that state should be checked to see whether such is allowable.

In medical malpractice cases it is well established that damages may be awarded for pain and suffering. Both physical and mental suffering are compensable. The mental suffering must have some connection, however, with the physical suffering. Some courts are reluctant to award such damages when the patient is an animal and the client has been affected only mentally. Some state courts, however, have allowed such when dogs were involved. Unless there is a state policy, either established by statute or court holdings, that such damages are not recoverable or there are limitations on such recovery, the better view would be that such an award can be made and the veterinarian's liability insurance should cover it.

☐
Veterinary practice acts—some significant features

In the following sections are listed some provisions that appear in all state veterinary medical practice acts.

Licensing

Because the prime purpose of practice acts is to license and thus exert some control over the professions, all acts provide a veterinary licensing board or similar body to administer examinations and issue licenses under provisions contained in the practice act. Details about qualifications for applying for licensure vary somewhat, though all acts require a minimum of 2 years of preveterinary education and a degree from a 4-year professional college.

License renewal

Either the practice act or rules developed under it provide that licenses shall be renewed at stated periods, normally yearly or biennially, for the payment of a stipulated fee. About half of the states in the United States require some continuing education before allowing renewal of a veterinary license.

Definition of practice

All practice acts contain a section defining the practice of veterinary medicine and stating that one who performs any of these acts without a license is violating the law. Definitions vary, but surgery, diagnosis, and treatment for disease or deformity and sometimes for mental conditions are included. There are many gray areas, some of which may be covered by specific rules or regulations and others left to conjecture until a court speaks.

Exempt persons and activities

Practice acts generally exempt people engaged in educational or research work and state- and federal-employed veterinarians so long as these people are engaged in their activities and are not moonlighting. Particular activities may also be exempt — castration of food animals, dehorning cattle, and artificial insemination, for example.

Cause for revocation of license

All acts state either in general terms or with much specificity causes that exist for revocation or suspension of a veterinarian's license. Regardless of how stated or implied, gross malpractice, violation of controlled substances laws, practicing with an unlicensed person, and fraud either in procuring a license or in making reports of animal disease testing are cause. Others included in many state laws are failure to keep the premises in a sanitary condition, chronic inebriety or habitual use of drugs, a conviction of cruelty to animals, and failure to meet continuing education programs if such is provided in the act.

A hearing process in revocation and suspension cases

Either in the practice act itself or in a general provision of state law, there will be described the process to be used when action is taken to revoke or suspend the veterinarian's license. The purpose of such a provision is to make certain there is due process, namely, that the veterinarian be informed of the charge, given time to respond, and given an opportunity to appear with counsel if so desired, to bring witnesses, and to cross-examine witnesses brought by the licensing board. After a hearing and the ruling of the board, there is generally a right to a rehearing and always the right to have the board's finding reviewed in a trial court and to take appeals from such.

Preventing unlicensed practice

All acts provide that practicing without a license is a violation of law for which a person can be prosecuted through the usual criminal law channels. Many states, however, provide that the state's attorney or attorney general shall seek to enjoin such practice after a petition from the veterinary licensing board, a veterinarian, or any interested person.

Incorporation of a veterinary practice

Commencing more than 20 years ago, state after state enacted laws permitting professional persons to incorporate and create either a professional corporation or a professional association. These are special incorporation laws apart from a business corporation act. Important features of them are as follows:

1. Only licensed professionals in a single profession can be members of the corporation.
2. The veterinarian-client relationship between a member of the corporation and the person whose animals are treated is not affected, so a malpractice action will proceed as it would if there were no corporation.
3. Members of the corporation who are not involved in an alleged negligent act by a member of the corporation are not liable in a malpractice action. Only the veterinarian involved and the corporation itself can be sued.

There are some fringe benefits from being incorporated such as the ability to buy insurance, create retirement plans, and cover the veterinarians with workman's compensation insurance.

Continuing education

Many states now require that for relicensure a veterinarian complete a stated number of hours of continuing veterinary medical education. Programs are administered by the veterinary licensing board that establishes rules and conditions on programs that qualify, on hours required, and on the method for reporting performance.

Assumed name

Either in the practice act or in a separate state law, there is likely to be a provision that a veterinary corporation or partnership that uses a name that does not indicate the veterinarians' names included in it shall file with a county or circuit clerk court, or possibly at the state level, a statement showing who the veterinarians are in the partnership or corporation. The purpose of such a law is to provide creditors or others who deal with the partnership or corporation the names of the true members.

Display of license

Many practice acts require that the veterinarian display the license in the waiting room of the clinic. The renewal certificate should also be displayed.

Registration of license and address

Some state laws require that the veterinarian register the license with the recorder or similar officer in the county where the practice is located or register it with the appropriate state agency. These laws may also require that when the veterinarian changes address, he must notify the state agency within a given length of time and reregister the license in the other county.

Reciprocity

Most state laws provide, though requirements vary, that veterinarians in good standing and licensed in another state may be licensed by reciprocity, providing the veterinary board of the state where they wish to practice finds that requirements for licensure in the state from which they are moving are substantially the same as those in the state where they wish to practice. There has been some relaxation in these requirements because in many states the national board examinations are used and there is now a common factor for judging competence of veterinarians.

Disposing of unclaimed animals

Most practice acts provide that if an owner does not reclaim an animal after being notified a veterinarian can inform the owner through registered mail, or in some cases by publication if an address cannot be found, that unless the animal is claimed within the time specified in the law the veterinarian will dispose of it as provided by law. One should have specific and current information before disposal of any animal.

Veterinarians' lien

A minority of states have provided specifically for a veterinarian's lien on animals treated. When there is a specific statute, it generally provides that the lien can be perfected by filing and is not lost because the veterinarian yields possession of the animal. Some provide that the veterinarian's lien takes priority over all others. In the absence of a specific veterinarian's lien it is possible that veterinarians could legally establish a claim against an animal to force payment under a general state law providing for a lien on services to or storage of personal property or under a lien that gives one who pastures, yards, feeds, or has custody of the animals for hire a lien for payment, as long as possession is retained (an agisters lien).

□
Summary

What laws are of most importance to the average practicing veterinarian? After receiving a veterinary degree, the first contact will be with the licensing provisions in the practice act of the state where one intends to practice and with the rules and regulations of the board administering the examination and notifying applicants of the results.

A second contact will be with those provisions of the practice act that impose certain duties: registering the license, displaying the license, informing about address, registering an assumed name (if this is involved), and if required, preparing to meet continuing education requirements.

A third contact encompasses the veterinarian's position as an employee or a partner or possibly as a member of a veterinary professional corporation. Should one sign a covenant not to compete? What are the rights and duties as an employee, partner, or corporation member? For a young veterinarian important considerations arise in this area.

A fourth contact with the law has to do with client relations. The veterinarian–client relation is a contractual one, and each party has certain rights and duties until the contract is legally terminated. The veterinarian should have a general knowledge of some of the legal issues that may stem from this relationship, especially as it relates to malpractice.

A fifth contact concerns the employment of clinic personnel, the veterinarian's legal obligation to them, and the legal obligation to clients or to third parties for their actions.

A sixth area of legal concern may exist when the veterinarian owns or is a part-owner in the clinic or when he decides to locate and build a new establishment. Zoning laws, building codes, permit requirements, and the common law nuisance theory may need to be considered.

A seventh area involves drugs and controlled substances and implies knowledge of the laws and regulations that affect procurement, storage, use, and accountability.

An eighth area encompasses the animal disease laws and regulations of both the federal government and state and implies a knowledge of those laws that pertain to one's practice.

Chapter 16
□
Patient death and dying

Laurel S. Lagoni
Suzanne Arguello
Stephen J. Withrow
Connee Pike

□
The human – companion animal bond

Throughout the many thousands of years that our companion animals have lived with us, they have assumed a variety of roles. In addition to filling the roles of companion, confidant, and trusted friend, they have been hunters, protectors of property, predators of pest species, and beasts of burden. Companion animals have also been cast in the roles of teaching aids in medical and veterinary schools and experimental subjects in many areas of research.

Each of these roles, however, has changed in recent years. New utilitarian functions for animals have been created with the advent of assistance dogs for the handicapped and hearing dogs for the deaf and hearing impaired. The concept of animal rights has also changed the way in which animals are now used in teaching and research. Multiple recovery surgeries in veterinary schools have generally become procedures of the past. Researchers in all areas of science have performed much needed reevaluation of their investigations and attitudes toward their animal subjects. The benefits of the emotional bonds between people and animals have been explored and put to use in many different settings. Pet-facilitated therapy programs have been established in a variety of institutional settings including human hospitals, nursing homes, rehabilitation centers, prisons, and psychiatric facilities.

With over 48 million families owning one or more companion animals, the greatest impact emerging from the human – companion animal bond is on the family.[1] Pets are considered to be a part of the "extended family network."[2] It is becoming a widely accepted fact among theorists and researchers that the majority of pet owners consider their animals to be family members, with "people status" within their families (Fig. 16-1). Evidence in support of this indicates that one or more family members talk to their pets as they would to a person, carry pictures of their animals, allow their pets to sleep on the bed, and celebrate their pets' birthdays.[3] Professionals in human medicine, psychology, family therapy, and other human service fields are beginning to recognize the important positions companion animals occupy within their clients' lives. Veterinarians are now beginning to recognize it too.

Breaking the bond

People living alone, the divorced, the never married, and the elderly are growing in numbers. Nontraditional families, those headed by single parents, stepparents, and dual-employed spouses, are also on the rise. Life-style changes are restructuring the family. In response to these changes, people are altering their social support systems, and companion animals are playing increasingly significant roles in this adaptation. People of all ages, in numerous living situations, are turning to pets for companionship and social support. In fact, it is estimated that 60% of American families share their lives with one or more companion animals. Substantial evidence is available to indicate that the majority of both dog and cat owners consider their animals to be family members.[4,5]

Acting as family members, pets often take on roles essential to family functions.[6] In the lives of nontraditional families, pets are seen as more important, more like friends, children, protectors, or comforters.[7] They also serve many other purposes such as providing sources of fun, exercise, protection, love, and companionship. In nontraditional families the basis of the human-pet bond corresponds with the human-human bond, which means attach-

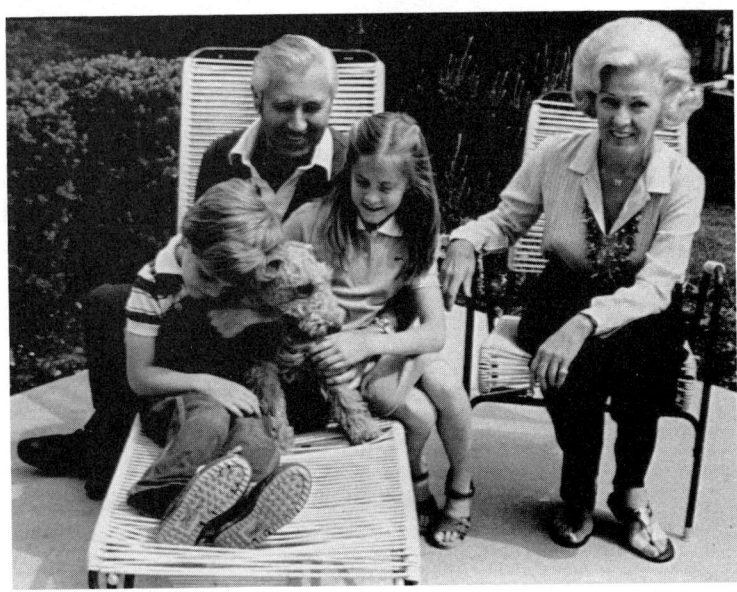

Figure 16-1. *Pets as part of the extended family network (Courtesy of Pets Are Wonderful Council, Chicago)*

ments to companion animals are very high and dependencies very strong.[7]

It is to be expected, then, that the death of a pet can be painful and traumatic and evoke a grief response comparable to the response to the death of a human family member or friend (Fig. 16-2). The significant difference, however, in grief for humans and grief for pets is that society does not generally accept grieving the death of a pet.[8] Consequently, there is a lack of available support and understanding for the bereaved. In our culture, there is no acceptable way of mourning a pet.[9] Grief for a dead pet is often considered inappropriate by others because the pet can be replaced.[10]

Veterinarians are unavoidably confronted with issues of loss and behavioral changes during the diagnosis, treatment, and death of their clients' pets. Frequently pet owners turn to their veterinarians as sources of support, comfort, and understanding after the death of their pet. This is due, in large part, to the caregiving role veterinarians play during the lives of animals. This places veterinarians in a role they may not be fully comfortable in and demands they have knowledge and training typically outside the boundaries of traditional veterinary medicine. In light of this, the areas of animal behavior, human bereavement, and grief therapy, as they relate to pet loss, are becoming increasingly more relevant to veterinary medicine.

The purpose of this chapter is to educate veterinarians about grief responses to pet loss

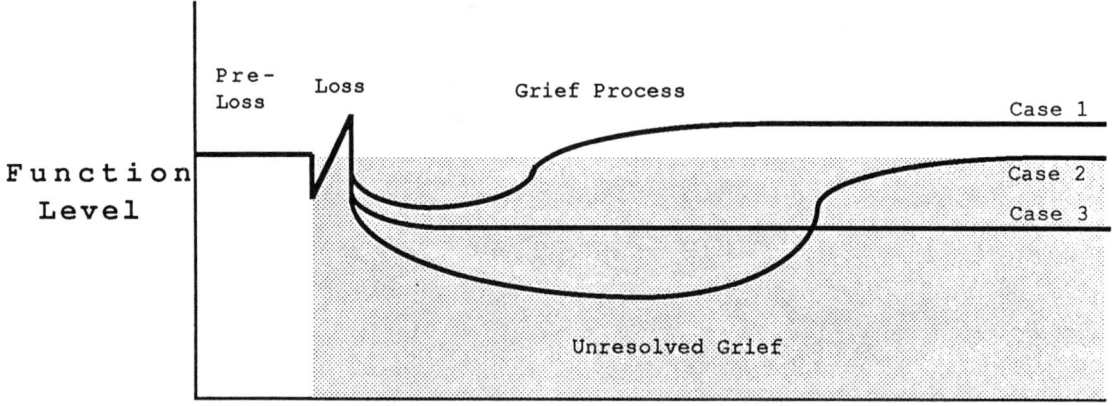

Figure 16-2. *Three responses to loss. People operate daily at normal levels of functioning unique to them as individuals. Since crises are perceived differently by each person, the degree that individual function drops at the time of a loss is also unique. Symptoms of a drop in functioning level may include shock, denial, forgetfulness, confusion, withdrawal, as well as other physical, intellectual, and emotional changes. As people move through the grief process, they accomplish grief work tasks with varying degrees of competency. Thus, recovery also varies. Some return to previous functioning levels (case 2), some learn from loss and achieve higher levels of functioning (case 1), whereas others remain below the level that was at one time normal for them (case 3). This latter scenario accounts for many cases of unresolved grief.*

and to offer a framework from which they can develop further expertise in support counseling. The goal is *not* to transform veterinarians into therapists but rather to complement their existing help-giving skills.

Loss and grief

Loss is present in every kind of change that people experience. Small losses, like misplacing a favorite sweater, and large losses, like filing for bankruptcy or learning of a friend's death, have one thing in common — they are catalysts for grief.

Pet owners experience change and its subsequent feelings of loss frequently throughout their companion animals' lives. Puppies become dogs, kittens become cats, and horses grow too old to ride. Often amputations and chronic illnesses contribute to shifts in normal interactions between pets and owners. For example, daily walks are suspended, greeting patterns disappear, and care-giving or playtime routines change. Odds are high that most companion animals will die before the people they live with do, yet few pet owners prepare themselves for this inevitability. Even after an animal has been diagnosed as terminally ill by a veterinarian, many pet owners continue to say *"If* my pet dies" rather than *"When* my pet dies."

The grieving process is important because it insists that people acknowledge that a loss has occurred. Once the emotional pain and physical sensations associated with loss have been experienced, the bereaved can adapt their lives to the changes brought on by loss. The bereaved person can then begin the process of drawing a closure to the old relationship and reinvesting in new ones. Grieving is a normal, natural, and healthy way to cope with loss, and it is important to remember that each person experiences grief in a uniquely different way.

Normal grief may last from a few weeks to several years, with emotions and sensations accompanying it that are often confusing and awkward. The emotional changes can be eased if those involved in facilitating a loss know what to expect. For example, during the course of normal grief, many people report feelings of sadness, anger, guilt, anxiety, loneliness, tiredness, helplessness, shock, and depression. Physical sensations reported include crying, hollowness in the stomach, tightness in the chest and throat, weak muscles, a dry mouth, appetite and sleep disturbances, and fatigue. After the death of a pet, it is common to be preoccupied with thoughts and memories of the pet and to imagine and fantasize they are still alive.

These responses to loss occur naturally whether the death is the result of disease, an unexpected accident, or an acute illness. The main difference faced by people coping with loss due to the latter are the demands made upon them to make life-and-death decisions at the same time they are experiencing the full range of grief responses.

How veterinarians assist pet owners in handling normal animal life span losses from birth to death depends on their own beliefs and values. Veterinarians who value privacy and a "get-on-with-life" attitude may encourage clients to grieve alone at home or not at all. Those who value the growth experience stimulated by loss and who have been trained to recognize symptoms of grief will validate the significance of any loss in a relationship and encourage clients to find effective support networks within which to sort out their feelings. To them, no loss will seem unimportant.

□

Progressive illness and euthanasia

The loss of a loved person is as traumatic psychologically as being severely wounded or burned physically.[11] The same could be said for the loss of a pet. The *grieving process* is the period of healing that is necessary to recover from the injury. This healing process enables individuals to adjust to the permanent loss of their loved one. Whether the loss is the death of a person or a pet makes no difference to most. Grief must be felt for life's equilibrium to be regained.

Many theoretical frameworks have been developed to explain the grief process people experience after a loss. Elizabeth Kubler-Ross's five stages of grief make up one of the most popular models: (1) shock or denial, (2) anger, (3) bargaining, (4) depression, and (5) acceptance.[12] An all encompassing grief model has been described, however, that is more easily adaptable to the field of veterinary medicine. This model describes three phases of the psychological manifestations of grief:

1. *Avoidance phase* consisting of shock, denial, and disbelief
2. *Confrontation phase* consisting of highly emotional stages (like anger, depression, sadness, guilt, and relief) wherein the grief is most intense and the psychological reactions to loss are felt most acutely
3. *Reestablishment phase* consisting of gradual declines in the symptoms of grief (like withdrawal, sleeping and eating disorders, fatigue, and loneliness) and the beginnings of emotional and social reentries back into the everyday world[13]

Anticipatory grief

Sometimes the grief response begins before the death of a pet and is known as *anticipatory* grief. Anticipatory grief often accompanies a diagnosis or the decision to euthanatize an animal. Owners begin to anticipate what life will be like without the presence of their pet.[14] They begin to say *"When* my pet dies" rather than *"If . . . "*

During this time, feelings imitating the actual bereavement process begin in varying intensities and durations. These feelings are tentative and are not substitutes for those after a death. They do, however, provide an opportunity to experience some of the responses before death as a way of preparation.

Anticipatory grief is also based on the number and significance of prior losses or deaths. Past experiences affect not only how people view a new loss but also the repertoire of coping skills available to them. Prior losses can be positive strengths if people have learned from them, but they can also be negative obstacles if not dealt with previously. Bereavement overload can occur if a series of losses (that serve to deplete the person's resources and coping mechanisms) occurs.[15]

Anticipatory grief is often in evidence with people who are dealing with the progressive illness of their pet. Many begin to withdraw from friends and family, which compounds their feeling of helplessness, loneliness, and isolation. Others feel compelled to talk through their rising feelings of grief and seek out any and all who will listen or aid them in their many necessary decisions.

Euthanasia

Anticipatory grief is perhaps most in evidence during the difficult decision-making process surrounding euthanasia. This is a time when pet owners are asked to be clearheaded and compassionate when in reality they feel confused, sad, and angry. Euthanasia is one of the most controversial issues to be dealt with during the illness and impending death of a companion animal. This is due to the complexity of the issue and the potentially conflicting factors that must be taken into account before final decisions can be reached.

The decision-making process regarding euthanasia has many steps. The first to be considered is the medical status of the animal. Although the decision is a painful one at any time, most owners faced with a pet who is in obvious pain with no chance of recovery will elect euthanasia with a minimum of conflict. The decision becomes much more difficult, though, when options are available for treatment, especially when treatment courses have different outcomes, success rates, and varying financial costs. For owners to make rational decisions they must fully understand each alternative; thus, before clients can arrive at the decision to euthanatize, most must be convinced it is the best option for them and for their pet. This process may entail several soul-searching conversations with their veterinarian and may require a veterinarian to patiently repeat the alternatives over and over again. This is normal when it is manifested in a grieving client. Many clients who are experiencing anticipatory grief are still numb from the shock of hearing their pet's diagnosis. Patience and repetition will help them face reality.

What is best for the animal is not the only factor operating in the euthanasia decision-making process. Clients have concerns, reactions, and emotional needs that must also be addressed before they can arrive at decisions. Ignoring these needs and attempting to persuade them to make what the veterinarian feels is the "right" decision can result in the client and veterinarian assuming adversary roles. This is to no one's benefit.

Knowing what to expect from clients can help break the tension during this difficult struggle. Typically, clients may need to

1. Know they have done everything possible for their animal. This can often only be accomplished by reviewing the facts several times.
2. Have time to say goodbye to their pet, even if this means taking the animal home for a brief period. Taking an animal home frequently acts as the deciding key because the owners realize the extent of their pet's deterioration.
3. Have help in deciding what to do with the body. All options including burial, cremation, and disposal should be thoroughly discussed.
4. Have someone with whom to review their pet's life and to talk to about what life will now be like without the pet. This can be a friend, family member, veterinarian, or therapist.
5. Be able to count on someone who will offer sensitive, sincere validation of their feelings.
6. Hear repeated reassurances that they will indeed feel better in time and begin to live with their feelings of grief and loss.

When choosing to euthanatize, owners are being asked to take the responsibility of choosing death for a cherished friend. Clients may sometimes ask the veterinarian to make the decision about euthanasia for them or ask the veterinarian what they would do if the dying animal were their pet. These requests may reflect the client's need to have someone else shoulder at least part of the responsibility for the death of their animal. Rather than be drawn into the trap of assuming responsibility, veterinarians can empower clients by gently reminding them that the bond existing between owner and pet entitles no one but them to make that decision. It is also appropriate for veterinarians to share experiences regarding their own personal euthanasia decision-making processes.

Once clients have decided to euthanatize their pets, they again have several options: (1) be with the animal during the euthanasia, (2) be absent during the euthanasia but view the body afterwards, or (3) leave the animal with the veterinarian for euthanasia as well as disposition of the body. Traditionally, many veterinarians have discouraged clients from being with their pets during euthanasia. They felt the owner's presence might upset the animal, or the owner would not be able to cope with the animal's physical reactions. Many have assumed also that seeing a pet die would be too painful for an owner to endure. Although these concerns are not without merit, many unprepared veterinarians have used them as excuses to avoid dealing with their clients' emotional feelings.

Denying clients' abilities to make decisions and choices about the euthanasia of an animal has several important ramifications. Clients can feel insulted when their wishes are not respected, guilt ridden about being forced to "abandon" their pet when the animal needs them the most, and helpless to provide themselves with a final sense of closure to the relationship between them and their trusted friend. Allowing clients the opportunity to be present at a euthanasia can alleviate these obstacles blocking the necessary process of grieving.

Veterinarians can lower anxiety levels in clients by preparing all involved for what to expect during the euthanasia process. Clear, specific descriptions of the procedure should be offered and concrete words like *death* and *die* should be used. Euphemisms like *put to sleep* only perpetuate clients' denial systems and can also be frightening for children because they do not understand figurative language.

Clinical experience has shown that the owner's presence does not, in most cases, upset an animal during euthanasia. People generally stroke their pet gently and talk quietly to it, soothing the fears of all in the room. If veterinarians are apprehensive and convinced this may be a problem, however, the animal can be lightly tranquilized before euthanasia.

To make the procedure as easy as possible for the client, animal, and veterinarian, it is recommended that an intravenous catheter be inserted before allowing the client in the room. This way, the drug of choice can be given smoothly and with a minimum of trauma. If at all possible, an additional professional (veterinarian, veterinary technician, or a human service professional) should be present along with the primary veterinarian and client. This allows the veterinarian to focus solely on the animal while the assistant is there to focus on the client.

Much of the resistance to allowing client participation in a pet's euthanasia seems to be fear of the unknown. Once veterinarians have permitted clients to be present and have observed the experience to be a comforting, gratifying one with no untoward affects, much of the resistance disappears. It is not recommended that clients be required to be present at a euthanasia but rather that they be given the option and freedom to decide for themselves.

Last, a few simple procedural steps can be taken to facilitate the euthanasia process. Euthanasia should be scheduled during a relatively quiet time of day when few other clients are present, and financial matters should be settled beforehand. Private areas should be provided for clients to collect themselves before driving home, and back exits should be made available so distressed clients do not have to pass through busy reception areas. Clients should be encouraged to bring a friend or family member with them to provide assistance and support, and last but certainly not least, facial tissues should be readily available. Symbolically the facial tissue gives clients permission to cry and to express their feelings of grief honestly and openly. Clients should be given ample time alone with their pet both before and after the euthanasia so they can say and do all of their "final business" in private. A euthanasia procedural checklist (Fig. 16-3) and euthanasia decision-making checklist (Fig. 16-4) are provided for information and reference before the euthanasia process.

□
Facilitating client grief

Whether a companion animal's death occurs as the result of a sudden accident or a prolonged disease, the impact is the same. The

Euthanasia Procedural Checklist

Once euthanasia has been elected, there are several steps veterinarians can take to facilitate the procedure for both themselves and their clients.

□ Have you offered the clients the option of being present during the euthanasia? Clients will feel more respected if you allow them to choose what is best for them rather than making that decision yourself.

□ Have you explained the procedure to all involved so they will know what to expect?

□ Have you assured your clients that they will be allowed to view the body and say good-bye to their pet in private after the euthanasia is over?

□ Have you scheduled the euthanasia during the relatively quiet time of the day?

□ Have you settled financial matters beforehand?

□ Have you encouraged clients to bring a friend or a family member along to support them during and after the euthanasia?

□ If the clients have chosen to be present during the euthanasia, have you

    Given the animal a mild sedative?
    Catheterized the animal for easy injection?
    Covered the animal with a blanket or towel?
    Enlisted another professional (counselor, technician or staff member) to be present to attend to clients while you attend to the animal?

□ Have you made facial tissue readily available in the room?

□ Do you have a stress management plan or "debriefing" procedure to help deal with your own emotions?

□ Have you written a condolence card or letter?

Figure 16-3.   Euthanasia procedure checklist

death creates a crisis from which the pet owner may or may not ever fully recover. The Chinese word for crisis means danger and opportunity. This is an apt description for the choices veterinarians face at the time of pet loss. Discussions of pet loss and grief response are often uncomfortable, and most people feel threatened by them. Sometimes talking openly and honestly about death feels like venturing into dangerous territory.

Veterinarians who feel threatened by helping clients deal with grief will typically choose (either consciously or unconsciously) to avoid their clients and discussions of grief. Avoidance is displayed in comments such as "I am too busy to deal with them right now," "I am

not good at these things, I never know what to say," "Time will heal" or in behaviors like walking away, judging crying clients to be hysterical clients, and refusing to consider the facilitation of the grieving process to be a veterinarian's responsibility.

Veterinarians who view a client's loss as an opportunity, however, will choose to facilitate grief responses and attend to the physical, emotional, and psychological manifestations of grief mentioned earlier in this chapter. Attending to grief is displayed in comments like "I feel sad now, too, because I knew Pepper for several years and cared about him just as you did," or "Would you like some time to be alone with Pepper so you can say good-bye?"

Euthanasia Decision-Making Checklist

Here are ways veterinarians can help clients move through the decision-making process regarding euthanasia. Even after doing all of these things, clients may not make the decision you would like them to make, but at least you will know you did your best to facilitate the process.

☐ Has the pet's medical status and prognosis been thoroughly explained to all?

☐ Are the treatment alternatives, including euthanasia, understood by all involved in the decision?

☐ Have you patiently (and repeatedly) attended to the clients' emotional needs and concerns?

☐ Have you provided education about the normal grief responses to be expected at the death of a pet?

☐ Have you helped clients identify their support networks so they will know who to turn to for guidance and reassurance?

☐ Have you helped clients decide how to dispose of their pet's body? Have all options been discussed?

☐ Have you encouraged clients to say good-bye and "finish business" with their pet? Sometimes the decision is easier to make after pet and owner have spent some special time together.

Figure 16-4. Euthanasia decision-making checklist

Attending behaviors are also in evidence when veterinarians' behavior and actions enable clients to confront their losses directly. This is displayed when veterinarians allow clients to be present at euthanasia, send a condolence letter or card after death, and take time to listen to and comfort crying, grieving clients.

If attending to grief is the choice veterinarians make at the time of loss, there are several helping skills they can develop that will be useful to all involved. Ten of these helping skills are explained in the text that follows.

☐ Ten grief facilitation skills

Education

Veterinarians can be vital sources of information for clients who are concerned or confused about the grief process. If veterinarians themselves are knowledgeable about grief responses, they can help clients understand that the emotional, physical, and psychological symptoms they are experiencing are all normal manifestations of loss.

Education can also be an important tool for those wondering about how soon to get a replacement pet, how to tell young children about the impending death of a pet, or how to help friends draw a closure to loss experiences so that they may once more invest in new relationships. Sponsoring classes or support groups and making grief-related books and brochures available to clients are ways to begin the education process within veterinary hospitals and private practices.

Acknowledging the loss

Recognizing that loss has occurred helps people adjust to an environment in which the deceased is missing. Acknowledgment can take many forms, from a comforting arm around a shoulder to condolence calls and letters. Perhaps the most useful kind of acknowledgment happens when veterinarians encourage their clients' open displays of emotions. By saying out loud, "You have a right to feel sad and to cry," veterinarians acknowledge the devastating effects of loss and show they understand normal grief responses.

Validating feelings

To validate means to lend credibility to another's words and behaviors. Veterinarians who are educated about loss and grief can let clients know that their emotions, thoughts, and behaviors are legitimate.

Normalizing grief responses

The grief process is unique to each individual, yet certain responses are predictable. Veterinarians trained in the area of loss and grief can educate clients about normal grief responses and predict phases of the grief and recovery processes. This can serve to prepare clients for a loss as well as let them know they are not alone with their feelings of grief.

Empathizing and self-disclosing

Empathy is different from sympathy. If veterinarians empathize with their clients, they can put themselves into their clients' situation and understand what they are feeling. In other words, if a client feels sad, the veterinarian can also access feelings of sadness and "be with" the client in experiencing that emotion.

If veterinarians *sympathize* with their clients, however, they feel sorry *for* them as opposed to *with* them. No one likes to be pitied, and this approach is rarely constructive to the grief process.

Self-disclosure is a valuable tool to use to demonstrate empathy. By disclosing information about oneself, a veterinarian can "join" with a client and share personal feelings, stories, and thoughts relevant to the situation at hand. This technique should be used sparingly, though, so that the focus does not stray from the client.

Giving permission

Clients often need to be told by someone (whom they perceive to be in authority) that it is alright for them to take certain actions. For example, they may need "permission" to say good-bye to their pet, to arrange a funeral ceremony, to openly show their emotions, or even to contact a professional for further grief therapy. The veterinarian is often the person they look to for this permission because of the relationship usually established between them. Permission often extends into other areas as well because many clients need to feel they have the right to end treatment, to euthanatize, and even to form new relationships with subsequent replacement pets.

Listening

Listening is perhaps the most overlooked skill in the health services field. Medically trained people are taught to have answers and explain complicated issues to people with little or no medical background. Because of this, veterinarians often err at the time of a loss by saying too much. The goal of grief facilitation is not to "fix" a problem or to "take a feeling away," but rather to allow feelings to be felt and "run their course."

Grief is a natural, normal response to loss, and most often clients will want to know first and foremost that someone cares enough about them to actively listen to what they need to say.

Providing structure

When people experience loss, most view the loss as a crisis and drop naturally to a lower level of functioning (see Fig. 16-2). This is due to the sensations of shock and feelings of denial that arise at the time of loss. Due to this change in functioning level, clients often "forget" to make plans, "forget" to take care of themselves, and "forget" to let others know they are in need of help. Veterinarians can help provide structure to their clients' lives by reminding them to make necessary arrangements. They can also help by urging clients to find ways to honor the memories of their pets in ways that are appropriate for them. For instance, veterinarians might suggest that clients create memorials like scrapbooks; bulletin boards, slide shows, or even funeral ceremonies to use as tools to begin the grieving process.

Assessing needs and making referrals

Occasionally veterinarians will encounter clients who are in need of grief therapy and who could benefit from professional intervention of some kind. Veterinarians who are well informed about their local human services network will know of the appropriate agencies, programs, and people to whom clients can be referred. Referral procedures vary, and veterinarians should become knowledgeable about the various programs available to assist them. Referral networks can include local hospice groups, clergy, grief therapists, and other mental health programs. Many universities, animal hospitals, and private practices have specific programs in place to deal with pet loss. Colorado State University, The University of Pennsylvania, and The New York City Animal Medical Center are three of the most well known and developed programs.

Clients who are suspected of being suicidal are special cases and ultimately need to be handled by trained crisis counselors. Veterinarians should be certain they know who to contact if faced with a suicidal situation and certain they are proceeding with the referral in a way that is timely and legal.

Debriefing

Veterinarians need support just as their clients do, especially when the loss is one that impacts on their personal lives. Veterinarians are encouraged to talk openly about their feelings of grief to friends, family members, and others in their profession so that they might form a "debriefing" support group for themselves. Stress is an inevitable part of the veterinary field, but a workable plan to manage the stress can help veterinarians cope with daily losses.

Further information about these grief facilitation techniques can be gleaned from a variety of resources. References are included here as a starting point for those interested in learning more about how to deal with client grief and patient death and dying.

□ References

1. Beck AM: Animals in the city. In Beck AM, Katcher A (eds): New Perspectives on Our Lives with Companion Animals. Philadelphia, University of Pennsylvania Press, 1983
2. Bowen M: Family psychotherapy with a schizophrenic in the hospital and in private practice. In Borzormenyi-Nagi I, Framo JL (eds): Intensive Family Therapy. New York, Harper & Row, 1965
3. Voith V: Attachment of people to companion animals. In Quackenbush J, Voith V (eds): Symposium on the Human–Companion Animal Bond, Veterinary Clinics of North America, Small Animal Practice. Philadelphia, WB Saunders, 1985
4. Cain A: Pets as family members. Pets Family— Marriage Family Rev 8:3, 1985
5. Voith V: Attachment between people and their

pets: Behavior problems of pets that arise from the relationship between pets and people. In Fogle B (ed): Interrelationships Between People and Pets. Springfield, IL, Charles C Thomas, 1981

6. Veevers J: The social meaning of pets: Alternative roles for companion Animals. Pets Family — Marriage Family Rev 8:3, 1985

7. Salmon PW, Salmon IM: Who owns who? Psycholgical research into the human-pet bond in Australia. In Katcher AN, Beck AM (eds): New Perspectives on Our Lives with Companion Animals. Philadelphia, University of Pennsylvania Press, 1983

8. Bernbaum M: The veterinarian's role in grief and bereavement at pet loss. Cornell Feline Health Center News 7, 1982

9. Neiberg H, Fischer A: Pet Loss: A Thoughtful Guide for Adults and Children. New York, Harper & Row, 1982

10. Cowles K: The death of a pet: Human responses to the breaking of the bond. Pets Family — Marriage Family Rev 8:3, 1980

11. Bowlby J: Attachment and Loss, Vol 3. Loss, Sadness and Depression. New York, Basic Books, 1980

12. Kubler-Ross E: On Death and Dying. New York, Macmillan, 1969

13. Rando T: Grief, Dying, and Death: Clinical Intervention for Caregivers. Champaign, IL, Research Press Company, 1984

14. Quackenbush J, Graveline D: When Your Pet Dies: How to Cope with Your Feelings. New York, Simon & Schuster, 1985

15. Kastenbaum R: Death, Society, and Human Experience. St Louis, CV Mosby, 1977

Chapter 17

□

Practice stress, burnout, and rustout

Eugenia G. Kelman

Work stress and *burnout* are new concepts in human history. In past times when life was short and cruel, people did not worry about achieving personal satisfaction from work. The prehistoric hunter did not return of an evening to his cave and complain of the repetitious boredom of his job. The slaves who built the pyramids did not reproach their overseers about the lack of job satisfaction. The oarsmen who powered ancient vessels across the sea did not consider a career change because the management did not appreciate them enough. Workers expected only to survive by means of their labor. A full belly and protection from the cold were enough. It is a luxury of modern times that we can think about "finding ourselves" through pleasant interpersonal relations at work or about developing our personalities and self-esteem through a career.

□
What is stress?

Stress is a perception of something threatening in the environment. Imagine one of our early ancestors strolling through the woods. He sees a large carnivorous animal. Not much relishing the idea of becoming this creature's dinner, our forebear experienced fear. His central nervous system went into high gear and set off his sympathetic nervous system, which, in turn, activated the endocrine and musculoskeletal systems. He was ready to fight or run. After either winning the fight, or the race to escape, he would have used up the energy released by the original emotion. He might be tired, but he no longer felt stress. He was probably just happy to be alive.

In the modern professional work setting, the major environmental threats are usually other people. For veterinarians they are clients, colleagues, employers, or employees. The sharp teeth of carnivorous animals are no problem: they can be clamped down with a muzzle. But the sharp tongues of their owners may be frightening. The client or boss cannot be muzzled. The desire to punch the living daylights out of some irritating person must be suppressed. Running away is usually not a reasonable option, either.

The essential problem of modern-day work stress is our belief that work should bring us satisfaction, and when it does not, we must stay put and be reasonably polite no matter how hurt, angry, scared, or depressed we feel. But, while a little smile is pasted on your face, your nervous and endocrine systems are churning away according to that primitive genetic plan. All that energy gets displaced somewhere else. If it happens over and over, the excess energy can cause serious problems. An outline

of stressors for veterinarians and the strain responses is found in Table 17-1.

Although some physical danger exists in veterinary work, most stressors are either threats to the veterinarian's self-esteem or are due to poor business practices or the lack of time management.

What drives one person crazy does not at all bother another. An individual must be vulnerable to a particular stressor to experience strain. Professionals are thought to be especially vulnerable to stress related to self-esteem because of the educational system through which they tracked to obtain their degrees. Young people cannot achieve access to graduate and professional education unless they compete successfully for high grades and demonstrate other desirable personal characteristics. These personal characteristics include attention to detail, absorption in work, social respectability, and the ability to focus on those activities and ideas that get them successfully admitted to college, professional

Table 17-1
Stressors and strain response for veterinarians

Stressors for Veterinarians: Human Contacts Including

Boss (conflicts with, unappreciated by)
Clients (angry, dissatisfied, unappreciative, mercenary, cruel, dishonest)
Employee (untrustworthy, incompetent, late, forgetful)
Family (complaints about not spending time with, quarrels)
Physical Challenges (inadequate equipment or facilities, handling difficult animals)
Mental Challenge (financial problems, paperwork, keeping up with new ideas, concerns about accuracy, competency, overload schedule)
Job Status (ambiguity, uncertainty about duties, promotion, future)

Strain Response Can Be

Behavioral (smoking too much, doing drugs, drinking too much, forgetfulness, daydreaming, withdrawal, biting fingernails, having accidents, tics, stuttering)
Emotional (variations on the themes of hostility, anxiety, and depression)
Physical (headaches, sleeping disorders, backaches, rapid heart rate, high blood pressure, excessive perspiration, trembling, low resistance to infection, peptic ulcers, colitis, jaw clenching, and other unpleasant things)

school, and finally, the profession. Most pre-veterinary and veterinary students perceive themselves as "on trial" throughout this long period. Their probationary status and compe-tition for grades condition an overly anxious person subject to worries about failure and class status. The long, demanding educational program leaves little time for the development of leisure activities.

When this generally "nervous" person is given the responsibility for the welfare of others, often for life or death of a patient, a situation develops that can lead to extreme stress. The professional person is also exposed to the joy of making a special contribution to the health and happiness of others, feelings of self-esteem, and a sense of power.

Most people are unaware of stress until symptoms of strain appear just as they are blissfully ignorant of a viral infection until the symptoms become a problem. The virus usually infects a person some days before ex-periencing the fever, sore throat, or nausea of a cold or flu. It is the same with stress. When the way a person copes with a stressor stops being a satisfactory solution, sooner or later symp-toms appear. The symptoms are clues that a better coping method must be found to pre-vent stress or relieve strain.

The stressor–stress–strain model suggests three possible approaches to the problem:

1. Try to prevent or reduce stressors in your life.
2. Change the way people and events are perceived to reduce stress.
3. Learn to become more physically re-laxed, even in the presence of people and events that were formerly found threatening.

All of these approaches work. The question is what combination of coping strategies applies best to any particular problem?

☐
Dealing with stressors

Dr. Brown was a young veterinarian who forced herself to go to work in the morning. She felt sick and tired, overworked and under-paid. After nearly 6 months in a new position, she had a formidable list of complaints against her employers, a partnership operating a mixed animal practice. She had taken the job with the understanding she would be able to work with some equine cases because she wanted eventually to be an equine practi-tioner. But she was assigned an entirely small-animal caseload. She was on call too many nights and weekends. Having to be available most of the time for after-hours calls made it difficult for her to develop any social life in her new location. The promised pay raise "if ev-erything worked out" had never come. They were taking advantage of her. She felt sad when she thought of being trapped in this un-fair situation much longer, and she felt angry when she thought about how the owners were treating her. On top of everything else, she could not seem to shake an upper respiratory infection that had plagued her for months. She liked her clients and knew she was handling her cases well, but she was seriously consider-ing a change of career. She had always dabbled in artistic endeavors. Maybe she should get out of veterinary medicine and try her luck and talent in that new direction?

Dr. Brown is in a stressful situation that is taking its toll on her emotional and physical well-being. Her problem is primarily one of conflict with her employers over hours, salary, and the type of cases referred to her.

In any conflict situation there are numerous possible solutions, and they all start with bet-ter communications. The "no-lose" system of checking out potential options is a good place to start. First, Dr. Brown would identify the needs of each person involved in the conflict, that is, define the problem. She wants a raise, more free time evenings and weekends, and more equine cases, but how do her employers see these issues? She should prioritize each of these goals. Before presenting them to her employers, she should also generate a list of possible solutions to each defined problem. At this point, she is free to brainstorm possible solutions. She has discovered one: become an artist. There are several other options at least as usable. She could look for another job within the veterinary medical profession, one with more regular hours or that allowed her to work with horses. She could request a half-time position and study art with the time that then becomes available. She could discuss all three major issues with her employers, or she could limit herself to trying to resolve just one problem at first.

Before she actually sets up the meeting with her employers, she needs to evaluate each potential solution and estimate the possible risks associated with each of them. For example, how long would it take to become an artist? How much would this cost? How would she earn a living as an artist?

She must select a solution that is consistent with her goals and has an acceptable level of risk. If Dr. Brown decides her present employers will probably be unwilling to accommodate her on any of her concerns, then she must be prepared to look for a job elsewhere. After evaluating that possibility, she decided it was a risk worth taking. She concluded that if they refused and she had to change jobs she would not be any unhappier than at the present time, and there was a good probability of finding a better job. If her employers did not value her contribution to their clinic enough to make staying more attractive to her, she really should leave.

After evaluating her alternatives, she set up a meeting with her employers to request a salary increase and less emergency duty. They refused. She did look for a new job and found one where she could work with horses at regu-

lar hours. The salary was not much better, but two out of three is not bad, and she is much happier now. As soon as she decided to deal effectively with her problem, her cold was "miraculously" cured. She is continuing to develop her career and, in the process, has learned something about her personality. Thinking about her career crisis in retrospect, she decided she had a pattern of being too agreeable to the demands of other people and needed to develop better problem-solving and communication skills to take better care of herself in conflict situations.

As more and more veterinarians are moving toward group practice, communication problems increasingly become a stressor. Clear communication is essential to a smoothly functioning group practice, and poor communication can quickly lead to tension. Issues that require clear lines of communication in a partnership are purchase of new equipment, definition of case duties and responsibilities (especially if more than one partner takes care of the same animal), maintaining complete records so that colleagues can take over a case if necessary, decisions about raises or profit sharing, decisions about hiring staff and personnel management (hiring, firing, training, instructing), and dealing with differences of opinion about the medical management of a case.

Time should be set aside specifically for partners to talk about how things should be done and to solve small problems before they become big ones. A regular weekly meeting, perhaps at a meal, is a good idea. In dealing with problems, respect for the ideas of your partner and a willingness to work toward solutions all can live with, at least temporarily, will make these weekly sessions work. Here are some suggestions for collegial problem-solving sessions:

1. Identify the problem. Pinpoint it accurately enough to be able to write it down.

2. Brainstorm. Ask everyone to think of as many possible alternative solutions as they can. Do not criticize any offering. Just think of as many as possible. Be imaginative about possible solutions. Consider minimizing (take something away, make smaller, eliminate something). Consider maximizing (add something, make something bigger). Consider reversing present procedures. Consider how other people or practices would solve this problem: How would Sylvester Stallone, Ronald Reagan, Great-aunt Harriet, or your child solve this problem? Loosen up!

3. Evaluate the options. Brainstorming can be fun, but some options are not very desirable, probably, or likely to succeed. Sift through and select an option or combination of alternatives your group is willing to try for a while, perhaps until your next meeting.

4. Form a plan of action based on costs/ benefits assessment.

5. Get group commitment to this plan of action.

The best way to make working with people easy is to develop excellent communication skills: to listen well; to show empathy and understanding for the other person's point of view; to give clear, acceptable instructions; and to be appropriately assertive (not aggressive!) when necessary.

Conflicts are resolved most readily by talking together, and the best communicators usually listen more than they speak. Effective and active listening prevents many problems involving interpersonal relations. Understanding the wants or needs of the other person, whether it be a client or a colleague, provides you a better basis for problem solving and action.

Good communicators convey a helpful attitude. Body language that silently says "I'm listening" includes a posture oriented toward the speaker and facial expressions and gestures that say "I'm interested in you." You can draw out the other person's ideas with open-ended questions: What are your thoughts about this? Would you like to talk about this? Can I be of help?

The other person can be encouraged to continue talking by noncommittal acknowledgement such as "I see," "Yes," or "Um-hmmm," which indicates that the line of thought is being followed. The other person's ideas do not need to be interrupted by interjecting your own, at least not until he or she has completed the entire expression. The other person's ideas can be clarified or developed into a deeper layer of thought by reflecting back what was heard, for example, "You seem concerned about what will happen if. . . ."

Communication skills are not inherited like the color of our eyes. They are learned just as all skills are learned. These skills can be learned from other people who are excellent communicators or in the classroom. If getting along with people is a work stressor, then consider some formal class work to learn about the meaning of body language, to be an active listener, to define and discuss a problem effectively, and to be respectfully assertive. Such classes are offered by colleges and consultants for a fee. Perhaps your state or local veterinary medical association would be interested in contracting with a consultant to offer communication workshops specifically for the veterinary medical work setting. The "live" training of a class is best because it offers the opportunity to practice and to receive feedback on your own performance. If a workshop or class is not available, specific references could be reviewed that will provide additional insight.[1-9]

□
Pressed for time

Feeling pressured by time is an important stressor for the busy professional. This is the case for Dr. Green. His life consists of three things — work, work, and work. He spends 70 hours a week at the clinic and then takes book work home because he cannot get to it during the day. His wife complains he does not pay enough attention to her and their children and also does not pay attention to her complaints either. He has tried a few times to get away from work by taking trips out of town, but it was hard to keep his thoughts away from work. When he returned to find that work had piled up waiting for him, he said, "Vacations are not worth it." He believes the additional overtime before or after the vacation does not make them worthwhile. He is a successful professional. He has achieved the American dream: a busy practice and a nice house, cars, and some luxuries for his family. While his wife and children are developing interests and relationships in which he has no part, he thinks only of his work. Dr. Green is a workaholic whose life is out of balance. He believes the time demands of his profession are the problem. In fact, his inability to set priorities and to better manage his time is the problem.

If he does not become more efficient about getting his work done, he may find that the American dream has turned into a nightmare. He could arrive home late (as usual) one night to find a sad note of farewell from his departed wife. His body may rebel by having a heart attack, or he may have a full-blown "mid-life crisis" and cast aside most of what he has worked to gain.

There is plenty of time to work and also to achieve goals not associated with work. About 1 out of every 3 days is available to most people for meaningful leisure. One third of the time is free with the typical schedule of time away from work: 52 weekend days (either Saturday or Sunday), 7 special holidays, 14 vacation days, and 50 week days off per year provide a total of 123 days or one third of a year. This also means the remaining 242 days are work days.

Being able to enjoy time away from work depends on using the work time efficiently.

According to the Pareto principle, people spend 80% of their time doing tasks that are related to only 20% of total job results.

How well do you manage your productive time? Priorities must be set on a daily basis, with as much of the drudgery as possible delegated to technical staff and other support staff. The multiple roles, long and irregular hours, and unclear definitions of responsibility in a practice can be all-consuming. The result will be a lack of control over scheduling, reduced efficiency (after 60 hours of work a week, no one is working very efficiently), strained interpersonal relationships on the job and at home, lower levels of creativity, and worsened physical and mental health.

Time scheduling is the first rule of good time management. Time is already fairly well scheduled for a busy practitioner. If paperwork is routinely carried home after a long day at the practice, an hour *within the workday* for paperwork needs to be scheduled. When some of the work does not get completed within the confines of a reasonable workday, the problem may be perfectionism, failure to delegate, not defining job responsibilities in the practice properly, or all of the above.

Most employees will blossom when given more responsibility. When necessary, delegate some authority too. Giving a competent employee full authority over a project or an area of the practice will give that person a strong motive to produce and pride in the results. When the work is properly done, it is essential to reward the employee with due notice of a job well done. When employees fail to produce, more training may be required. If additional training still does not get the job done, then the employee should be dismissed and replaced with someone who can be of assistance in achieving the professional goals. Continuing a poor employee – job match is not good for the practice or the employee. Additional information concerning personnel management may be found in Chapters 3 and 14.

Getting things done is a question of prioritizing. Set three goals for each day and put them in order of priority. Be sure to always accomplish the number one–priority task each day. The lower-priority tasks should always be attempted, but do not feel badly if they cannot be completed. Remember that the top-priority job was accomplished. By following this golden rule of time management faithfully, 242 high-priority goals will be accomplished every year.

If your daily schedule does not reflect your professional goals, you should analyze how your time is being spent. The first step in this analysis is to chart how time is used, perhaps in half-hour chunks, throughout the day. Do this for at least a week — or longer if a week would not be a representative period of time.

You will begin to use your time better as soon as you start this charting project. Time wasters in the practice will be quickly identified. At the end of the baseline record-keeping period, calculate how much time you spent in major categories: business management, examinations, surgeries, client communications, traveling on calls, with your spouse, with your children, with your friends, reading and learning, exercising, and just relaxing. Then decide: are you spending your time according to your life priorities? Dr. Green's category totals would show almost no time spent in an enjoyable way with his wife and children. Maybe he does not like his family and will be happier away from them. If that is the case, he is spending his time properly. But if he values having a family, wants to get to know his children before they grow up and leave home, and really wants a wife who is a friend for life, then he must reallocate his time before it is too late. What percentage of your time is spent working, developing a personal support system, and developing personal interests?

People say silly things like "I never have time to read or to write letters." We all have the same amount of time — 24 hours a day, 365 days a year. We have a great deal of choice about how to spend it. Time is nothing more or less than life itself. Time is also money. If more leisure time is a priority for social and personal development, then a reduction in work and income may be necessary to attain this goal.

Some people do not really want to do anything but work. In that case, an overloaded schedule is not a stressor. It is an unimaginative way to spend a lifetime, but it is not stressful. Successful time management requires decisions about what is important and then action on those decisions. You are feeling stress from lack of time management when you feel rushed all the time, feel tired or listless, feel you did not get enough done during the day, constantly miss deadlines, do not have enough time for rest or for personal relationships, feel overwhelmed by demands and details, or do unpleasant tasks most of the time. Here are some tips on saving time.

Limit telephone conversations to 3 to 5 minutes.

Cut food preparation by eating more foods that do not require cooking (or cook a big batch on the weekend and eat from it for a few days).

Only watch television when there is a special program — and schedule it just as any other prioritized activity.

If you travel long distances by automobile, dictate correspondence, use audiotapes to learn new skills, or get a car telephone and make client calls.

Learn to speed-read.

Keep lists and check off things as they are completed.

Minimize interruptions at work (ask your secretary or receptionist to prevent interruptions by inquiring "Can someone else help you?" or have the problem referred to a technician).

Throw away junk mail without opening it.

Put very low priority items into a "future" basket; it is amazing how many do not *ever* need to be done.

Do high-priority items immediately.

Handle each piece of paper once (do not keep looking at it and then returning it to your work basket).

Get up earlier (most people are very efficient early in the day).

Start meetings on time; if you are not in charge of the meeting, ask the chairperson to start on time.

Learn to say *No* to low-priority requests.

To summarize what can be done to reduce time pressure: (1) define the job duties, authority, responsibilities in your practice; (2) monitor how time is spent; (3) schedule time according to priorities; (4) list tasks to be accomplished in order of priority and get rid of one each day: and (5) delegate!

For more information on time management please refer to Chapter 13 and/or review the material by Douglass and Douglass and Lakein. [10,11]

□
Changing the job

Work stressors sometimes require changes in the work setting rather than in the individual. Consider changing the work setting by shifting job or hours, moving nearer or farther from work, changing job responsibilities, or changing jobs within the profession. Consider reorganizing the work setting or redecorating or redesigning your office or clinic. Get a partner (if you do not have one), time share for a while, rotate services, use an emergency service for out-of-hours calls, or train employees to do some management tasks.

Sometimes changing jobs works, sometimes not. It is partly a matter of personality and partly luck. If the new job is more interesting and allows development in a new career

direction that rekindles enthusiasm, the change was obviously a good one. If a change just replaces one set of faces and problems for another set of the same, you will soon be back in the same dilemma. Leaving the profession can be an act of desperation and a sign of defeat. In any case, be assured that every job and every vocation has stressors and problems to solve.

□
It's (almost) all in your head

If problem solving, job hopping, and time management cannot improve how you feel about your work environment, consider changing your feelings. It is a common fallacy that feelings cannot be changed. In fact, it is relatively easy to change perceptions and emotions, and you will be a more even tempered person ever after for having learned this skill.

Think of two people you know. Recall someone who is very excitable, whose emotions run the roller coaster from the heights of joy to the depths of despair. This person can be a lot of fun on the upside of the ride but is very depressing when things take a dip for the worse. The downhill ride will usually have a stronger effect. There is such a thing as having too many feelings. They can be a pain in the clavicle to the overly emotional person as well as to everyone else within earshot. You probably also know someone who is emotionally steady. No matter what happens, this person remains fairly calm. This is a friend with whom almost anything can be discussed. No topic will cause a storm of emotion. Some people control how they feel; others do not.

Learning how to change thoughts and feelings is not a new idea. The ancient Greek philosopher Democritus pointed out that it is not events that trouble us but rather how we think of them. You may have heard the sensible prayer: "Lord, grant me the serenity to accept the things I cannot change, courage to change the things I can, and wisdom to know the difference." An event that might make one person feel suicidal could be accepted by another person as a good learning experience from which to profit in the future.

People can learn to be more objective and less emotional observers of events in their own lives. Behavioral scientists call this attitude adjustment treatment "cognitive behavior management" or, more simply, thought control.

Therapists who specialize in thought control intervene in the middle of the three-part sequence of stressor-stress-response. They teach the importance of being less extreme in interpreting the meaning of an event.

Here are some popular thoughts that can cause unpleasant emotional responses:

1. I need to be liked, appreciated, or approved by all my clients and colleagues all the time.
2. I must prove myself thoroughly competent, adequate, and achieving in everything I do.
3. It is terrible when things do not go the way I would like them to go.
4. People who do not share my values and opinions are stupid, mean, or both.
5. Things should go better at work than they do, and it is terrible if I cannot find an immediate solution to every problem.
6. Other people cause all my miseries.
7. Events over which I have no control cause all my problems.
8. I cannot change my feelings.
9. I cannot make a mistake.
10. My thoughts and feelings are determined by past events that cannot be changed (after all, they are in the past).
11. My clients (colleagues, employees, children, and so forth) should behave better than they do.
12. I should feel very concerned and upset over my clients' (colleagues', patients', employees') problems.
13. Every problem has a perfect solution, and I must find it (and I will not do anything about this problem until I do).
14. I should never let my clients (colleagues, employees) discover that I have any weakness.
15. My happiness depends on being appreciated by each and every client (colleague, employee).
16. I cannot stand certain clients.
17. I cannot stand certain habits of my partners (employees, colleagues).
18. I must be available for all emergency calls of my clients.
19. I am responsible for the happiness of my clients (employees, family).
20. I cannot stand being interrupted by emergency calls.

These negative, dysfunctional thoughts can be reduced to a few categories and then associated with problem personalities. The anxious person exaggerates the dangers or possible negative effect of any situation, for example, "Not getting this promotion is the worst thing that could happen to me" or "I'll never get over having made that mistake in diagnosis." Any daily newspaper illustrates the fact that people recover from far more difficult situations than either of these.

The "I can'ts" make a difficult situation even worse. Frequently people say, "I cannot stand my job" (boss, hours, clients, and so forth), when, in fact, they have "stood" it for years (complaining all the while) and will continue to bear it for many more years. It is rare to have the power to change other people, certainly not clients in the brief time of interaction with them. You are extremely unlikely to change their basic values about caring for their animals. Wishful thinking about how they ought to behave does not help deal more effectively with their actual behavior.

Dysfunctional thoughts cause you harm, get you into trouble with other people, are untrue, or keep you from accomplishing your goals. The most painful of all dysfunctional thoughts is not to have faith in yourself or in your ability to eventually solve your problems, to be competent, to be likable. It is a gross overgeneralization to think that if one person does not like you or if you make a mistake you are therefore worthless. Deciding that other people are worthless (because they disagree with you or do not behave the way you wish them to) will only make it more difficult to deal with them.

Consider the case of Dr. White. Dr. White is a good veterinarian, and he makes an excellent living as a small-animal practitioner. But he wants out of practice. The reason he is willing to give up a successful career is that he cannot stand to hear the phrase "It's only a dog" one more time. This terrible situation occurs when he has conducted an examination on a sick dog and discusses his treatment plan with the client. Sometimes the client does not want to pay for an expensive treatment and justifies this decision by saying, "After all, it's only a dog." When he hears that hated phrase, Dr. White feels worthless.

Dr. White spent many long, hard years to learn how to diagnose and treat this dog's problem. If the owner does not think the animal is worth the cost of treatment, it signifies to him that all his training and his whole life as a practitioner are as worthless as the life of that dog. When this event occurs, as it does with predictable regularity, his day is ruined. He goes home feeling depressed. It does not matter that he earns a good income. Nor does he think of the many clients who are devoted to their pets and appreciate his services. He has considered returning to graduate school for an advanced degree that would lead to a job in a research laboratory where he would never again have to hear anyone say "It's only a dog."

Dr. White is the victim of stressful, distorted thinking. Some time in his past he learned from parents or other teachers that his self-worth depends on the value other people place on what he can do. There is a kernel of truth in the thought, but he has exaggerated it out of proportion. His friends might tell him; "Hey, stop doing that to yourself! You are a good veterinarian. Most of your clients appreciate you and your service. Being a bench researcher in a laboratory probably has its hassles too." This might work, but chances are he has heard all that before and still feels bad every time he hears that phrase.

Specialists in thought control have found it helps to train their clients to go through a complete four-step logical analysis of how their thoughts in particular situations cause bad feelings and stress. This four-step process can be recalled by an A, B, C, D format as follows:

A. They identify the *activating* event, the situation in which the dysfunctional thought occurs. For Dr. White, this is when a client does not want to assume the financial burden of treatment and says, "After all, it's only a dog."

B. They identify the person's *beliefs* about that event. Dr. White associates that statement with worthlessness. He says to himself, "If this client does not want to pay for treatment of his pet, my profession is worthless. Since I have invested so much of my life in a worthless profession, I am worthless."

C. Believing he and his work are worthless leads to a negative consequence — feeling depressed. Experiencing this very unpleasant emotion repeatedly at work leads him to the further thought that he should leave his career as a practitioner.

D. Rational-emotive or cognitive-behavioral management (changing your feelings through changing your thoughts) suggests that Dr. White should *dispute* his self-talk in a systematic way.

First, he should ask himself, "Is my thought true? Is it accurate to say that if a client does not want to pay for treatment then my professional practice is worthless?" There is a germ of truth in most useless thinking, so usually an additional question needs to be answered: "How often?" If all or even 90% of his clients made that statement, he probably would be wise to consider a career change. Only a few clients, however, refused to agree with the suggested treatment. Perhaps he heard the dreaded statement only once a week. Possibly as many as 95% of his clients were pleased to pay for good care for their pets. To be accurate, the question is then rephrased, "Is it true that if 5% of clients do not choose expensive treatment for their pets my life's work is worthless?" The answer is clearly No. A 95% success rate in gaining clients' agreement for treatment is certainly good.

Even if there is some truth to the belief, there is a second question to ask: "Is this thought useful in my situation?" Sometimes a negative thought is true enough, but dwelling on it only makes an inescapable situation worse. For example, in veterinary practice, some patients will die. That is an inescapable fact. Most veterinarians would prefer that their patients live. A veterinarian who thought constantly of all the animals whose lives he could not save would become depressed and disillusioned with the profession. This would lead to talking to those clients who have terminally ill animals in a despondent manner. This veterinarian might not make the best effort to help the animal because he knows the work will be in vain, even if the client wishes to have every possible treatment. At the end of the day, this veterinarian remembers the animals who were not cured rather than those helped by his med-

ical skill. Therefore, even though it is true and inevitable that many patients will die, it may not be useful to emphasize that thought.

The final question to ask is "Does thinking this help me achieve my goals in life?" If Dr. White's goal is to feel better, to be a calm, even-tempered professional, he must stop thinking that his job satisfaction depends on his being appreciated by everyone or knowing that everyone shares his values and opinions. These thoughts will ensure dissatisfaction in any profession and work setting.

Dr. White must then decide whether he wants to get rid of the dysfunctional or irrational thought. If he is ready to commit himself to change, then he can begin systematically to replace the useless thought pattern with one that is more true, more useful, and that helps him achieve his goals. He needs to identify counterthoughts at this point. Some possible counterthoughts for him might be

- "Most people appreciate my services; I can tolerate the small minority who will not give their animals what I consider to be proper care."
- "People are different; I do not expect everyone to share my views on the value of animal life; I can set a good example of my own value system and hope that the best of what I have to offer is helpful and remembered by most clients."
- "Many animals never receive any health care; if this animal does not receive what I consider to be optimal health care, it will at least have some help (relief of pain)."
- "I have been able to help many people and animals today; I have been able to offer a useful service to many who needed it."

This A-B-C-D method of thought analysis can be applied to any belief. If the thought turns out to be true and useful, then you need to consider one of the problem-solving strategies described earlier.

"On-call syndrome" could be diagnosed as

a case for thought control. The activating event is the telephone ring. The doctor believes, "Oh no, it is going to be another disaster, and I will not be paid." The emotional consequence is likely to be some slight hostility toward the caller. The behavioral consequence might be an abrupt, hasty treatment of the case and possibly the loss of a client if the hostility and hurried manner are too obvious. It is not awful to receive an out-of-hours call. It is an expected part of any medical profession. Emergency calls, unless you use an emergency service, are a part of medical practice. To complain about them is like complaining about the weather or the rising and setting of the sun. The negative consequences illustrate the uselessness of this thought. Possible replacement thoughts are

- "This is what I planned to do with my life."
- "This is a standard part of medical practice."
- "I knew I was on call tonight, and I planned to be interrupted."
- "Perhaps this will be a good future client for my practice."
- "I really want to help this client and patient."

The emotional and behavioral consequences of the replacement thoughts are more likely to be positive for the client, practitioner, and practice building.

Learning to regard life events from a more reasonable perspective gets rid of irrational perception of stressors in the environment. Additional information about cognitive stress intervention may be found in the references.[12-16]

□
Worrying

Worrying is a special kind of dysfunctional thinking. Worrying is usually not really thinking at all — more like a needle caught in a pho-

nograph record so that the same phrase repeats and repeats in your head without getting anywhere. Worrying can be time-consuming and unproductive and leads to negative emotions and behaviors. *Planning,* on the contrary, is goal oriented. A plan has an identifiable result and steps to attain that goal. A good test of whether mental preoccupation is worrying or planning is to schedule a time for it and then to write down the steps needed to solve the problem. Worrying cannot be scheduled because worry is rather unconscious, uncontrolled behavior that occurs when the mind is not deliberately focused. Planning, however, can be scheduled. Plans can be described on paper. Schedule a particular time to deal with a major concern. If you cannot concentrate on this problem and can't identify a goal connected with it and set out some steps to achieve that goal, it is probably just useless worrying related to a dysfunctional thought pattern such as "This is terrible, awful, catastrophic, and I'll never survive it," rather than "This is inconvenient, unpleasant, or disadvantageous, but I will manage to deal with it."

□
Stopping the strain response

The third approach to dealing with stress involves alleviating the strain response.

Behavioral symptoms such as eating disorders, sleeping disorders, nailbiting, or excessive use of tobacco, alcohol, or other drugs suggest a behavior modification therapeutic technique. Specific behavioral treatments can be individually designed by a therapist for any unwanted, undesirable behavior. There are also many books about how to stop smoking, eat more sensibly, drink less alcohol (or stop altogether), or achieve control over any behavior. The basic principles of all behavior change programs are similar: (1) identify the problematic behavior, (2) study the present practice with regard to that behavior (get a baseline), (3) identify the desired change goal and set up a schedule to achieve that change, and (4) implement the schedule.

If the schedule is not followed, analyze what thoughts or events interfered and establish a subroutine to eliminate the interference. Additional information on behavior change systems can be found in the references.[17,18]

□ Relaxation

Learning to relax will alleviate most of the physiological strain symptoms. Just as the mind, perceiving threat, starts a chain of physiological reaction that can cause physical illness if it becomes chronic, so also can the mind be used to soothe the body and make it less tense. There are many mental techniques to achieve physical relaxation. These techniques use either mental imagery or the repetition of certain words in a quiet manner to achieve this result. They are all a kind of self-hypnosis, which just means the attention becomes narrowed and focused on achieving a quiet, relaxed state.

Relaxation techniques are especially helpful for those who have high blood pressure, headaches, muscular tension that causes any bodily pain, or tension-related habits such as stuttering, tics, squinting, scowling, and jawclenching.

□ Progressive relaxation

Progressive relaxation is probably the easiest technique to learn. Audiotapes are available with simple instructions to attain a state of deep relaxation. The instructor will ask you at the outset to assume a supine position so that all parts of your body are supported, either on a mat, couch, bed, or floor. In a systematic way, you will be asked to first tense and then to relax specific muscles. The exercise will start

with the muscles of the hands or feet, slowly progress through the body, and conclude with the muscles of the face. When the exercise has been completed, all the muscles of the body will be relaxed. This system of relaxation teaches you to be more aware of the difference between muscular tension and muscular relaxation. Many people do not realize they are tense until a pain develops in the neck, head, or shoulders. Through systematic relaxation training, attention is focused entirely on each set of muscles, first tensing them, then holding the tension briefly, and finally releasing the tension and feeling it flow away as the muscles relax. By the time the entire body is relaxed, usually in about 15 to 20 minutes for beginners, a fresh, relaxed, and rested feeling will be experienced.

□ Meditation

There are many forms of meditation. Some seem exotic or are accompanied by a religious or philosophical set of beliefs such as transcendental meditation, Zen, and yoga. Others, like the system used by Dr. Herbert Benson of Harvard University, simply ask that attention be focused on an object or a word to force all other thoughts and distractions from the mind. Dr. Benson describes a simple relaxation technique[19]:

1. Find a quiet place.
2. Close your eyes.
3. Deeply relax your muscles by starting at the feet and working up to the facial muscles (this part is like systematic relaxation but is abbreviated).
4. Breathe in through your nose.
5. While breathing out, silently say the word *one*.
6. Continue doing this for 20 minutes.

Most forms of meditation have four essential elements: Meditate in a quiet environment;

use a mental device such as a word or phrase that is repeated over and over, or concentrate all attention on a physical object; adopt a passive attitude (let everything go) and sit in a comfortable position.

Medical researchers have found that practicing meditation techniques regularly will lead to decreased oxygen consumption, decreased respiratory rate, decreased heart rate, increased alpha waves in the brain, decreased blood pressure, and decreased muscular tension. All of these physical conditions are signs of relaxation and of an emotionally calm state.

The great advantage of most meditation techniques is that a skilled meditator can use them anywhere, even in a public place, without being especially noticeable. The relaxation effect comes very quickly with practice, and no special equipment is necessary.

☐
Biofeedback

Biofeedback is popular, especially for specific problems such as headaches. The two most common forms of biofeedback measure temperature and electrical conductivity in muscle nerves. Temperature feedback is used for people with migraine headaches. They are asked to make their hands and feet warmer, that is, to have the blood flow more toward their extremities and away from the head. An electromyograph (EMG) will provide either auditory or visual signals of the level of muscular tension. The trainee attempts to reduce the level of sound or visual feedback by relaxing target muscles. When attached to the frontalis muscles of the head, EMG training can be used to reduce or eliminate tension headaches. Biofeedback can also be useful to eliminate jaw clenching (which causes headaches and serious temporomandibular joint problems) or reduce muscular tightening of the lower portion of the back, which leads to pain in that area.

☐
Autogenic training

Autogenic training combines the principles of relaxation training and meditation. Like meditation, it involves the use of close concentration and mental images to produce specific bodily changes associated with relaxation. Like systematic relaxation, the images proceed systematically over the whole body position. As with meditation and relaxation training, a comfortable body position must be assumed. You are asked to concentrate your attention on a particular part of the body, perhaps the hand. You are to think of your hand becoming heavy. You maintain this image of your hand becoming increasingly heavy by repeating that thought silently. You maintain this image of your hand feeling very heavy. Then you may be asked to think of your hand becoming warm. Finally, you will feel that hand as very heavy and very warm. You progress through various parts of the body with instructions that will make you feel very relaxed all over. Autogenic training can, with practice, be done in a crowded room, on an airplane, or wherever there is a quiet place to sit. Other people need not be aware of what you are doing. The technique requires no equipment, just imagination and the ability to concentrate and focus your own attention.

When feelings of nervousness and time pressure build up during the workday, it is easy to become hasty or abrupt with people. The solution might be to build into the schedule a daily 15- to 20-minute break when no interruptions would occur and one of these proved relaxation techniques could be practiced. Most people experience the sense of well-being that comes from relaxation for about 2 hours afterwards. If, for example, a period of tenseness starts about 2:00 PM on busy days, a scheduled relaxation training break at that time would probably smooth out the rest of the day.

Good scientific discussions on the aforementional techniques and their benefits can be found in the references.[19-23]

Audiotapes can be purchased that will provide guidance in the relaxation technique until it is mastered.

☐
Physical exercise

Recall the example of the prehistoric human and his encounter with a predatory animal at the beginning of this chapter. He took care of the physiological products of stress by fighting or fleeing. Though we really cannot fight or run away from contemporary stressors, many of us can and do run for exercise. Vigorous exercise can be a substitute for that primitive urge and has somewhat the same physical effect: we get so tired that we become relaxed. A planned, systematic exercise program could be described as "artifiical fight or flight." The physiological results of lowered blood pressure, lowered heart rate, and so forth are the same as for planned, systematic relaxation. Regular exercise becomes a healthy addiction substituting for less healthy addictions like overeating and drugs.

☐
Burnout: the professional's problem

Burnout is a special kind of stress that occurs most for those in the "helping" professions, that is, people who deal with other people's problems, which includes all the medical professions. Burnout comes from caring too much. In fact, it is a specialized form of the dysfunctional thought: "I am totally responsible for the happiness and well-being of my patients and clients."

What characterizes professions, as distinct from other occupations, is the personal contact with people who have problems or concerns about important matters. Whether it is their finances, a legal problem, their mental or physical health, or the health of their animals, people expect to bring their serious problems to someone else for resolution. This can become an emotional burden for the professional worker.

Though most veterinarians begin their professional careers with noble aspirations and the desire to help people by caring for their animals, the gap between their expectations and their measurable accomplishments can become painful and frustrating. If veterinary medicine is entered with the expectations of always being able to accomplish miraculous cures and of being beloved by clients, the reality may be very difficult to accept. The early rosy glow of veterinary school may fade and die if the daily routine is watching animals die or go untreated because the owners will not or cannot have them treated. This is burnout.

Some of the signs of burnout are not wanting to keep doing what you are doing, feeling frustrated and unappreciated, feeling disinterested in clients or patients, losing idealism and energy, and feeling mentally overburdened and not wanting to go to work.

Some behaviors associated with burnout for a veterinarian might be looking and acting tired or bored, making cynical remarks about clients or patients, sounding irritable, cutting corners in diagnosis or treatment (not giving each patient full time and attention), taking unnecessary risks, handling patients more roughly than necessary, speaking abruptly to clients or employees, and doing anything else indicating partial withdrawal from work. The burned-out professional feels used up and has little left to give.

Dr. Black's career is a good illustration of the stages of professional burnout. As a new graduate just beginning his career in practice, Dr. Black had high hopes of making a special contribution through his veterinary skills. He met his clients with enthusiasm. He worked up each case with meticulous care. He rushed around to get everything done that needed to be done at the clinic. He hated to see a patient die, and the grief of the animals' owners was felt as his own. He arrived at work early and left late.

Little by little, as he realized his limitations, some of the zest went out of his work. Patient death became routine. He felt less. He sympathized less with the grief of others. He kept plugging away at the job, but with less idealism, less interest in developing his professional skills, and more interest in how he spent his leisure time. He dreaded seeing certain difficult clients or cases that required special care. He felt anger toward animals with difficult behavior. He had dropped the burden of caring.

At the end stage of burnout, Dr. Black was not very interested in getting up in the morning to go to work. He ate breakfast grumpily. He arrived at work at the last possible minute, sometimes even late. He looked around the clinic and saw nothing but problems — facilities that need repair, mistakes made by the kennel worker, equipment that should be replaced. He dawdled at his desk after the time for his first appointment. He didn't really want to see this client. He was abrupt with her and hurried through the examination to get it over as quickly as possible. He described the client as a "whiner" to his assistant. He forgot to check up on the patient's progress. He was glad when the day was done and he could go home. At home, he might have been moody because he had to spend his days unhappily.

He was once enthusiastic about his work and showed interest in his family, employees, clients, and patients. Now he mainly wants to be alone, and he has little positive to say about anything.

What happened to dull Dr. Black's earlier glow? The zest for work, and even for life, fades when people feel that their efforts are useless or unappreciated. Dr. Black had a solo practice, so he did not have the opportunity to hear a respected colleague say, "You did a wonderful job on that fracture repair." Clients can be grateful, but they are more likely to be grateful for kindness than for clinical skills, which they do not usually understand well enough to appreciate. Dr. Black was never a very verbose person. He tended to say only what was necessary to others to get the job done, so he got little verbal feedback from them. They did not tell him he was helpful.

Since the chief source of burnout is the feeling of being unappreciated, consider some strategies for having a helpful attitude noticed and for getting collegial support:

1. See fewer clients and spend more time with them. In all helping professions, it is the client's or patient's perception of being attended to and cared for that counts more than the actual service itself. When the animal's medical problem cannot be improved, the owner can still be helped to make an adjustment to the animal's illness or death. The patient's life may not be saved, as in the case of terminal cancer, but the owner can be helped with the grieving process. Owners who feel everying possible has been done for their animals are more likely to express appreciation. When euthanasia is necessary, the procedure can be worked out in a way that is respectful of the client's emotions. Making a friendly follow-up telephone call or sending a card expressing sympathy will demonstrate to the client the "I care" personal touch. Another helpful technique is to call owners of animals who were successfully treated and returned to their homes, "just to be sure that Fifi is recuperating well." Medical skills are not so much appreciated by clients as are the human relations skills. Services are judged more on what clients perceive rather than what they receive.
2. Keep a thank-you file. Collect and retain

all the letters from grateful clients including those from children. When you feel a bit unappreciated, read through the file. In the oncology unit of the Colorado State University Veterinary Teaching Hospital, the walls are papered with letters from clients expressing their appreciation of the kindness of the staff toward their pets and toward themselves. Because they were all suffering from cancer, most of these pets died, either during treatment or shortly thereafter. Though their owners were saddened by the loss of a beloved pet, their lives had been enriched by the caring atmosphere of the clinic, and they sent cards, letters, and even photographs of their pets to express their gratitude for help in time of trouble. The oncology unit is a warm, pleasant place, even though it necessarily deals with serious cancer cases and with death.

3. If in a solo practice, form a regular discussion group with one or two congenial local colleagues to discuss cases. If in a group practice, have regular "rounds" where difficult cases can be shared for comments and ideas. In these collegial discussions, positive feedback can be given and received on case management in addition to support and advice when there is uncertainty about diagnosis or treatment.

4. Appreciate the people who work in the practice. Make it a point to catch employees doing something right. Thank them for a job well done. Or if the overall job was not especially well handled, thank them for some part of it that was. The effects of positive verbal reinforcement are well established. *You* get burned out when you do not receive it, so be sure to let colleagues and employees know that you appreciate their efforts. People, and even some animals, have been found to work harder for praise than for more tangible rewards. Insincere or inappropriate praise, of course, will be received for the counterfeit coinage it is. Luckily, it is not hard to spot someone doing something praiseworthy fairly often, and the more often noticed, the more it will occur. Personal warmth and supportiveness are contagious to others: "You will receive as you give."

5. Savor the sense of having helped a client or patient, even if you don't receive a formal expression of appreciation. When most people think back over their own lives, they can remember many people who helped along the way. Have you always taken the time and effort to thank these people who meant so much to you? Probably not. Yet after many years, you still remember and appreciate them. Those clients, colleagues, and employees who do not freely express their satisfaction now will one day be in that same position. They will think about your helpfulness, though they said nothing special about it at the time. Recognize and accept that most people do appreciate your efforts, though they may fail to acknowledge it to you at the time.

6. Decide to go out of our way to help someone at least once a day. Veterinarians have many opportunities each day to perform some small (or large) extra service in a spirit of helpfulness to others. On the way home from work, think about how much that person was helped. It gives the day an added value.

7. Earlier it was noted that delegating authority would save time. One should also delegate authority to help colleagues and employees develop themselves professionally and to promote a team approach that makes work more enjoyable for everyone. Everyone wants to develop self-esteem through work whether it be a kennel person, receptionist, student ob-

server, or veterinarian. The veterinarian has the power to help others learn new skills and to grow as human beings just as the staff members have some power to make the veterinarian's work more rewarding. Clients will sense the resultant aura of respect and goodwill in the practice and will benefit from the positive atmosphere.

8. Recognize that there is a difference between *accepting* another person's problem, which you do by listening, giving professional advice and treatment, and having a helpful attitude, and *assuming* the problem yourself. The problem remains the client's. It is definitely not callous to mentally refuse to assume the burden of the client's problem. The job of a professional veterinarian is to give the best possible medical advice and treatment in a caring manner. When you cannot distinguish between your own professional responsibilities and the emotional problems belonging to the client, solving the true professional problem becomes more difficult. Burnout can result.

If professional burnout is a potential problem, more understanding and ideas for coping can be found in the references.[24]

□

Rusting out

Rusting out is being bored. Too little stress can also be a problem. Life without any uncertainty or pressure is not very stimulating. Out of sheer boredom some people may take unnecessary risks, drink or gamble too much, quit their jobs, or leave their families. When this happens in middle age, it is called *midlife crisis.* Middle age is the prime time for rustout because earlier the professional was too busy struggling to succeed to become bored and

older people perhaps expect to slow down a bit.

Rustout is usually more of a problem for people who work in bureaucracies or on production lines than for those in professions. It is possible to have your professional life so well organized or so routine in the way patients and clients are handled that rustout can occur.

Hans Selyé, the famed expert on stress, has identified a concept he calls *eustress* or *positive stress.* Selyé states that people sometimes suffer from a lack of sufficient tension.[25] We all need some stress in our lives to help us grow, adapt, change, and move ahead. The trick is to have an optimal balance between tension and relaxation, the ideal level of stress. The ideal level is somewhere between being overloaded with work, having too many expectations to meet and not enough time, and doing repetitive tasks that lack challenge, learning, growth, and development. Though rusting out is less likely than burning out for most veterinarians, it is still possible for a busy practitioner to feel that life is measured in distemper shots. When a you start feeling that you could go through the workday on automatic pilot, you probably need some eustress in your life. To avoid rustout, a positive decision; must be made to raise the level of challenge. Here are some ideas for lighting your fire and adding some excitement to professional and personal life:

1. Expand the practice. Add new services, for example, pet nutrition for your conscientious pet owners, animal training classes for people whose pets have behavioral problems, or "producer nights" for the equine, bovine, or porcine owner.

2. Learn something new. Become more of an expert on equine nutrition, mastitis control, pet nutrition, animal behavior management, and so forth in order to offer new practice services. Or learn a foreign language to plan an international

trip; learn to draw or paint or to take photographs of what is beautiful or especially interesting to you. Some hobbies can also be enjoyed at the clinic. Drawings, paintings, woodwork, and photographs can be used to decorate the clinic and will be interesting to clients. There is *always* something new to learn!

3. Specialize. Become an expert in a specialty area and work toward board certification in the American Board of Veterinary Practitioners.

4. Develop interpersonal communication skills. This will not only improve the practice in many ways it will also add interest to life in general. People will become more interesting as new communication skills develop and important personal matters are discussed.

5. Become more involved in community activities (school board, town council, any citizen's advisory board), a club, or a charitable organization. Community service organizations and clubs put you in contact with many different people who may become friends and clients.

6. Set aside an hour (or at the very least a half hour) every day "just for fun." No day should go by without some pure enjoyment. It can be something as brief as making it a point to enjoy a beautiful sunrise or sunset to something as grand as going to an opera or the theater. Choose what turns you on to life, but just be sure to take time to do it every day.

Each person needs to find the optimal activity level, the range where there is enough challenge to be kept alert and busy, but not so much that the mind and body become exhausted.

A bell curve depicts the full range of activity level/stress from rustout to stress or burnout (Fig. 17-1). The goal should be to remain in the comfort zone most of the time.

To keep in the eustress comfort zone, be sure to

1. Use time well.

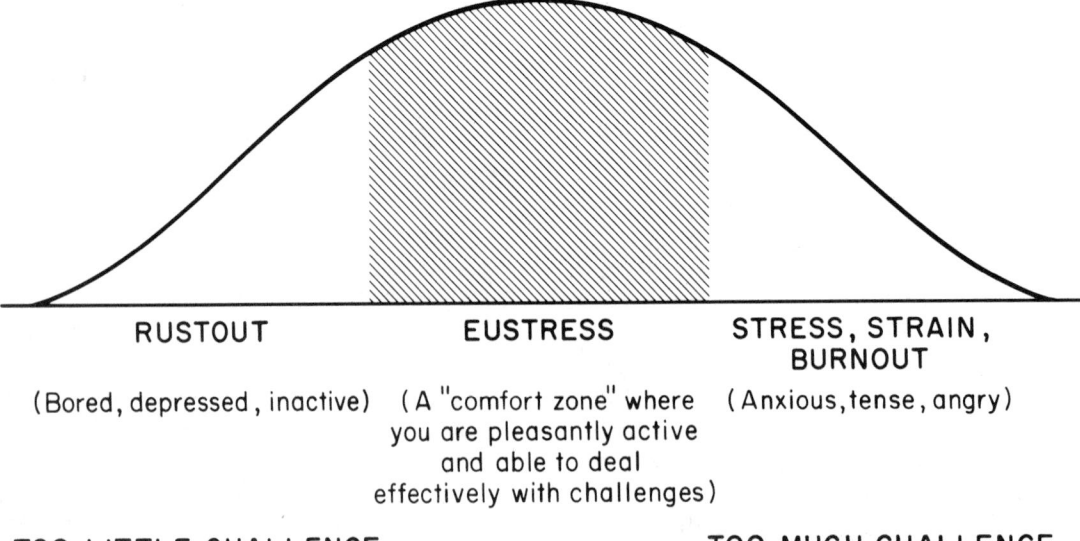

RUSTOUT	EUSTRESS	STRESS, STRAIN, BURNOUT
(Bored, depressed, inactive)	(A "comfort zone" where you are pleasantly active and able to deal effectively with challenges)	(Anxious, tense, angry)

TOO LITTLE CHALLENGE ←   TOO MUCH CHALLENGE →

Figure 17-1. *Potential activity from rustout to burnout*

2. Reduce physical tension (by learning to relax or through physical exercise).
3. Analyze thoughts (eliminating dysfunctional thinking and keeping in a rational, problem-solving mode most of the time).
4. Improve your ability to communicate well with family, friends, clients, colleagues, and employees.

Understanding the causes and responses to stress, burnout, and rustout is the first step toward achieving the right balance between pressure and tedium. You are the person who can make yourself happy. If help is needed, remember that there are professionals who specialize in stress management.

□
References

1. Bullmer K: The Art of Empathy. New York, Human Sciences, 1975
2. Carkhuff R: The Art of Helping. Amherst, MA, Human Resource Development, 1972
3. Carkhuff R: The Art of Problem Solving. Amherst, MA, Human Resource Development, 1973
4. Carkhuff R: How to Help Yourself. Amherst, MA, Human Resource Development, 1974
5. Egan G: The Skilled Helper. Monterey, CA, Brooks/Cole, 1975
6. Enelow A, Swisher S: Interviewing and Patient Care. New York Oxford University Press, 1971
7. Fensterheim H, Baer J: Don't Say Yes When You Want to Say No. New York, Dell, 1975
8. Smith M: When I Say No, I Feel Guilty. New York, Dial Press, 1975
9. Strayhorn J: Talking It Out: A Guide to Effective Communication and Problem Solving. Champaign, IL, Research Press, 1977
10. Douglass M, Douglass D: Manage Your Time, Mange Your Work, Manage Yourself. New York, AMACOM, 1980
11. Lakein A: How to Get Control of Your Time and Your Life. New York, Wyden, 1973
12. Burns DD: Feeling Good. New York, William Morrow, 1980
13. Ellis A: Growth Through Reason. Palo Alto, CA, Science and Behavior Books, 1971
14. Ellis A, Harper R: A Guide to Rational Living. North Hollywood, CA, Wilshire Books, 1961
15. Greenberg D: How to Make Yourself Miserable (A Vital Training Manual). New York, Random House, 1966
16. Maultsby M: Help Yourself to Happiness. New York, Inst. Rational–Emotive, 1975
17. Azrin N, Nunn R: Habit Control in a Day. New York, Pocket Books, 1978
18. Robbins J, Fisher D: How to Make and Break Habits. New York, Dell, 1976
19. Benson H: The Relaxation Response. New York, Avon Books, 1975
20. Albrecht K: Stress and the Manager. Englewood Cliffs, NJ, Prentice-Hall, 1979
21. Brown B: Stress and the Art of Biofeedback. New York, Bantam Books, 1978
22. Jacobson R: You Must Relax. New York, McGraw-Hill, 1962
23. Pelletie K: Mind as Healer, Mind as Slayer. New York, Dell, 1977
24. Pines A, Aronson E, Kafry D: Burnout. New York, Free Press, 1981
25. Selyé H: Stress Without Distress. Philadelphia, JB, Lippincott, 1974

Chapter 18
☐
Inventory, prescriptions, and equipment

Stuart D. Forney

☐
Inventory control

Having an adequate inventory and supplies is essential in any veterinary practice. Although discussion here will focus on pharmaceuticals and biologicals, you must also stock materials needed in a number of other areas. Included would be surgical supplies (gauze, tape, blades, suture, cotton, and so forth), nutritional items (dog and cat food, grain, alfalfa), radiology items (film, contrast media, chemicals), laboratory or diagnostic supplies, disinfectants, janitorial items, and office supplies. One can readily surmise that a poorly managed inventory not only leads to anxiety and compromised treatment and diagnosis but also can be a major practice expense when supplies are excessive. A properly managed inventory is even more important in those practices generating a large portion of their gross revenue from sale of patient health products.

Monitoring inventory

Whether you periodically assess the inventory level manually or use the computer to provide immediate inventory status, you must have a means of determining replacement needs. With proper monitoring frequent "outs" can be avoided as well as excessive stock of individual items, thereby keeping the total inventory value at a minimum.

Continually being out of stock is a real detriment to a practice. Besides lost sales, obtaining urgently needed items is costly. Additional inventory expense occurs with poor utilization of manpower (interruption of normal work routine, special check-in procedure, special handling), long-distance telephone calls, transportation fees, and a higher purchase price for special items plus additional costs for processing a special order.

Having an excessively large inventory results in lost revenue from having capital committed to inventory. Using 10% as an average investment return results in $100 annual personal income loss for each $1000 invested in inventory. If one is purchasing inventory with borrowed capitol, each $1000 of inventory is costing the practice an additional $100 to $150 in interest expenses.

Determining optimal inventory levels

Ideally it would be nice to receive replacement stock immediately after the emptying of a container; however, replacement time depends upon the time it takes the vendor to receive and fill the order and the time required for the order to reach the practice. A practice cannot wait until exhausting the present supply to reorder, so future supply needs must be estimated. What may appear to be a month's supply of an item may be used in a few days or may sit on the shelf for several months.

In general, most practices will find that in the typical pharmacy inventory 20% to 25% of the items stocked will account for 75% to 80% of the total annual purchases. These fast-moving or expensive items must be monitored closely because they greatly affect inventory turnover. All practices regardless of location or large-quantity (discount) buying should "turn" their inventory at least four times per year. Inventory turnover is calculated by the following formulas:

Inventory Turnover =

$$\frac{\text{Total Inventory Purchased During Year}}{\text{Average Inventory}}$$

Average Inventory =

$$\frac{\text{Year's Beginning Inventory} + \text{Year's Ending Inventory}}{2}$$

Practices located near major vendors may easily increase their inventory turnover to six times a year. With computer assistance a practice may approach an inventory turnover of eight, but considerable effort is usually required. One reaches a point in attempting to further reduce the inventory when the cost of closely monitoring and maintaining the inventory becomes greater than the cost of carrying the additional inventory.

□
Ordering drugs and supplies

Establishing inventory levels

The first year in a new practice is certain to be the most difficult for maintaining proper inventory levels. Even with good drug usage records, future needs can only be estimated. In the absence of accurate usage information a practice should only stock limited amounts of essential items, monitor usage frequently, and increase stock levels for high-use items. Avoid "deals" or quantity discount purchases until the practice is well established.

The new practitioner needs to be aware of the initial order plan offered by several veterinary suppliers. To provide incentive for practices to initially stock and continue to stock their products, tremendous discounts are offered on the first order placed. Although savings may be significant, one must exercise good judgment to avoid purchasing low-use items when cash flow may be critical.

If service from a vendor is good, a 1 month's supply is a reasonable quantity to stock. For some items having sporadic use or from vendors with poor delivery service, a larger quantity can be justified. For inexpensive low-use items from a vendor rarely used, you may order a 3 to 4 month's supply rather than generating a small order more frequently. The usage of some items such as calf electrolyte solutions, vaccines, and equine anthelmintics will vary seasonally and require additional stock during certain periods of the year. Another consideration for specialty items or unique combination bovine vaccines would be to avoid stocking such routinely. Clients could be informed that a special order could be placed for lower-use items.

Ordering costs

Whether you mail an order to a supplier, place the order through the sales representative, or simply call an order into the vendor, personnel and expense costs are generated. Ordering, receipt, and payment records are necessary. The received order must be checked for breakage, accuracy, dating, and proper billing before being merged into existing stock. If discrepancies or problems are found, considerable effort may be required to correct the situation. All these expenses related to replacing stock, including the purchasing price of the item, are called *acquisition costs.*

Figure 18-1 shows the relationship of various inventory costs. A practice ordering daily may maintain a small inventory with minimal carrying costs but would have major acquisition costs. Besides significant labor cost the purchase price would be at the highest unit price. In contrast, if one placed only one major order each year, the acquisition costs would be minimal due to quantity discounts and reduced order processing. The carrying cost, however, would be prohibitive. The practice objective is to place orders that will result in the lowest *total* inventory cost. Note, the total cost equals the acquisition costs plus the carrying costs. The order value that will produce the lowest total inventory costs is termed the *economic order value* (EOV). It is usually found when you are taking advantage of some quantity discounts by reducing the number of

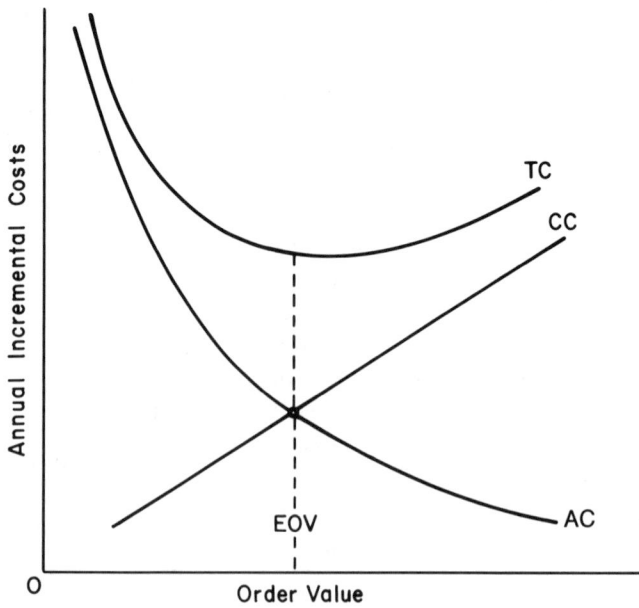

Figure 18-1. Relationship of various inventory costs (TC, total cost; CC, carrying cost; AC, acquisition cost; EOV, economic order value)

orders and processing costs while still maintaining an awareness of carrying costs.

Suppliers

Although a practice can purchase supplies from several different sources, there are primarily two types of suppliers: major manufacturers and wholesalers, with either type specializing in either human or veterinary products. Because human medical manufacturers and wholesalers do not usually deal with veterinary practices (except by arrangement in unique circumstances for frequent large orders), our discussion will be limited to veterinary suppliers.

Wholesalers purchase a wide variety of products (i.e., pet food, surgical instruments, instruments, pharmaceuticals) from numerous manufacturers or other vendors for resale to the veterinarian. Their prices are usually competitive because they purchase in large quantities and sell with little markup. Some manufacturers sell their products only through wholesalers, whereas others sell only to veterinarians. A few companies sell both ways.

The major advantage in dealing with wholesalers is a reduction in the number of small orders to individual vendors. In addition, problems with orders can be corrected more readily because a close relationship usually exists between practice employees and wholesaler's personnel. One other significant advantage of using a wholesaler is the single payment each month regardless of the number of orders.

For those major manufacturers who do not sell their products through wholesalers you must deal with them directly to obtain their unique products. While placing an order for essential items, you should review the company's product list for other needed items because discounts may be offered if a certain dollar volume is met.

Veterinarians occasionally need products intended for humans that may not be readily available from common veterinary suppliers. In some parts of the country human drug wholesalers welcome the veterinarian's business. Most human medical wholesalers, however, restrict their sales to retail and hospital pharmacies. By using the closest metropolitan yellow pages, the practitioner can identify drug wholesalers in their area to determine their sales policy to veterinarians.

Retail pharmacies can be a real asset to veterinary practices. Not only can they fill prescriptions for many human drugs but they may special order human items needed in veterinary practice. Drug, product, and price information can also be obtained through a helpful pharmacist.

There are large mail-order houses throughout the country from which veterinarians can buy nearly anything including vaccines, surgical supplies, equipment, and even controlled substances (with proper order forms). Unless you are specific about the product ordered, it is not uncommon to receive a slightly different product, perhaps somewhat inferior and sold a little cheaper than purchasing through normal channels. Returning these products, especially once they are opened and tried, may be a difficult, timely, and costly chore.

Selection of products

Attempt to limit inventory to items truly essential to the practice. The practice manager must determine exactly which steroids, antibiotics, anthelmintics, and so forth will be used routinely and which ones are more of a luxury. It is far better to be thoroughly knowledgeable with a limited inventory than to have a vague pharmacological understanding of the vast number of products on the market.

When satisfied with a product, veterinarians are encouraged to continue using it even though new products with new claims become available. If problems are experienced with a product, however, others should be evaluated.

Certain products commercially available may be unique and only obtained through a single source, leaving no other alternative. For most items there will be alternatives, either as generic equivalents or therapeutic equivalents. Note that generic equivalent products may meet established standards but may *not* be bioequivalent. In selecting equivalents the practitioner must not only consider price but also quality, service, and the company's contribution to veterinary medicine. Some companies are only in business for a profit and contribute little toward the profession through research, continued education, and service.

Placing and logging orders

Inventory records

Although some effort, time, and expense are required to maintain inventory records, it is likely that poor, inadequate records are more expensive. Good inventory records will provide the following information:

1. Usage of item
2. Items on order but not yet received
3. Quantity on order
4. Approximate time required to receive
5. Vendors from which the item has been ordered
6. Past purchase price(s) of the item
7. Date ordered/date received

Several manual inventory record systems are available through office supply outlets although you can create your own using a card file or loose-leaf notebook. Figure 18-2 is an example of an inventory card that features the type of information most often needed. Note that this card has an area to record quantity issued and balance on hand. Most veterinary practices would probably not use the issued or on-hand portions because recording the nu-

merous withdrawals of doses given could not be justified. For movement of stock from an inactive storage area to an active one, however, the issued portion of the card may have application.

The use of the computer has not only made the task of record keeping easier but it also provides additional, more accessible information. Most computer programs available keep a running inventory of each item and reduce the levels as each dose given is charged to the client. Although there may be a few doses of frequently used items that do not get recorded, which causes some discrepancy, records are usually accurate enough to warn when the stock falls below a certain preestablished minimal level.

With a computerized system, usage can be monitored more closely for trends or seasonal fluctuations. Computerized inventory control may allow deals or quantity buying, perhaps saving enough to justify the purchase of a computer system.

Identifying stock shortages

Computerized inventory control allows simplified monitoring of the entire inventory usage. If the practice wants to stock a 1- or 2-month supply of an item, the average monthly quantity can be easily calculated and a reorder point established. Some programs will actually maintain inventory of each item in "days' supply on hand" by dividing the amount on hand by the average used per day. Thus if usage increases, the number of days' supply would be recalculated and, not only reduced, but automatically altered. These lows or "shorts" could be displayed on the computer each morning or evening for reordering.

Without computer assistance more effort is required to maintain desired inventory levels. One suggestion is to take a rough inventory each month of the 20% to 25% of the items in inventory that account for the 75% to 80% of

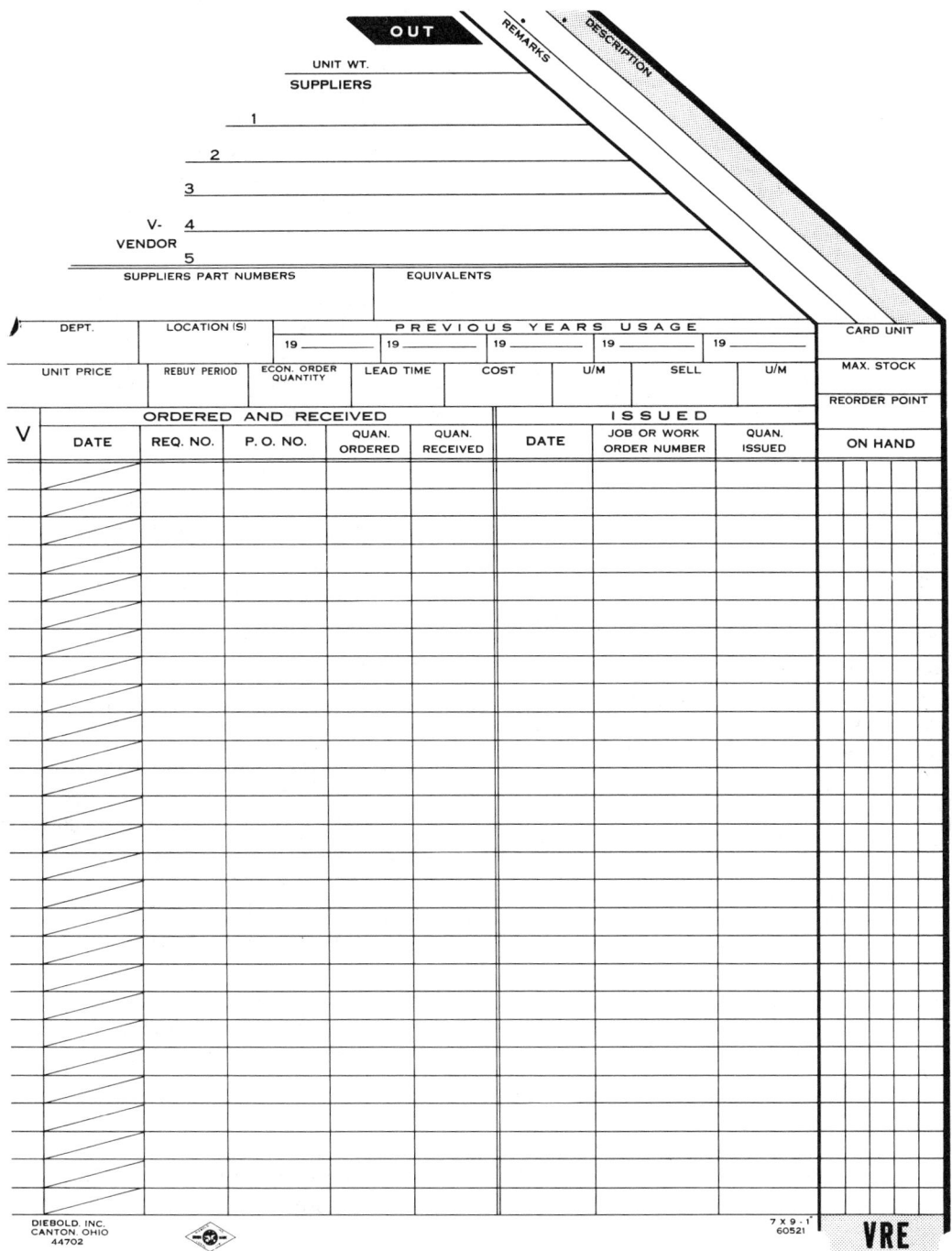

Figure 18-2. Inventory control card

the dollar volume. A sample inventory sheet is shown in Figure 18-3. For major vendors it is suggested than an inventory count sheet be used for all items purchased from that vendor rather than just the fast-moving ones. The task of taking counts can be assigned to a veterinary technician. Inventory counts can be taken on all items monthly or divided into portions weekly.

A "want book" is an essential. It should be kept in one location so that personnel can easily and immediately jot down items that should be considered for reorder. Another simple method for noting items needing reorder is to designate a convenient area (portion of a shelf, countertop, or box) for placing empty containers, cartons, or samples of items needing ordering. Throwing a syringe, tongue depressor, or an empty rabies vaccine vial in a box is simple to do even when busy. Reorder of these items can then be done when time permits.

For a few select items it may be beneficial to take special measures to avoid running out of stock. Special items can be monitored more frequently, but a simple method is to identify the last two or three containers on the shelf with a special marking or tape. Upon entering a marked container, the user is reminded to reorder.

Placing the order

Several methods for ordering stock exist. Perhaps the simplest and fastest is placing an order by telephone. Other ways of ordering include mailing orders or placing them with professional sales representatives. Some vendors can also receive orders from electronic transmission devices or computers via the telephone line. Regardless of the means used, a written or computer copy of the order should be generated and kept in a suspense file until the order is complete.

Receipt of orders

Vendors should have adequate stock to fill the entire order but may occasionally have to backorder certain items until they become available. Sometimes the availability of these items is so indefinite that the vendor may cancel and ask for a reorder after a certain date.

Quantities of items received should be recorded and dated on the order copy. In addition, quantities received and the purchase price should be recorded on inventory cards if such are used. If the purchase price is significantly different from previous ones, it may be necessary to adjust the selling price and make appropriate notations.

For computer-assisted inventory maintenance, similar information would be entered upon receipt of stock. Some programs may automatically adjust selling prices when price changes occur or at least prompt consideration of such.

Records of completed orders

Until an order is complete either as originally requested or as adjusted by additions, deletions, or price changes, it should be kept in an open-order suspense file. Upon completion of the order, the order copy should be dated and marked *complete*. These completed orders may be kept in the open-order suspense file until matched with invoices for payment. Upon payment, all invoices, packing slips, and receipts should be attached to the order copy, with the check number, date paid, and amount noted. These completed orders should then be filed by vendor for future reference. Minor vendors can be kept together in an "other" vendor file.

Inventory control personnel considerations

Because of the importance of inventory control, it is best to designate one person in the

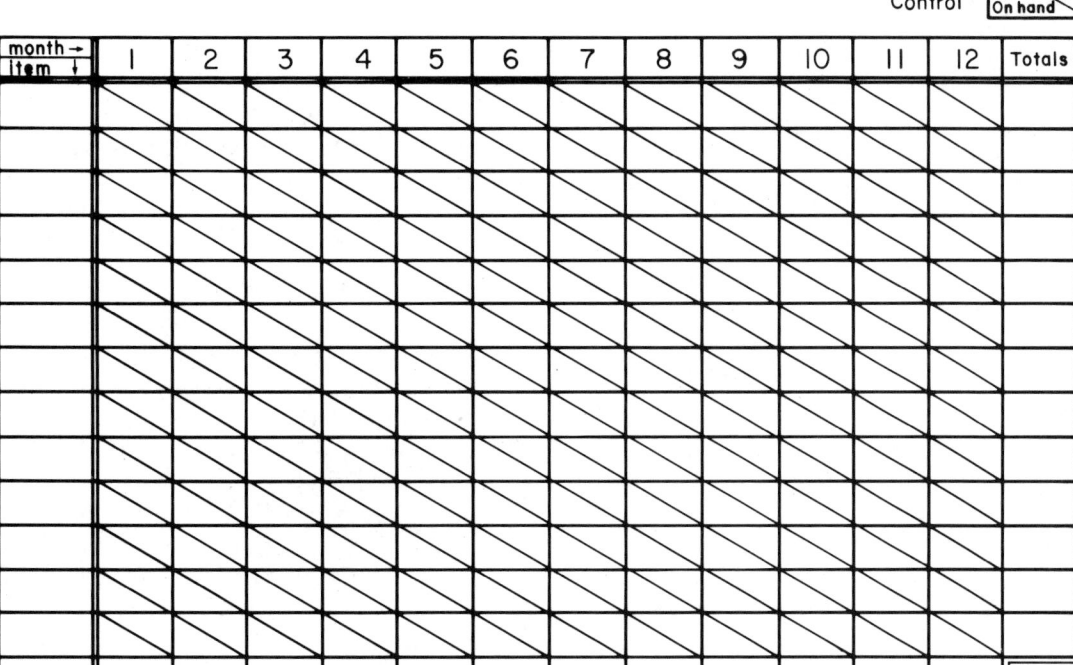

Figure 18-3. *Inventory sheet*

practice the specific responsibility for inventory monitoring, maintenance, and reordering. Others in the practice should have a general understanding of the system and must assist by identifying items needing to be ordered. With one person responsible and accountable, any shortages or "outs" should have a legitimate reason. The individual must monitor problem orders of critical supplies and seek alternatives when appropriate.

The following are some benefits of having one person responsible and accountable for inventory control:

1. Excessive stock should be avoided.
2. Duplicate orders should be avoided.
3. The status of an item can be determined easily from the individual.

4. "Outs" or shortages should be minimized and legitimately justified.
5. Problem orders for critical items are monitored closely.
6. Problem vendors and less-than-satisfying products can be identified easily.
7. Duplication of inquiries or long-distance telephone calls on orders can be minimized.

A purchasing specialist can become a valuable resource person who knows or identifies sources or alternative sources. In addition, such a specialist may reduce acquisition costs by being aware of vendor specials or purchasing programs.

There are few disadvantages of having one person ordering, provided the responsible individual has the interest or ability to do the job. The individual does not have to be a veterinarian. A highly motivated technician may have more time and greater interest in maintaining adequate stock. The major disadvantage of having one purchasing specialist is the practice's dependence upon his presence. When he is sick, on vacation, or even out for lunch, the handling of certain problems or questions may be compromised. The termination of such a key individual could be a real detriment to the practice; therefore it is essential for another employee to have at least a working knowledge of the ordering process (perhaps having some responsibility for receiving and posting orders) to provide some continuity.

☐
Arrangement of inventory

Possible arrangements

The possibilities for organizing inventory within the clinic pharmacy are

1. Alphabetical
   a. Generic
   b. Brand name
2. Therapeutic use or drug classification
3. Dosage form
4. Level of use (highly active, active, inactive)

There is no "best way" because each has advantages as well as disadvantages. Each practice is encouraged to develop a combination arrangement that will work best for that practice.

An organizational arrangement to consider would be to identify those items having frequent use and place them in the most accessible area (i.e., ophthalmic items in the ophthalmic examination tray, atropine and acepromazine near surgery, vaccines near or in the examination room). Infrequently used items could be kept in a remote area or even with bulk backup supplies if space is limited.

Arranging items by dosage form offers the advantage of placing all the tablets and capsules near the counting area, the liquids near a pouring area with a sink, the injectables near syringes, needles, and alcohol wipes, and so on. In addition, excellent utilization of shelf space occurs when the pharmacy is organized by dosage form.

The following dosage forms are suggested for categorizing:

1. Oral solids (capsules and tablets)
2. Injectables of 100 ml or less
3. Injectables greater than 100 ml
4. Oral liquids less than 1 gallon
5. Gallon section
   a. Internal
   b. External
6. Other externals (ointments, aerosols, topical powders, etc.
7. Other oral preparations (boluses, paste, granules)
8. Ophthalmics
9. Otics
10. Miscellaneous

To use a pure alphabetical arrangement would not only promote poor space utilization (i.e., gallon bottles next to 1-ml ampules) but also compromise convenience. However, alphabetizing items after splitting them into categories is desirable.

Rather than alphabetizing only by the generic name, popular brand names used commonly by the practice may be merged into the order. The brand name items should be kept to a minimum, perhaps restricting them to combination products or products not yet generically available. Using an excessive number of brand names leads to duplication of stock because one may not realize that a different brand was recently purchased while a reorder was made from the former vendor.

Regardless of inventory arrangement, some items will require special storage conditions such as refrigeration or security (see the section dealing with controlled substances).

Since vaccines will constitute a major portion of refrigerated items, it may be helpful to separate them from the pharmaceuticals. For practices requiring considerable refrigeration space, an industrial refrigerator with drawers is suggested because items are easily accessible and space efficiently used.

Location coding

To assist employees, especially new or relief help, in locating stock it is helpful to designate location sections with an appropriate *inventory location index*. Sections can be as small as a drawer, but most generally a shelving unit or a larger specific area is identified. Sections can be designated by number, with further divisions using letters if necessary (i.e., lettering shelves by beginning with an *A* as the top shelf).

Although there are several means for labeling cabinets and shelving units, embossing tape is simple without being too offensive. It is helpful to then prepare a map or a rough general floor plan identifying sections by their code.

If you have a master list of the inventory (e.g., a price list), location codes can be easily added. Most computer programs have a field for location in the drug data base. Even without a specific field, the computer can easily generate a hard copy of the drug list to which locations can be added. When a master list is not available, location codes placed on inventory cards will provide a means for locating stock.

☐
Pricing drugs

There are no simple formulas for establishing selling prices on inventory. These comments are offered only for consideration in establishing prices.

For most practices it is better to "sell" one's professional services than to rely on the merchandising of drugs and supplies. Although some practices are able to generate additional revenue through the sale of professional products, most will find the market quite competitive. Practitioners who merchandise must contend not only with other private practitioners but also lay veterinary outlets, retail pharmacies, and mail-order houses.

Most clients will readily pay what they consider a reasonable price for quality and service, but few will tolerate being exploited. Trying to make excessive profits on prescription drugs will likely result in lost clients. Being honest with clients is always good policy. When clients ask about pricing, they should be given an open explanation that a fair pricing schedule is used to recover overhead. Specific items, however, may be slightly higher than at other sources due to discount volume purchases. On items available through pharmacies, offer to give them a written prescription and allow them to shop elsewhere, especially for long-term, expensive drugs.

Although competition is a major factor in determining the selling price, it is not necessarily always wise to try to meet the cheapest prices in the area. This is especially true when competing with unethical cut-rate individuals. Most such individuals will not be around long because they too must make a profit to stay in business.

For items commonly available, you should not expect more than a 50% markup, with 25% probably being more reasonable. For some prescription drugs, a 50% to 100% markup for infrequently used items is not unreasonable. Developing a general markup policy for over-the-counter items and another for prescription drugs is suggested. The entire inventory, however, must be reviewed item by item with exceptions being identified and adjusted accordingly.

Regardless of the method used for establishing a selling price, it must be used by everyone in the practice to maintain consistency. Unless everyone is charging the same price, there will be constant turmoil. Selling prices must, therefore, be conveniently available and current to ensure proper charging.

Selling prices can be marked directly on the container, either coded or uncoded. Having selling prices on inventory cards is all right for a backup measure but not usually convenient for routine use. Typing a master list of the inventory with prices and location is a laborious task initially but, once the list has been completed, it will find extensive use. Computer programs incorporate selling prices into the charging system so that when quantities of drugs used or dispensed are entered charges are generated automatically. Also an additional hard copy can be produced by the computer for review or use elsewhere.

It is not uncommon to charge a fee for each transaction or administration and thereby reduce the per-item markup. Transaction fees can vary depending on the means of administration or the dispensing of repackaged vs. original-container drugs. Minimum fees are also common and may be established for different types of transactions.

□

Dispensing medications

Containers

"The Poison Prevention Packaging Act is administered and enforced by the Consumer Product Safety Commission of the federal government. The purpose of the law is to decrease the chance that children may obtain access to poisons."[1] The act identifies certain hazardous substances as well as most drugs intended for oral human use.

Although federal law may require that only a few veterinary drugs be dispensed in child-resistant containers, state laws may require the use of safety closures. Whether required by law or not, however, it is suggested that child-resistant containers be used whenever possible. Since all pharmacies and most veterinary

practitioners are using child-proof containers, it is reasonable to assume that if an accident involving the use of non–child-resistant containers did occur the practitioner using such would be found negligent.

If clients do not want their medication dispensed in a child-resistant container, you should have them sign a form indicating their desire for a regular closure. For certain containers where safety closures are not available, written permission from the clients should be obtained to reduce liability. Note that concern is directed primarily to products for oral use or external preparations that would be hazardous if taken internally. Although most injectables, ophthalmics, otics, ointments, and powders should be regarded as potentially hazardous, dispensing them in their original non–child-resistant container would be common.

Certain oral drugs may be highly sensitive to light or moisture, and therefore, require light-resistant or "tight" dispensing vials. Since these containers are priced similarly to regular containers, it is wise to use these special containers routinely. Envelopes should *never* be used for dispensing loose tablets or capsules and should be used with judgment when dispensing individually wrapped tablets (i.e., Clavamox [Beecham Laboratories, Bristol, TN], Ovaban [Schering Corp, Kenilworth, NJ]).

Labeling—over-the-counter vs. prescription drugs

Drugs for veterinary (as well as human) use fall into two major classes: over-the counter (OTC) and prescription drugs. The classes are established by federal law although state law may require certain OTC products be dispensed only by prescription. Veterinary prescription drugs bear the legend CAUTION: Federal law restricts this drug to use by or on order of a licensed veterinarian. Human prescription drugs have the legend CAUTION:

Federal law prohibits dispensing without prescription.

Prescription drugs are primarily those drugs that the typical layman would not know how to use properly. In fact these are drugs for which it is impossible to write adequate directions that would permit the layman to use the drug safely and for the purpose for which it was intended.[2] Adequate directions would have to address the following product concerns:

1. When indicated
2. When to discontinue
3. What hazards or risks exist
4. Special technique required to administer

Investigational drugs without adequate information on safety and efficacy are also classified as prescription drugs.

Veterinarians, physicians, dentists, pharmacists, and other licensed practitioners have been made custodians of these drugs to protect the public from their misuse and abuse. Veterinarians dispensing or prescribing legend drugs must have a valid client–patient relationship. An appropriate veterinarian–client–patient relationship is defined as existing when

1. The veterinarian has assumed responsibility for making medical judgments regarding the health of the animal(s) and the need for medical treatment, and the client (owner or other caretaker) has agreed to follow the instructions of the veterinarian; and when
2. There is sufficient knowledge of the animal(s) by the veterinarian to initiate at least a general or preliminary diagnosis of the medical condition of the animal(s). This means that the veterinarian has recently seen and is personally acquainted with the keeping and care of the animal(s) by virtue of an examination of the animal(s), and/or by medically appropriate and timely visits to the prem-

ises where the animal(s) are kept; and when
3. The practicing veterinarian is readily available for follow-up in case of adverse reactions or failure of the regimen of therapy.[2]

The FDA's Center for Veterinary Medicine (CVM) has recently increased its action against the illegal distribution, sale, and use of veterinary prescription drugs by gaining assistance of state agencies. Because states are primarily responsible for laws and regulations governing dispensing and prescribing, the CVM is looking to states to investigate, educate, and take regulatory action against firms or individuals when appropriate.

OTC preparations must be labeled as well as packaged properly for lay use. The label of any drug sold over the counter must bear a

1. Statement of the identity of the commodity
2. Statement of the place of business of the manufacturer, packer, or distributor
3. Statement of net quantity of contents
4. Statement of ingredients
5. Statement of adequate directions for safe and effective use
6. Statement of any habit-forming drug contained in the prescription
7. Statement of any cautions and warnings needed for protection of the user

Since labeling requirements for OTC drug products are quite detailed and specific, it would be unwise for an individual to engage in repackaging these medications. A practitioner, however, can repackage OTC drugs legally if they are treated as prescription drugs and labeled as a prescription.

Labeling prescription drugs

The label requirements for prescription drugs are most likely found in the state's pharmacy laws and regulations. These of course will differ between states, but will most likely require the following:

1. Name, address, and telephone number of clinic/hospital
2. Name of practitioner
3. Date filled
4. Name of client
5. Patient (species required for controlled drugs)
6. Adequate directions for proper use

Most generally you will find the identity (name and strength) of the drug on the prescription label (Fig. 18-4), although it may not be required by state law. Some practitioners may not want the client to know the drug being used, but this practice was much more popular in the past. When dispensing several prescriptions to one patient, placing the identity of each item on the label seems most prudent.

Supplementary labels (i.e., shake well, refrigerate, expiration date, external use only, and so forth) if not required by law are advised. A controlled drug (see the section on records in this chapter) must bear the following: CAUTION: Federal law PROHIBITS the transfer of this drug to any person other than the patient for whom it was prescribed.

Pharmacies are usually required to place a unique prescription number on the label that corresponds to the written prescription so that the identity and quantity of the prescription can be easily determined. Because most veterinary clinics do not use prescription numbers, they should have some means of identifying the drug dispensed for refill requests or more importantly for accidental poisoning. The date can be used provided the prescription was logged in the patient's record and only one prescription was dispensed on that date for the particular patient.

□
Prescription writing

Prescription writing has been greatly simplified with trends toward the use of English, the metric system, and the wide variety of commercial dosage forms commonly available. Veterinarians do, however, need to learn how to write prescriptions properly and take the responsibility seriously because poor prescriptions can have disastrous results.

The form

Most small commercial printers welcome the opportunity to work with a practice to develop their prescription order form (Fig. 18-5). Besides reviewing sample forms, graphic designers can be consulted for a special layout and clinic logo that could also be used on stationery, and other printed items.

The typical prescription order form measures 4 × 5¼ inches. Pads of 50 are conve-

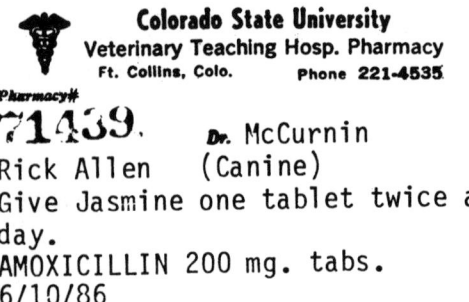

Figure 18-4. Prescription label

Colorado State University
VETERINARY TEACHING HOSPITAL
300 West Drake
Fort Collins, Colorado 80523

Phone: 221-4535

Date _____

Client _____ Patient _____

Address _____

℞

Refill _____ times

Please Label _____ D.V.M.

DEA# _____

Figure 18-5. Prescription order form

nient, although you may wish to obtain loose forms with an attached carbonless copy. With a copy filed in the patient's record or in a separate prescription copy file, you can review exactly what was initially prescribed. Such copies are especially helpful when clients call for refills or bring their animals in for rechecks.

The clinic name, address, and telephone number should be preprinted on prescription forms. Most will also include the full names and state license numbers of the clinicians in the practice. Printing Drug Enforcement Administration (DEA) registration numbers (see the discussion of controlled substances in the section on records) is discouraged because controlled drugs are more easily obtained if prescription forms are stolen from examination rooms.

The procedure

In writing the heading of the prescription it is helpful if the veterinarian indicates the client, client's address, date, and patient information (animal's name or species). Any information on the prescription (including the DVM's signature) omitted, intentionally or unintentionally, by the prescriber can be completed by the pharmacist since pharmacists can receive the entire prescription via telephone (Schedule II controlled substances are exceptions).

In the body of the prescription the first information given following the symbol *Rx* ("take thou") should be the name of the drug and dosage form desired (e.g., prednisone, 5 mg tabs). You may use either the brand name or generic name when requesting a drug. (Caution: *NEVER* abbreviate drug names because no national standard exists.) In most states pharmacists are permitted to substitute for a generic equivalent product unless the practitioner indicates by notation on the prescription to dispense only the brand requested. Statements such as "do not substitute" or "dispense as written (DAW)" are commonly used. Note that these are not valid if preprinted on the prescription form. Prescriptions can, however, bear preprinted statements like the following: "Dispensing by generic name permitted UNLESS checked here □." Checking the box would require the pharmacist to dispense only the brand requested. If the prescriber desires the name and strength of the drug placed on the prescription label routinely, a statement to the pharmacist should be preprinted on the prescription order form. As mentioned previously, the identity of the drug on the label is not usually required by law but is a good and common practice.

Although uncommon, if specific directions to the pharmacist are necessary, these should appear next on the prescription order. Such directions might state, "Dilute to 1:10 mixture" or "Add prednisolone to make 0.25%." Compounding instructions to the pharmacist was once routine before commercial dosage forms became common.

Directions that are to instruct the client on how to properly use the medication should occur next in the body of the prescription. Preceding the directions the latin abbreviation "Sig." for *Signa* ("mark thou") should appear. Although practitioners are encouraged to use English terms, the following abbreviations are frequently employed in prescription writing:

a.m.	morning
b.i.d.	twice a day
c	with
cap	capsule
Gm.	gram
gr.	grain
gtt.	a drop
gtts.	drops
h	hour
IM	intramuscularly
non rep.	do not repeat
o.d.	right eye
o.s.	left eye
o.u.	each eye
p.o.	by mouth
p.r.n.	as needed
q. a.m.	every morning
q.i.d.	four times a day
q. 4 h.	every four hours
q.o.d.	every other day
q. p.m.	every evening
q.s.	a sufficient quantity
Sig.	instructions to patient
SC	subcutaneously
tab	tablet
Tbs.	tablespoonful
t.i.d.	three times a day
tsp	teaspoonful

Note: s.i.d., which is commonly used in veterinary medicine, is not used in human medicine. Unfortunately errors have occurred when pharmacists have attempted to decipher s.i.d. It is recommended that the English term *daily* be used.

The pharmacist is responsible for interpreting the instructions and placing directions on the label so that the client understands how the prescribing veterinarian wants the medication used. Neither the pharmacist nor the client should hesitate to call the veterinarian if questions exist concerning proper use.

The quantity of medication to be dispensed usually appears in the upper right in the prescription body. It is suggested that the practitioner wait to determine the quantity needed until after the directions for use are written. If the directions for use are written first, the quantity necessary for the treatment period can then be easily calculated. Using markings such as *Disp.* (dispense), *Amt.* or # before the quantity are helpful in separating it from other prescription information.

The practitioner is encouraged to review each prescription for completeness and accuracy and then affix his signature. If the item prescribed is a controlled substance, the clinician's DEA registration number should be inscribed.

Although telephoning prescriptions into pharmacies may be convenient for the practitioner as well as the client, one must be mindful that the potential for error is much greater. With verbal prescriptions it is best to have the pharmacist restate the prescription back to ascertain correctness.

In calling in prescriptions veterinarians need to state their identity, state the client's name and the patient (either by name or species), identify the product to be dispensed, state the quantity, and give directions for proper use. One may also authorize refills by phone. Note that schedule II controlled substances cannot be called in to a pharmacy except in a bona fide medical emergency. Even if one can substantiate a valid veterinary emergency for Schedule II drugs, a signed written prescription must be received by the dispensing pharmacy within 72 hours.

Refills

The refilling of veterinary prescription drugs is prohibited without specific authorization of the clinician. Refill authorization may be indicated on the original prescription, or the pharmacist may obtain authorization by phone. It is recommended that the prescriber designate a specific number of refills (if any) or authorize refills for a certain period of time. Such refill instructions as *ad lib.*, *as requested*, or *p.r.n.* are not encouraged because they may lead to unmonitored misuse. In fact, many states now place time restrictions on prescription refills, usually limiting refills to a maximum of 1 year. Federal law prohibits refilling of prescriptions

for Schedule II controlled substances and restricts refills on other controlled substances to five refills, with no refills permitted 6 months after the original prescription order. For patients requiring maintenance therapy with controlled substances (i.e., phenobarbital as an anticonvulsant), pharmacists may treat refill authorization by telephone as a "new" prescription without requiring the practitioner to provide a new written prescription.

Responsibility

Although mentioned previously, the responsibility of prescribing prescription drugs (either new orders or refills) must be taken seriously. Indiscriminate refill authorization not only violates state and federal criminal law but also subjects you to civil litigation from owners or clients when their animals develop complications from unmonitored drug treatment. Patients receiving steroids, even ophthalmic drops, need to be examined occasionally even though lifetime therapy may be required. Liability is even greater in treatment of food animals with the potential of drug residues.

☐
Controlled substances

The DEA was established in 1973 from a merger of several federal agencies to combat drug diversion through enforcement of the Controlled Substances Act of 1970. This comprehensive piece of legislation identifies those individuals, businesses, or instructions that may legitimately handle those substances having abuse potential. Handlers may include manufacturers, importers, distributors, prescribers (MDs, DVMs, and so forth), pharmacies, hospitals, researchers, or educators, as well as clients and patients for which controlled substances have been prescribed. The intent of the act is to provide a closed system authorizing legitimate handlers through licensing and to monitor movement of these drugs through required records.

All controlled drug preparations are divided into five classifications depending primarily on their potential for abuse.

Schedule I

Drugs within this classification have no accepted medical use in the United States. Heroin, marijuana, LSD, peyote, and mescaline are but a few examples of drugs in this class with the highest abuse potential.

Schedule II

Drugs in this schedule have the highest abuse potential of all controlled substances ap-

proved for medical use in the United States. Most include either an opiate, stimulant, or depressant as the sole active ingredient in the dosage form. Examples are morphine, codeine, meperidine, oxymorphone, amphetamine, phenobarbital, etorphine, phencyclidine, and cocaine. A few combination products such as fentanyl and droperidol (Innovar-Vet, Pittman-Moore, Inc., Washington Crossing, NJ) are also found in this schedule.

Schedule II products are monitored and controlled much more extensively than those found in Schedules III, IV, and V. Practitioners are required to use special DEA order forms (DEA Form 222, Fig. 18-6) when purchasing Schedule II preparations. Telephoned prescriptions for Schedule II drugs are not permitted. (Note: there are exceptions for bona

See Reverse of PURCHASER'S Copy for Instructions		No order form may be issued for Schedule I and II substances unless a completed application form has been received, (21 CFR 1305.04).		OMB APPROVAL No. 1117-0010
TO: *(Name of Supplier)* Tri-City Pharmaceutical Co.		STREET ADDRESS 328 5th St.		
CITY and STATE Anytown, NY	DATE Dec. 22, 1987	**TO BE FILLED IN BY SUPPLIER** SUPPLIERS DEA REGISTRATION No.		

L I N E No.	TO BE FILLED IN BY PURCHASER					
	No. of Packages	Size of Package	Name of Item	National Drug Code	Packages Shipped	Date Shipped
1						
2						
3						
4						
5						
6						
7						
8						
9						
10						

2 ◄ NO. OF LINES COMPLETED	SIGNATURE OF PURCHASER OR HIS ATTORNEY OR AGENT	*John L. Doe*, DVM

Date Issued 2/16/87	DEA Registration No. AZ 1234567	Name and Address of Registrant
Schedules 2, 2N, 3, 3N, 4, 5		Doe, John L., D.V.M. 321 Main Street
Registered as a Practitioner	No. of this Order Form 8700112340	Anytown, NY 10110

DEA Form -222
(Jun. 1983)

U.S. OFFICIAL ORDER FORMS - SCHEDULES I & II
DRUG ENFORCEMENT ADMINISTRATION
SUPPLIER'S COPY 1

28333142

Figure 18-6. DEA order form

fide emergencies, but in veterinary medicine these would be extremely rare.) In addition prescriptions for Schedule II substances cannot be refilled.

Order forms for Schedule II substances come in booklets of six and may be requested when making the initial application to the DEA for registration. Additional booklets may be obtained by mailing form DEA 222A, which is attached to the booklet of order forms. These forms are in triplicate and require certain information from both the purchaser as well as the supplier. The veterinarian (purchaser) retains the last copy of the order and, upon receipt of supplies, enters the number of packages and date received in the section provided on the form. The original portion of the form is kept by the supplier who forwards the other copy to the DEA.

Schedules III, IV, and V

Drugs in Schedule III have less abuse potential than those in Schedules I and II. Such may be products with single active agents like thiopental or thiamylal or may contain limited opiates, stimulants, or depressants in combination with noncontrolled substances. Examples of this latter class would be hydrocodone/homatropine (Hycodan, Du Pont Pharmaceuticals, Wilmington) and pentobarbital/phenytoin. Schedule IV substances with less abuse potential include diazepam, phenobarbital, and chloral hydrate. Those products in Schedule V have the least abuse potential and consist primarily of antitussives or antidiarrheals with small quantities of certain opiates. Products found in this class are diphenoxylate/atropine (Lomotil, Searle Pharmaceuticals, Inc., Chicago) and guaifenesin/codeine.

Although no special order form is required when ordering Schedule III, IV, or V drugs, you must be registered with the DEA and have an assigned two-letter, seven-digit number (i.e., AB7654321). It is advisable to place this number on all written orders and provide it upon request for all verbal orders. Vendors may occasionally request a photocopy of the practitioner's DEA registration certificate to make certain the purchaser is currently registered.

Registration

Any veterinarian intending to order, administer, prescribe, or dispense controlled substances must be registered with DEA. (Note: *each* veterinarian in a practice prescribing, administering, or dispensing controlled drugs must be registered.) To apply for registration the veterinarian must complete Form DEA224 (Fig. 18-7), which may be obtained by calling a DEA field office or requesting a form from the Drug Enforcement Administration, Registration Unit, P.O. Box 28083 Central Station, Washington, DC 20005. When inquiring about an application you should also request a helpful booklet the DEA supplies without charge entitled *Physicians Manual.*

A DVM must be licensed in at least one state before submitting an application. When completing the application, the veterinarian should check "Practitioner" under registration classification rather than "Hospital/Clinic." It is also suggested all boxes under "Schedule" be checked even though you may not intend to use all. You would, therefore, have approval to use any scheduled drug should the need arise. The practitioner may also request forms for ordering Schedule II substances by checking block 4 on the application. Processing of the application takes approximately 8 to 10 weeks. Reregistration is required annually.

Records

Federal law requires practitioners to keep complete records of all controlled substances acquired for a period of 2 years. In addition, the federal act requires one to keep records for

Form **DEA** – 224 (Apr. 1984)   OMB No. 1117-0014

NEW
APPLICATION FOR REGISTRATION
UNDER
CONTROLLED SUBSTANCES ACT OF 1970

Please PRINT or TYPE all entries.

No registration may be issued unless a completed application form has been received (1301.21, CFR 21).

CITY   STATE   ZIP CODE

RETAIN Copy 3. Mail Orig. and 1 copy with FEE to:
UNITED STATES DEPARTMENT OF JUSTICE
DRUG ENFORCEMENT ADMINISTRATION
P.O. Box 28083
CENTRAL STATION
WASHINGTON, D.C. 20005
For INFORMATION, Call: 202 254 - 8255

See "Privacy Act" Information on reverse

THIS BLOCK
FOR DEA
USE ONLY

REGISTRATION CLASSIFICATION: Submit Check or Money Order Payable to the **DRUG ENFORCEMENT ADMINISTRATION** in the Amount of **$ 20.00.**

1. BUSINESS ACTIVITY: (Check ☑ ONE only)   (Specify Medical Degree, e.g., DDS, DO, DVM, MD, etc.)

● **FEE MUST ACCOMPANY APPLICATION**

A ☐ RETAIL PHARMACY   B ☐ HOSPITAL/CLINIC   C ☐ PRACTITIONER   D ☐ TEACHING INSTITUTION *(Instructional purposes only)*

2. SCHEDULES: *(Check ☑ all applicable schedules in which you intend to handle controlled substances. See Schedules on Reverse of Instruction Sheet.)*

SCHEDULE II	SCHEDULE II	SCHEDULE III	SCHEDULE III	SCHEDULE IV	SCHEDULE V
1 ☐ NARCOTIC	2 ☐ NONNARCOTIC	3 ☐ NARCOTIC	4 ☐ NONNARCOTIC	5 ☐	6 ☐

3. ☐ (Y) CHECK HERE IF YOU REQUIRE ORDER FORMS.

4. ALL APPLICANTS MUST ANSWER THE FOLLOWING:

(a) Are you currently authorized to prescribe, distribute, dispense, conduct research, or otherwise handle the controlled substances in the schedules for which you are applying, under the laws of the **State** or jurisdiction in which you are operating or propose to operate?

☐ YES - **State** License Number(s) _____

☐ NOT APPLICABLE   ☐ PENDING

(b) Has the applicant ever been convicted of a felony in connection with controlled substances under State or Federal law, or ever surrendered or had a CSA registration revoked, suspended, or denied?   ☐ YES ☐ NO

(c) If the applicant is a corporation, association, partnership, or pharmacy, has any officer, partner, stockholder or proprietor been convicted of a felony in connection with controlled substances under State or Federal law, or ever surrendered or had a CSA registration revoked, suspended, or denied?   ☐ YES ☐ NO

IF THE ANSWER TO QUESTIONS 4(b) or (c) is YES, include a statement using the space provided on the REVERSE of this part.

● ATTACH CHECK HERE

Print or Type Name Here - Sign Below   *Applicants Business Phone No. (Optional)*

SIGN HERE ▶ _____   _____
Signature of applicant or authorized individual   *Date*

Title (If the applicant is a corporation, institution, or other entity, enter the TITLE of the person signing on behalf of the applicant ((e.g., President, Dean, Procurement Officer, etc....))

5. CERTIFICATION FOR FEE EXEMPTION

☐ (E) CHECK THIS BLOCK IF INDIVIDUAL NAMED HEREON IS A FEDERAL, STATE, OR LOCAL OFFICIAL.

The Undersigned hereby certifies that the applicant herein is an officer or employee of a Federal, State or local agency who, in the course of such employment, is authorized to obtain, dispense, or prescribe controlled substances or is authorized to conduct research, instructional activity or chemical analysis with controlled substances, and is exempt from the payment of this registration fee.

Signature of Certifying Official   *Date*

Print or Type Name

Print or Type Title

Name of Institution or Agency

WARNING: SECTION 843(a)(4) OF TITLE 21, UNITED STATES CODE, STATES THAT ANY PERSON WHO KNOWINGLY OR INTENTIONALLY FURNISHES FALSE OR FRAUDULENT INFORMATION IN THIS APPLICATION IS SUBJECT TO IMPRISONMENT FOR NOT MORE THAN FOUR YEARS, A FINE OF NOT MORE THAN $30,000.00 OR BOTH.

Mail the Original and 1 copy with FEE to the above address. Retain 3rd copy for your records.

Figure 18-7. DEA application for registration

all narcotics *dispensed* but not those narcotics *prescribed* or *administered* in the lawful course of their professional practice. Dispensed is defined as "to deliver controlled substances in some type of container to the client."

There appears to be an inconsistency in the Controlled Substances Act because it requires complete usage records for all nonnarcotic scheduled drugs (i.e., thiopental, diazepam, and others). All records of receipts as well as deposition should be kept for a period of 2 years.

Practitioners should be familiar with their state's laws governing substances of abuse be-

cause state laws may be more stringent or include products not found in DEA schedules. The American Animal Hospital Association (AAHA) recommends to its members that separate records for the receipt and usage of each controlled substance be maintained.

An initial inventory of all controlled substances is required on the first day a new practice opens or when a practice changes ownership. In the event that no controlled substances are stocked at the time of opening, an initial inventory of zero should be recorded. An inventory is required every 2 years after the date of the initial inventory. This inventory date may be changed with prior approval from the nearest DEA field office. Inventory records are to be kept at the address appearing on the registration certificate for at least 2 years.

Inventory records must contain

1. Name, address, and DEA registration number of the registrant
2. The date and time the inventory is taken, i.e., opening or close of business day
3. The signature of the person or persons responsible for taking the inventory
4. Names, strength, and quantities of all controlled substances, with Schedule II drugs being separated from all other controlled substances.

Security

Veterinarians are required to keep controlled substances in a securely locked, substantially constructed cabinet or safe. After-hours alarm systems are recommended by the DEA. Official Schedule II order forms (DEA Form 222) should also be kept secure. Access to the controlled substances storage areas should be restricted to the absolute minimum number of employees for proper control.

Breakage, waste, drug theft, and disposal

Any drug theft or suspected drug theft should be reported to the DEA field office and the local police department immediately upon discovery. The DEA will send the veterinarian a report form (DEA Form 106) for completion and return to the field office.

Notation should be made in usage records of any breakage or wasting of controlled substances. Such notations should be countersigned and dated by another employee who may have observed the incident.

For disposal of obsolete, contaminated, or otherwise undesired controlled substances, one must first obtain a DEA Form 41 from the nearest DEA field office. After completion of the form, four copies must be prepared, with two copies mailed to the special agent in charge under separate cover. One copy is to be enclosed in the shipment with the drugs, with the remaining copy retained for the veterinarian's records. Drugs should be shipped tape sealed by prepaid express or registered mail to the special agent in charge, DEA field office.

☐
Drug and product information

All veterinarians prescribing or administering medication are practicing pharmacology and should, therefore, have reference materials to practice knowledgeably. With the new references that have become available in recent years, drug information is more complete as well as more accessible. Table 18-1 provides a brief description of some of the more popular references. The classification is provided only as an aid because several references will fall in more than one category.

In addition to text references several other informational sources exist. Proceedings from symposiums, journal articles, and product literature from manufacturers will be helpful.

To make use of information available it is necessary to organize a good system for retrieval. For photocopies of journal articles, notes, handouts, and product literature, it is suggested two files be used. One file for information on specific drugs or veterinary products and the other file for articles or information by topic. Because drugs are frequently discussed by therapeutic class or an article on a specific disease may list several agents for possible treatment, it is suggested that broad general categories (e.g., anesthesia, gastrointestinal, antibiotic/antibacterials, food animal vaccines, and so forth) be used. You can further divide the category (e.g., antibiotics into penicillin, aminoglycocides, other antibiotics) if the need arises. Important useful ref-

Table 18-1
Outline of pharmacy library references

Title of Reference	Author	Publisher
Veterinary Disease and Treatment		
Textbook of Veterinary Internal Medicine	Ettinger	W.B. Saunders
Current Veterinary Therapy IX	Kirk	W.B. Saunders
Handbook of Small Animal Therapeutics	Davis	Churchill Livingstone
Current Therapy in Equine Medicine	Robinson	Saunders
Veterinary Medicine	Blood et al	Lea & Febiger
Veterinary Pharmacology		
Veterinary Pharmacology and Therapeutics	Booth and McDonald	Iowa State University Press
Drugs in Veterinary Practice	Enos and Spinelli	
Handbook of Clinical Veterinary Pharmacology	Upson	VM Publishing
Pharmacological Basis of Large Animal Medicine	Bogan et al	Blackwell
Veterinary Product Information		
Veterinary Pharmaceuticals and Biologicals	Aronson et al	VM Publishing
Human Product and Drug Information		
USP Dispensing Information	—	USP Convention, Inc.
American Hospital Formulary Service Drug Information	McEvoy, et al	American Society of Hospital Pharmacists
Drug Facts and Comparisons	Kastrup et al	J.B. Lippincott
Physicians' Desk Reference (PDR)		Medical Economics
PDR for Ophthamology		Medical Economics

erences can be cross-indexed between files or categories, but cross-indexing all materials would be of questionable value. It is also suggested that all information filed be stamped with a date stamp to facilitate in purging for file maintenance.

One additional suggestion is to have an alphabetically indexed loose-leaf notebook for recording certain unique information. Such might contain doses for certain drugs in unusual species, strengths or formulations for various compounded mixtures, supply sources for infrequently used items, as well as prices charged for rare procedures or mixtures.

□

Equipment

The purchase of equipment should be viewed as a practice investment that produces revenue or reduces operational cost. Poor business decisions to invest in expensive, infrequently used equipment, however, result in additional overhead and expense. One need not have a great deal of equipment to practice veterinary medicine, but without the aid of good diagnostic or patient support equipment the level of medicine practiced is restricted. As a result, income as well as job satisfaction is limited. Discussion within this section will focus on general basic equipment needs with some comment on enhancement considerations.

Equipment needs

Equipment needs will vary depending on the size and type of practice. A large-animal practitioner involved primarily in ambulatory and consultant activities may function well with only a well-equipped mobile unit. Although there may be a few small-animal practices or mixed practices that specialize or limit their practice to nonsurgical procedures, most practices will require surgical equipment as well as support equipment (i.e., autoclave, x-ray unit, and so forth).

Telephone

A good telephone system with adequate incoming lines and proper location of handsets is necessary. Added features such as speakers, intercoms, memory dialing, and call forwarding should be considered because these are inexpensive and provide time and cost savings to the practitioner. Time should be spent evaluating various features and services available to make the proper selection of equipment. Data and voice communication is one area to be aware of when considering phone and computer equipment.

Computer

Most veterinary practices will be using computers in the near future. Although there are sophisticated systems designed for complex practice situations, small personal computers have available software that is quite useful in private practice. Applications include

1. Record keeping: payroll, accounts receivable, orders and appointments
2. Word processing: correspondence, price books, and medical record comments
3. Check writing and accounting records
4. Data base: client information, vendor information, and product information.

Even though many practices will use personal computers, most will still require at least one typewriter for preparing labels and completing forms. Word processors will handle the routine text needs but a good reconditioned typewriter will still be necessary. A ready supply of used typewriters will be available as more offices convert to computerized word processors.

Radiology

Although there are basically three types of x-ray machines, most private practices will be using either a portable or mobile unit instead of the more powerful stationary unit. Portable units are commonly used in large-animal practices for examination of extremities. Mobile units, which may be mounted for small-animal use, provide flexibility for a mixed practice.

Most machines used with human patients are replaced on a regular basis before their useful life has ended, so good used machines are always available. Before purchasing used equipment, however, it is essential that it be checked by a qualified service technician, not only for safety and function but also for parts and future service needs. The purchase of obsolete equipment is not a wise investment regardless of price.

In addition to the radiology machine, a method of processing film will be required. Hand processing must be performed in a darkroom and requires a developing tank, rinsing tank, and fixer tank. These tanks (sinks) should be large enough to accommodate several 35 × 42.5-cm films. Having running water of the proper temperature in the rinsing tanks is ideal although, if not available, frequently changed water will suffice. Tanks of stainless steel facilitate cleaning and extend their life.

There are specialty businesses that will clean and replace solutions used for x-ray development. Another consideration would be to evaluate the possibility of having x-ray films developed by a medical practice (veterinary, chiropractor, orthopedic) in the vicinity that has an automatic processor.

Automatic film processors that are capable of processing film within minutes do offer convenience but require additional investment and regular maintenance. A steady volume of radiographs in a large clinic practice would be necessary to justify the purchase of one of these units. Smaller practices should consider the purchase of a desktop automatic processor, which has become more reasonably priced.

Surgery

In addition to surgical instruments and supplemental items necessary for sterile surgery (i.e., drapes, towels, bowls, trays), several expensive pieces of equipment are required. The major pieces of surgical equipment are (1) operating table, (2) overhead surgery light, and (3) anesthesia machine. Both the table and light have a relatively long period of usefulness and require little routine maintenance. Consequently one should consider the purchase of used equipment initially and plan for replacement when financially possible.

The other important piece of surgical equipment is an inhalation anesthesia machine. Although surgery can be done with only injectable anesthetic agents, gas anesthesia is safer and provides greater overall patient control. Anesthesia machines may also serve for administering oxygen in an emergency.

Since a wide variety of machines are available through numerous manufacturers, it is wise to do an in-depth investigation of the advantages and disadvantages of several units before purchase. Considerations would include nonrebreathing vs. rebreathing, specific-size patient vs. range of patient sizes, single anesthetic gas vs. those adaptable to more than one agent, ease in use, ventilation support, safety, cleaning, dependability, and of course cost.

For sterilization of surgical instruments and related items an autoclave is recommended. Various chemical agents can be used for cold sterilization, but all have their limitations and do not guarantee complete sterility. Through the use of an autoclave that provides saturated steam under pressure, complete sterility for packs and instruments can be obtained.

Autoclaves are available with different capacities and features that create a wide price range. Options include automatic timers, different temperature settings, and different cycles (i.e., slow exhaust for large-volume fluids, drying cycle for packs). It is possible to find used autoclaves, but exercise caution because autoclaves are fairly high maintenance items and require replacement parts. Having a used autoclave tested and inspected before purchase by an individual who may eventually service it is wise. Before the purchase of an autoclave make sure all instruments and instrument packs can be accommodated by the chamber.

Patient care and monitoring

Scales that accurately weigh patients seen in the practice are essential. This may only require a good set of bathroom scales for most dogs but a baby scale for cats and puppies. Other monitoring and patient care equipment, although somewhat expensive, will be found not only in large group practices but also in many single-person practices. Such equipment will include ECG monitors, digital electronic thermometers, fluid pumps, water blankets, oxygen cases (with or without controlled temperature and humidity), and whirlpool baths. The availability of local repair service is extremely important with this equipment.

A fiber-optic endoscope has become a valuable tool in veterinary medicine. Applications for large animals include examination of the upper respiratory tract, upper gastrointestinal (GI) tract, penis, uterus, rectal area, joints, as well as several other areas that may be made accessible by minor surgery. For dogs, similar examinations of the upper respiratory tract, upper GI tract, and uterus can be performed although the diameter of the endoscope and the size of the dog will limit utilization. Endoscopes do require care and proper cleaning after each use. Because of their diagnostic

value, however, more practices will be using them routinely.

Laboratory

A good microscope is the most important piece of laboratory equipment a practice can possess. With proper care it should last a lifetime. Proper care includes only using lens paper to clean the lenses, cleaning the oil off the oil immersion lens after use, and covering the microscope when not in use to prevent dust collection on the lenses. For veterinary clinical pathology a microscope with $10\times$ ocular objective, and $40\times$ to $45\times$, and $100\times$ oil immersion objectives should be adequate. Microscopes should be cleaned and serviced annually to ensure maximal life.

Other laboratory equipment such as a centrifuge or refractometer are helpful diagnostic tools. The use of commercial laboratories for more elaborate uncommon tests is suggested for reduced investment in laboratory equipment.

Pharmacy and supply

Few pieces of equipment are required in these areas although special storage is required for some supplies. A refrigerator for certain pharmaceuticals or biologicals is necessary. This unit need not be a commercial type, but if fitted with metal or plastic drawers, more efficient use of space can be obtained. Those veterinarians using controlled substances are also required to keep them in a securely locked area so that a substantially constructed cabinet or safe is necessary. An area to clean dirty instruments and reusable items is desirable, but specialized equipment is usually not necessary unless the work load becomes significant. An autoclave may be used to sterilize small fluid volumes or empty vials. In addition, a balance may be helpful for weighing chemicals and pet food as well as small patients such as hamsters, guinea pigs, and birds.

Miscellaneous equipment

Additional equipment will be required depending on the individual and type of practice. Those in large-animal practice will need stocks or chutes for restraint. Practitioners involved with birds or reptiles will have a need for special cages or tanks for housing these patients. Others having specialized interest in such areas as ophthalmology, dermatology, cardiology, or orthopedics are likely to acquire equipment to support their area of interest. The more specialized the equipment, the more important it becomes to evaluate the service, repair, and loaner status for the equipment.

Leasing considerations

For expensive equipment that is continually being improved leasing should be considered. Leasing provides the opportunity of evaluating expensive equipment without the investment, and most arrangements allow at least a portion of the lease payment to apply toward purchase. In addition, repair costs and routine maintenance expenses are usually the leaser's responsibility. Leasing also permits upgrading or downgrading of equipment depending on needs or use. Switching to more reliable equipment or suppliers is also an incentive for leasing.

A total-practice computer system would be an item that a practice might consider leasing. Some large group practices might do well to investigate leasing radiology equipment as well as other pieces of expensive diagnostic and monitoring equipment. Equipment lease agreements should not extend beyond 5 years. Agreements should be reviewed by the practice's attorney or certified public accountant.

Maintenance

Maintenance requirements differ, not only between pieces of equipment but between parts on the same unit. Although some equipment is low maintenance, no equipment should be completely neglected because all will function better and longer when properly and routinely maintained.

Arrangements can be made for certain pieces of equipment to be serviced regularly by equipment suppliers or independent service technicians. Some services contracts will include replacement parts in addition to routine maintenance. Except for extremely expensive or continuous problem equipment, however, service contracts are cost prohibitive.

Proper cleaning and lubrication, which may be all that is required for most equipment, can be done by personnel in the practice. The gas anesthesia machine is one item that should be inspected and cleaned at least monthly. All fittings, gaskets, hoses, valves, and other connections should be checked. In addition, vaporizer maintenance should be done by a qualified service technician annually.

Each refrigerator should have a thermometer that should be checked at the beginning of each workday to ensure proper function. Refrigerators also need to have their compressor vacuumed at least annually.

Steam autoclaves may require the routine addition of a sodium phosphate solution or other commercial preparation to prevent a buildup of scale on valves and pipes. Temperature indicators should be used with every load and included in every pack to ensure sterility.

Radiology machines come with specific maintenance and inspection checks for each model. It is essential that these be followed for patient and operator safety. Suspected malfunctions should be checked before continued use of the machine.

Other equipment mentioned in this section may have specific maintenance requirements that should be followed. With proper cleaning after each use as well as thorough routine maintenance, however, years of additional usefulness can be added to even low-maintenance equipment.

Maintenance record keeping

To aid the busy practitioner in keeping a record of maintenance on various equipment items, each piece of equipment must be assigned to an employee. As an example, the office equipment is assigned to the receptionist; the laboratory and surgical equipment are assigned to the surgical technician; the furnace, air conditioner, refrigerators, and water heater are assigned to the maintenance person; and so on. The equipment responsibilities should be listed in each person's job description.

Each piece of equipment is then tagged with a plastic-coated card that has the last service date, the name of the person performing the service, and the date of the next service. The practice manager can review the tags to determine the maintenance status of any piece of equipment. Certain pieces of equipment that cannot be tagged (i.e., endoscope, air drill, ophthalmoscope, microscope) can have a wall- or cabinet-mounted card next to the piece of equipment. These tags or cards will then serve as reminders to the responsible person.

Major repair vs. replacement

In the life of each piece of equipment there is a point at which replacement must be considered over repair. The specific point of replacement will vary with the philosophy of the individual making the decision. Some people trade cars every 2 or 3 years whereas others use a vehicle for 10 or more years. The dependability factor for a specific piece of equipment will often push the decision toward replacement. Other times, the cost of repair is just more than the value of the item.

When considering major repair to replacement you should weigh the following: (1) cost, (2) life expectancy, (3) dependability, (4) state of the art, (5) availability of future repair parts, and (6) warranty. Seeking the advice of others who are knowledgeable can also aid in the decision process. The important point is that each time repair is needed on an item the options are to repair, replace, or eliminate the item.

□
References

1. The United States Pharmacopeia, 21st revision. Rockville MD, United States Pharmacopeial Convention, p 1330, 1984
2. Stefan G, Beaulieu A, Ballitch E: FDA Regulation of Veterinary Prescription Drugs. JAVMA 189:513–517, 1986

Chapter 19
☐
Financial aspects of practice management

Marvin L. Samuelson
Joseph Barton-Dobenin
Frederick H. Rice

When you can measure what you are speaking about and express it in numbers, you know something about it.

Lord Kelvin William Thomson

Competent financial management is essential to the success and growth of any business. Due to the continuous significant increase in numbers of practicing veterinarians, practice competition is at an all-time high. As a result, understanding the financial aspect of a practice becomes a key part in successful practice management. It would be unrealistic to assume, however, that in a few pages one could explain all there is to know and provide the necessary guidelines for the best approach to financial management. Based on our experiences it takes many hours of hard work to accumulate basic accounting and financial knowledge, and it takes an additional major effort to learn how to profitably use it in one's practice.

The purpose of this chapter is to introduce the reader to some key concepts of financial management and present procedures on how to interpret information obtained from various statements developed by the accounting process. It is important to the future of any practice that the owner-manager be able to read and analyze the financial strengths and weaknesses of the practice, develop cash forecasts and, on the basis of the generated data, plan future actions or take corrective steps.

In the latter part of this chapter we will briefly discuss some of the hand-recorded accounting systems that can be used and some of the new computer systems and programs that are available. Finally, we will briefly indicate how the practitioner can use financial data to make sound decisions, what help and support can be obtained from a certified public accountant (CPA), and the possible use of a professional practice manager.

□ A look at financial statements

Today most well-managed practices are using an accounting system based on the double-entry concept. This approach provides at least two entries for each financial transaction and at the end of the accounting period summarizes the activities into two key financial statements. The *balance sheet* reflects the financial position of the practice, and the *income statement* provides a summary of revenues and expenditures and a final profit or loss figure.

The balance sheet

The balance sheet can be viewed as a financial photograph of a practice. It provides a picture of the financial position of the operation at a given moment in time (Fig. 19-1).

Every balance sheet has two major parts. The first part presents all items the business owns at a given time, (Total Assets in Fig. 19-1, $140,500). The second part illustrates the origin of the funds invested in the assets (Total Liabilities and Net Worth, again $140,500). If all the entries have been made properly, the two parts are equal and therefore the same — thus, a balance sheet.

Assets

Any item the practice owns that has monetary value is considered to be an asset. Assets are either current or fixed.

Current assets are assets readily convertible to cash and generally will be converted into cash during 1 year. In Figure 19-1 current assets are: cash, accounts receivable, and drug inventory.

Fixed assets are tangible, relatively long-lived items owned by the practice, which are indicated on the balance sheet at their cost. With the exception of land, fixed assets generally decline in value as they are used. This decline is reflected in the depreciation charges, and the individual items are shown on the balance sheet at their net, or depreciated value, which represents the cost of the item less accumulated depreciation (see Fig. 19-1).

Intangible assets are items that have only tentative value such as goodwill and practice name, which may increase in value over time, and organization costs or agreements not to compete, which may decline in value. Careful consideration should be given to these assets, especially when buying or selling a practice.

Liabilities

This part of the balance sheet indicates the claims of outsiders against the business.

Current liabilities are obligations due in the near future, usually no more than 1 year (see Fig. 19-1).

Long-term liabilities include debts that are not due to be paid within a year such as mortgages on properties or long-term notes.

Net worth or owner's equity

This section indicates the values of the contribution of the owner or stockholder to the business. The net worth may increase through earnings retention from profitable operation or may decrease when losses are incurred or earnings are paid out.

The income statement

The second important financial report is the income statement, sometimes called a profit-and-loss statement. It is related to the balance sheet because it shows the components of the final changes in retained earnings. The income statement has a major significance for the practitioner because it displays reasons for profitability or lack thereof insofar as can be reflected by accounting data. Important individual items on the income statement (Fig. 19-2) are *income*, which consists of profes-

John Smith, D.V.M.
Balance Sheet
December 31, 19--

Assets

Current	Value		Percent
Cash in Bank	$ 8,000	. . . .	5.7
Accounts Receivable	10,000	. . . .	7.1
Drug Inventory	13,000	. . . .	9.6
Total Current Assets	$ 31,500	. . . .	22.4

Fixed		Value		Percent
Land		$ 12,000	. . . .	8.5
Building	$80,000			
Less Accumulated Depreciation	−18,000	62,000	. . . .	44.1
Truck	$10,000			
Less Accumulated Depreciation	− 3,000	7,000	. . . .	5.0
Instruments & Equipment	$25,000			
Less Accumulated Depreciation	− 7,000	18,000	. . . .	12.8
Total Fixed Assets		$ 99,000	. . . .	70.5

Intangible Assets	Value		Percent
Goodwill	$ 10,000	. . . .	7.1
Total Assets	$140,500	. . . .	100.0

Liabilities

Current	Value		Percent
Accounts Payable	$ 2,000	. . . .	1.4
Note, Bank	6,500	. . . .	4.6
Current Mortgage, Bank	5,500	. . . .	3.9
Total Current Liabilities	$ 14,000	. . . .	9.9

Long Term	Value		Percent
Mortgage on Land and Building to Bank . . .	$ 54,500	. . . .	39.8
Total Liabilities	68,500	. . . .	48.7
Net Worth (also called owner's equity)	$ 72,000	. . . .	51.3
Total Liabilities and Net Worth	$140,500	. . . .	100.00

Figure 19-1. Sample balance sheet

sional income and profit from drugs sold for cash or credit that result in gross revenue. At times money may be refunded or credited to clients and is subtracted from the gross revenue. *Expenses* are all those costs incurred in the day-by-day operation of the practice. They range from labor expense, supplies, utilities, insurance, interest expense, and depreciation. One of the important elements of depreciation is that it is an estimate based on management judgment and can significantly affect the final profit or loss figure. A careful analysis of these entries should be made to ensure compliance with IRS guidelines for the accelerated cost recovery system, which spells out the normal expected life of various types of equipment.

Gross revenue less expenses indicates the net profit before income taxes, and that figure reflects the financial success or failure of the practice during a given period.

To determine the economic profit of a practice you must estimate the income (imputed salary for the owner operator) and the return on the owner's investment at current interest rates. This, in essence, is the income earned if you had worked for someone else and left your money invested in a financial institution. By subtracting these two amounts from the net income before taxes, the economic profit of a practice can be determined (see Fig. 19-2). These two values are important factors to consider when determining the goodwill or excess earning value of a practice. Additional information on how to buy or sell a practice is found in Chapter 7.

John Smith, D.V.M.
Income Statement
For the Year Ended December 31, 19--

Income		Value	Percent
Professional Time Income		$125,500	85.9
Total Drug Sales	$45,000		
Less Cost of Drugs Sold	(30,000)		
Profit from Drugs Sold		15,000	14.1
Gross Revenue		$140,500	100.0
Expenses			
Labor		$ 32,200	22.1
Payroll Taxes		5,500	3.8
Truck Repairs		2,500	1.7
Supplies		6,500	4.5
Dues and Travel to Meetings		900	0.6
Depreciation		14,000	9.6
Utilities		2,000	1.4
Telephone		700	0.5
Taxes and Licenses		800	0.6
Repairs and Maintenance		1,800	1.2
Accounting and Legal		2,000	1.4
Insurance		1,800	1.2
Interest		6,500	4.5
Total Expenses		$ 77,200	53.1
Net Income Before Taxes		$ 68,300	46.9
Income on Investment ($72,000 @ 15%)		$ 10,800	
Veterinarian Labor Income		30,000	
Economic Profit		$ 27,500	

Figure 19-2. Sample income statement

□
Financial statements analysis

The financial statements present to management the dollar figures reflecting the status and changes that have taken place during an accounting period. To better understand these results and to provide opportunity to compare past results with the current ones several approaches can be used.

Segregation of fixed and variable expenses

Depending on the nature of a practice the owners may be interested in segregating the financial data in more appropriate categories. Income may be subdivided on the basis of activities such as (1) medical, surgical, vaccination, laboratory, radiology, pharmacy, inpatient, outpatient, emergency, or country calls; (2) equine, bovine, or small animal; or (3) who generated it, doctor A, B, or C; or all three subdivisions can be combined.

Expense categories can be subdivided into fixed and variable or direct and administrative. In Figure 19-2 the fixed expenses are those that generally occur regardless of the volume of the activities and decrease as a percentage of gross income as the practice gross income grows. (In the example they are dues and travel to meetings, depreciation, utilities, telephone, taxes and licenses, repairs and maintenance, accounting and legal, insurance, and interest.)

Variable expenses generally change with gross income and reflect the movement up or down of the practice activities.

Percentage analysis of financial statements

One of the most relevant analyses is the comparison of individual accounts in both the balance sheet and the income statement with re-sults in previous accounting periods. These comparisons can detect positive or negative developments at any early stage and provide the owners with opportunities for appropriate actions. Comparison may be made by the month, quarter, 6-month, or 12-month periods.

Ratio analysis

The use of ratio analysis may provide the owners an additional financial picture of their operation and enable them to make important comparisons with other operations or with their profession as a whole. A ratio is computed by taking selected figures from the financial statements and expressing one figure as a percentage of another one.

The following sections include some of the ratios offering valuable information to the owner.

Return on investment

This ratio indicates the return on owner investment in the practice. It is computed by dividing the net profit by net worth (or owner's equity). The results are expressed in percentages (for data see Figs. 19-1 and 19-2).

$$\frac{\text{Net profit}}{\text{Net worth}} = \frac{\$68,300}{\$72,000} = 94.8\%$$

From strictly an economic point of view this figure should be relatively larger than the return the owner could obtain from investing his money elsewhere. The practitioner should receive a better-than-average return on the investment for the time, effort, and risk involved in owning and operating a practice. Our case indicates exceptionally good results in this area.

Net profit to revenue

This ratio indicates the net profit margin on each dollar of revenue and is computed by dividing the net profit by gross revenues.

$$\frac{\text{Net profit}}{\text{Gross revenue}} = \frac{\$\ 68,300}{\$145,500} = 46.9\%$$

This ratio is also favorable and indicates that the owner retains on an average 46.9% net profit out of each dollar of revenue. The ratio should be compared with past results for changes in performance and with those of the profession for future planning.

Inventory turnover

The inventory turnover figure indicates how fast the drugs and other items for distribution in the practice are moving and is expressed in the number of times the inventory was sold in the year. It is determined by dividing the cost of goods sold by the average inventory (beginning inventory plus the ending inventory for each month divided by 13); assuming that in our case the average inventory is the same as the ending inventory the computation is as follows:

$$\frac{\text{Cost of goods sold}}{\text{Average inventory}} = \frac{\$30,000}{\$13,500} = 2.2\times$$

Usually a turnover rate of 6× or more is preferred according to the *Troy Almanac of Business and Industrial Financial Ratios* published by Prentice-Hall. Our ratio indicates that in this case the owner for some reason turns his inventory about half as fast as normal. We should look into the situation to see whether there is room for improvement by either increasing sales or reducing inventory items that are not selling.

Current ratio

The current ratio is strictly a balance sheet ratio obtained by dividing current assets by current liabilities.

$$\frac{\text{Current assets}}{\text{Current liabilities}} = \frac{\$31,500}{\$14,000} = 2.3\times$$

The current ratio measures the ability to meet short-term obligations. A 2 : 1 ratio is generally considered good. Bankers or other lenders are always interested in this measure because it indicates how a practice can meet its current obligations.

Many other ratios can be computed, and only the individual practitioner with the help of a CPA advisor may determine the relevant measurements.

Other significant data may be compiled and used for important comparisons. Thus, for example, it should be of interest to compile data on average client charges, number of clients seen per day, and housing costs or comparisons of income and expense allocated to various activity centers in the practice. Such parameters may be tracked and used as measures of the financial soundness of the practice.

Where can additional ratio data be located? There are various sources of ratio data that can be used for comparison purposes. The following are some of the most reliable and well known:

- *Key Business Ratios.* Published annually by Dun and Bradstreet, Inc., 99 Church Street, New York, NY 10007. Free
- *Statement Studies.* Published annually by Robert Morris Associates, Philadelphia National Bank Building, Philadelphia, PA
- *DVM Management.* Published by American Veterinary Publications, Inc., P.O. Drawer KK, Santa Barbara, CA 93102. Publishes yearly analysis of various practice results
- *Troy Almanac of Business and Industrial Financial Ratios.* Published by Prentice-Hall, Inc., Englewood Cliffs, NJ

In Table 19-1 an operating expense guide is presented. Table 19-2 illustrates a brief financial status checklist, and Table 19-3 indicates some of the key strategies for profit improvement.

Table 19-1
Operating expense guide

Gross Income	*100%*
Expenses (Range Expressed in Percentages)	
Employee wages	12.0 – 17.0
Interest and depreciation	5.1 – 7.0
Drugs	8.2 – 12.0
Hospital supplies	4.0 – 7.0
Office supplies	1.4 – 2.0
Utilities	0.8 – 1.0
Telephone	1.1 – 1.5
Automobile	1.0 – 1.9
Commercial laboratory	0.5 – 1.0
Insurance	0.6 – 1.4
Taxes and licenses	2.0 – 2.3
Repairs and maintenance	1.1 – 1.6
Accounting and legal	0.8 – 1.1
Dues, subscriptions, continuing education, and professional meetings	1.0 – 1.3
Miscellaneous	1.0 – 1.6
Total expenses	40.6 – 59.7
Net Income	*40.3 – 59.4*

Data not additive vertically.
Source: Figures compiled by authors from research gathered in midwest United States.

Table 19-2
Financial status checklist (what an owner-manager should know)

Daily

Cash on hand
Bank balance
Daily summary of sales and cash receipts
Correct errors
Maintain a record of all monies paid out by cash or check

Weekly

Accounts receivable
Accounts payable
Review payroll for accuracy
Make sure all local, state, and federal taxes are paid

Monthly

Be sure that general ledger is posted
Review income statement
Review balance sheet
Reconcile bank statement
Balance petty cash account
Deposit all taxes
Age accounts receivable
Review inventory

Table 19-3
Strategies to improve profits

Reduce Expenses — Direct Plus Overhead

Reevaluate Fee Structure and Activity

Increase activities with larger profit margins
Adjust fees where profits are low
Improve efficiency and services
Polish client communication
Build client confidence

Use New and Innovative Marketing Methods

Advertising (institutional or individual)
   Direct mail
   Newsletters
   Radio
   TV
   Newspaper
   Specialty items
Public Relations — by doctors and staff
   Public speaking
   Community youth group participation
   Fair booth
   Fair judging
   Prizes or scholarships
   Pet show sponsor
   Public service announcements
   Write newspaper column

See More Clients per Day

Establish clinic hours that meet market needs
Book more elective calls on slow days
Mail out more specific reminder notices
Encourage early morning appointments

Improve Collection Methods

Carefully plan all patient discharges with specific follow-up
Ask for payment at completion of visit
Give discount for cash payment
Use major credit cards
Send bills out daily rather than waiting till the end of the month
Add interest to bills not paid after 30 days
File liens against property if payment is slow
Use a collection agency as a last resort
Review collection policy with attorney and accountant

□
Financial management systems

The selection of an appropriate accounting system for a practice will depend mainly on the patient caseload, the number of practitioners involved, and the type of services provided. For a one-doctor practice, a manual "one-write system" designed to handle up to 100 cases per day may be appropriate. For large multidoctor practices, a computerized system may be most appropriate.

Hand-recorded systems

One-write or pegboard systems are offered by several companies. Some programs can be used immediately, but others may need to be customized for special cases. Some firms are moving into computerized systems. The following firms provide various systems: Control-O-Fax, Box 778, Waterloo, IA 50704, (319) 234-4651; Safeguard, 455 Maryland Drive, P.O. Box 7501, Fort Washington, PA 19034, (800) 523-2422. Several others are advertised in current veterinary literature.

The major advantage of these and other record systems is the accomplishment of all necessary records in one single entry. Most of these systems also can be operated with the limited help of accountants or bookkeepers. They greatly simplify the work of producing financial statements and the summarization of internal financial information. Finally they provide formulas allowing balancing and proofing of all the entries. The key requirement for success is self-discipline and a desire to achieve financial control. For proper and accurate operation a CPA should be periodically consulted to ensure desired results.

Computerized service bureaus

Using computers in a practice can develop into a major problem when the practitioner is faced with a new "language" and a new technology. In the long run the effort expended, however, should return major benefits in efficiency and income.

To provide a less traumatic transition for all concerned a local computer service bureau can be considered in lieu of an on-site computer system. They can take the information generated by the accounting system in use and produce a broad range of financial reports. They can also take care of accounts receivable and payable and inventory control plus other valuable services.

The advantage of a service bureau is the development of valuable managerial and financial information for a modest charge and in the process a valuable exposure of all concerned to the basics of electronic data processing. The limitation of these services, however, may be in the restrictions of the programs these bureaus can provide. It is one thing to use computers or a computer service in a practice but quite another thing to have a completely computerized practice.

Direct use of computers

Increasing numbers of veterinarians are introducing computers into their operations. Major changes are taking place in this area because costs are declining, capabilities of the hardware and software are dramatically expanding, and the operations are becoming simpler and more user friendly. In Chapter 5 various aspects of computers are discussed in detail.

In the area of financial management the computer can be of great value as an efficient bookkeeper and provider of timely results for better decision making and future planning. The ratios discussed earlier, the percent analysis of financial statements, and comparisons with other operations can be continuously provided for better management. Regional or national veterinary medical associations can provide necessary advice on the latest developments in this field.

☐
The use of a CPA

Although practically anyone can provide accounting and financial advice for the veterinarian, a specialist in the field such as a CPA should be considered a member of the management team. Not only does a CPA hold a degree in accounting, he or she must have a minimum of 2 years of accounting experience, pass a competitive examination, and meet

Table 19-4
A guide to veterinary practice: financial management evaluation

Sustainable Practice: Sound Management	Average Practice: So-So Management	Marginal Practice: Weak Management
1. Have done considerable long-range planning for practice growth	1. Long-range plans are carefully thought out	1. Day-to-day activities involve you so much that there is no opportunity for advanced planning
2. Plans are developed in a budget covering receipts, expenses, margins, etc. Key employees assist in budget information	2. Plans are visualized but not developed in a budget. Key employees assist very little	2. No plan or budget
3. Continually compare actual results with budget projections	3. Compare actual results with budget projections as time allows	3. Never compare actual results with budget or no budget prepared
4. Accounting data supplied promptly in a form best adapted to its use by management	4. Accounting data not adequate in comparison with most modern concepts of control.	4. Accounting not highly regarded as a tool of management.
5. Prepare monthly income	5. Prepare a quarterly income statement	5. Prepare annual income statement or rely on income tax statement for profit figure
6. Prepare a monthly balance sheet	6. Prepare a quarterly or annual balance sheet	6. Do not prepare a balance sheet
7. Forecast working capital and cash requirements for planned practice volume and profit level	7. No forecast of working capital or cash requirements and funds not always obtained or used	7. Working capital and cash inadequate. No forward planning.
8. Calculate financial ratios and compare them with standard data of profession	8. Seldom review standard data of profession and calculate few or no financial ratios	8. Do not review standard data and do not calculate financial ratios
9. Keep additional data to use in calculating activities and operating ratios	9. Must spend some time developing additional data to use in calculating activities and operating ratios	9. Do not calculate activities and operating ratios. Do not keep necessary data
10. Have a written credit policy that is understood by clients. Credit is used as a management tool	10. Have credit policy but not written that is seldom understood by clients	10. Do not have a credit policy
11. Age accounts receivable monthly.	11. Age accounts receivable quarterly or annually	11. Do not age accounts receivable
12. Healthy financial status with favorable rewards for owners and employees	12. Struggle to maintain positive financial status sustained by hard work and moderate to low salaries for owners and employees	12. Financially declining. Sustained by long hours and low salaries.

continuing education requirements. Thus the CPA can help the veterinarian not only with all accounting aspects of the practice but also aid with tax planning and proper tax return preparation. Finally, a major contribution of a CPA could be in the area of management services. Here the CPA can periodically review and evaluate the financial results and suggest strategies to enhance future performance.

□
Summary and conclusions

Financial management is by no means an easy task but is one of the key activities for a veterinarian to master and practice consistently. It will provide the practitioner an in-depth picture of his operations and may answer questions of why certain results are as they are. Table 19-4 is a guide for a veterinary practice financial management evaluation that indicates some of the key areas of concern.

One can anticipate that future practice operation and management will change dramatically due to major changes in all components of veterinary practice.

People with special business training are serving in many of the larger practices, and in some instances a manager serves more than one practice. Practice managers who are not veterinarians function best when teamed with veterinarians who can appreciate sound business principles. The practice manager is discussed in Chapter 14. At least one veterinarian in each practice must take the lead to maintain a balance of good veterinary practice and good business.

We feel that John Naisbitt expressed it best in his *Megatrends* when he wrote: "Out of touch with the present we are doomed to fail in the unfolding future," and concluded "My God, what a fantastic time to be alive!"

□
Recommended readings

Hamilin F: Progress in the right direction. DVM Management, Vol 16, March 1985

Naisbitt J: Megatrends. New York, Warner Books, 1984

Opperman M: Veterinary Business Management. Media, PA, Harwal Publishing, 1983

Pratt PW: Veterinary Practice Management. Santa Barbara, CA, American Veterinary Publications, 1979

Wilson JF: Business Guide for Veterinary Practice. Princeton Junction, NJ, Veterinary Learning Systems, 1983

Chapter 20
☐
Referrals

Jack D. Henry, Jr.

The concept of referrals among medical clinicians is not new. As knowledge and expertise develop and grow, more individuals gain specific, specialized information that complement the general and routine clinical scene. To keep abreast of diagnostic and therapeutic changes and advancements veterinarians must avail themselves of every source of material for continuing education. Education ranges from newsletters and professional journals to seminars and personal consultations. The evolution of individuals with special training is a result of practitioners with a special clinical interest embarking on a personal program of self-study and then making observations and application of their new knowledge.

The general public is constantly being exposed to advances in human medicine through information on transplant surgery for heart, lung, and liver and dramatic reattachments of severed limbs. In addition, epidemiological concepts regarding nutrition and consumption of various drugs and foodstuffs, the harmful effects of smoking, and new treatment modalities against cancer and various infections are commonly reported. Occasionally an item appears in print about a surgical procedure that was performed on a zoo animal or on an experimental animal. Regardless of this broad coverage these advances appear isolated and unavailable. It is doubtful that the public is aware that these techniques are also available for animal patients. The general public has very little awareness about the background and education of veterinarians and essentially no knowledge about veterinarians who are specialty trained.

Apart from the animal owners who are aware of specialty-trained veterinarians there are a few clients who demand a higher level of medical care. For a great many families, the pet has become "equal" to other family members. Sometimes they are the only family members. In these cases financial considerations take a low priority. The owners are willing to consider any expense or even travel great distances as long as the best available veterinary care can be obtained.

Even though it is common for people to be referred from one physician to another, the majority of people are not aware that veterinarians with specialized knowledge exist. There is a paradox between wanting to provide the best possible health care to animal patients and holding it back by placing limits on what will be offered.

Fortunately, veterinary medicine has become more specialized since the 1950s. At first the specialists were mostly research and academic veterinarians. As more knowledge was acquired and it became increasingly difficult to maintain a proficient depth in every aspect of animal disease and therapeutics, clinical disciplines began to take on more definition. Some academicians resisted the fact that they could not know everything about veterinary medicine and were unwilling to accept that a particular specialist might have in-depth expertise in a specific area. On the other hand, more enlightened academic clinicians recognized and supported the idea of organized specialization. They recognized that it was no longer acceptable for veterinarians to be self-proclaimed experts but that guidelines needed to be set forth for an individual to acquire their expertise. Each specialty-trained individual should be examined by an austere body and given separate approval that they indeed possess the qualifications of a specialist.

The American Veterinary Medical Association (AVMA) recognizes specialists in the following disciplines: veterinary practitioners, toxicology, laboratory animal medicine, theriogenology, anesthesiology, dermatology, internal medicine, cardiology, neurology, microbiology, ophthalmology, pathology, preventative medicine, radiology, surgery, and zoological medicine.

□
Specialty training and examination

Basic training for a specialist requires that the trainee be exposed to academic and clinical courses and gain practical experience and expertise through specific apprenticeship, clerkship, internship, and residency positions. The intense, in-depth, postgraduate study can vary in length but generally will take no longer than 5 years. Two major advantages of individuals being subjected to such rigorous study are (1) the acquired discipline and (2) the recognition of one's own limitations. The trainee gains tremendous breadth as well as depth and therefore becomes very resourceful and proficient at directing others to sources that can provide answers to specific problems. Specialists gain a great appreciation for their own limits of expertise and will be the first to refer to colleagues who have either a greater depth of expertise or have access to specialized equipment that allows more technically precise and efficient procedural management.

The various specialty colleges have provisions that allow practitioners to quality for examination. In most instances, however, the practitioner will need to enter a formal training program. The American Board of Veterinary Practitioners is less stringent in that it allows a candidate to be examined by submitting acceptable credentials without having completed a specific academic training program. This provides for the recognition of veterinary practitioners who have, in fact, gained and demonstrated by examination a greater extent of knowledge in their area of practice than their fellow practitioners.

Specialty examinations are comprehensive and cover all phases of basic science and clinical instruction. The boards that are more academic and research oriented such as pathology and toxicology have less practical orientation. To sit for the examination the candidate must first be accepted by the credentials committee of the respective board or college and ultimately be accepted by the governing body such as the Board of Regents of the American College of Veterinary Surgeons.

The overall examination will usually be divided into the following portions: (1) written, (2) oral, and (3) practical parts. The written portion is comprehensive and covers both basic science and clinical science. In addition, it will have questions applicable to any or all of the domestic animal species. For example, the written examination could have 50% directed toward a small-animal species but would have enough physiological or pathological basis that a candidate predominantly trained in equine treatment could grasp the essence of the question and determine the correct answer.

The oral examination varies from college to college in format, but most have a general theme such as acid–base balance, metabolic diseases, wound management, or sterile technique. The questions are presented by the group of examiners and are often illustrated with slides. The purpose of the oral examination is to evaluate the candidate's clinical thought process. The practical examination might be more species or discipline oriented and even further refined to examine the particular group taking the examination. It is essentially presented as case material shown as a series of slides and establishes the candidate's ability to recognize specific clinical conditions.

Obviously, each specialty board or college is strictly autonomous, although each is recognized and functions under the auspices of the AVMA's Advisory Board on Veterinary Specialties. Therefore, each one totally governs its own group and writes its own examination. Some examinations are prepared by the respective board or college, whereas others enlist the services of the National Examination Service. Information about each of the specialty groups (objectives and qualifications needed to become a candidate for examination) is listed in the AVMA directory along with the list of members of each group and the member to contact for application information.

Members of the respective specialty boards are referred to as *diplomates.* A diplomate is an individual who gains admission to a scholarly body by examination. The correct pronunciation is in contradistinction to diplomat in which the *a* is enunciated with a short vowel sound. The word *diplomate* rhymes with the *candidate.*

The earliest specialty boards were established in the 1950s with the American College of Veterinary Pathologists and the American College of Veterinary Public Health. Although more boards were created in the 1960s, the individuals gaining diplomate status in these groups were predominantly in either veterinary colleges or private institutions such as The Animal Medical Center in New York City and Angell Memorial Hospital in Boston. In the 1970s and 1980s more board-certified specialists moved into practice encompassing the disciplines of radiology, clinical pathology, surgery, medicine (internal medicine, cardiology, and neurology), dermatology, and ophthalmology.

In 1978 the Board of Veterinary Practitioners was formed and drew attention to the need for highly qualified general practitioners. Entrance into the specialty group by examination allowed skilled practitioners to be recognized for their special expertise without having to separate from their practices to participate in a formal training program.

☐ Specialty referral

The practitioner who makes the decision to refer a patient to a specialist does not suggest a deficiency in his clinical skills. Generally, the more enlightened and progressive practitioners use area specialists as an active everyday component of their practice. Often, in working with the specialist, the veterinarian can collaborate closely with the specialist, particularly by carrying on management of the case once the specialist specifically defines the disease process and outlines a course of management. Even in those cases when it is best for the patient to remain for a period of time under the direct care and supervision of the specialist, the referring veterinarian can continue to maintain communication with the client.

How does the practitioner refer a clinical case? The referring veterinarian usually establishes a presumptive or perhaps even a definitive diagnosis. He would then discuss the approach to management with the client. At this point is when the referring veterinarian needs to be critical of his own knowledge and competence regarding the disease process under question. If he feels the symptoms are vague but can identify an organ system of involvement or make a specific diagnosis (such as diabetes mellitus complicated by ketoacidosis), then he could suggest a specialist in internal medicine. The internist would be recommended on the basis of his greater depth of knowledge and experience in handling this kind of medical problem. If the problem was a complicated fracture or a vague neurological disorder, the practitioner would inform the owner that the pet would be better managed by a board-certified surgeon or neurologist, respectively.

After being assured, that the client is interested in the expertise of the specialist, the practitioner would make phone contact with the specialist to discuss the case, perhaps discuss fees, and establish the best time to transfer the case. It is often best for the client to make the appointment directly with the specialist's office.

Pertinent case data including radiographs and laboratory data may be sent along with the client to be delivered to the specialist at the time of the referral appointment. If time of scheduling permits, these records could be sent by mail directly to the specialist.

Once the specialist has examined the referred patient and a plan of management is established, the specialist should call the family veterinarian to inform him of the initial approach to management. If it is necessary for the patient to stay with the specialist for a period of days, the referring veterinarian should be called by the specialist to update the patient's status, test results, and procedures. When the patient is ready to be discharged by the specialist, the referring veterinarian should be called to provide an update on the patient's condition and present the final diagnosis and instructions for the patient's care. If the patient is to be seen subsequently by the referring veterinarian for any reason (i.e., recheck exams, follow--up radiographs, bandage checks, or lab analysis), these visits should be discussed with the referring veterinarian.

Finally, the care should be summarized in a formal letter from the specialist. This summary might also take the form of a report (Fig. 20-1 and 20-2). The report could also include copies of test results, ECG tracings, radiographs, and other laboratory and clinical findings.

JACK D. HENRY, JR., D.V.M., M.S.

DIPLOMATE, AMERICAN COLLEGE OF VETERINARY SURGEONS

REFERRAL CONSULTATION REPORT

DATE _____ REFERRING VETERINARIAN _____ PHONE _____

PATIENT _____

OWNER NAME _____ PHONE _____

===
===

PRESENTING PROBLEM _____

HISTORY _____

_____

_____

_____

_____

PHYSICAL FINDINGS _____

_____

_____

_____

CLINICAL IMPRESSIONS _____

_____

_____

RECOMMENDATIONS - PLAN _____

_____

_____

_____

VETERINARY SURGICAL REFERRAL SERVICE, P.C.

MOON VALLEY ANIMAL HOSPITAL ▥ 13650 N. 19TH AVENUE ▥ PHOENIX, ARIZONA ▥ 85029 ▥ (602) 942-8850

Figure 20-1. Referral consultation report

ARIZONA VETERINARY SURGICAL SPECIALIST

13650 North 19th Avenue
Phoenix, Arizona 85029
(602) 942-8850

Jack D. Henry, D.V.M., M.S.
Diplomate, ACVS

DISCHARGE SUMMARY   DATE_____

PET NAME_____BREED_____CASE #_____

OWNER_____REFERRING VETERINARIAN_____

PROBLEM:_____

_____

_____

DIAGNOSIS:_____

_____

PROCEDURES:_____

_____

DIET: Normal____ Special____ _____

EXERCISE:_____

INSTRUCTIONS:_____

_____

_____

_____

_____

_____

_____

_____

_____

MEDICATION:_____

_____

_____

FOLLOW-UP:_____

_____

_____VETERINARIAN_____

White – Medical Record
Yellow – Referring Veterinarian
Pink – Client

Figure 20-2. Discharge summary form

□
Telephone consultation

Telephone consultations constitute a large part of the veterinary specialist's communication with referring veterinarians. The referring veterinarian may call to discuss a referral case or oftentimes seek advice about a patient currently being treated. This assistance could range from uncertainty about a diagnosis to advice about the most appropriate manner for definitive care of a problem. It is *critically* important for the sake of the client and patient that the practitioner be highly conscientious in the assessment of his understanding of the problem, application of a particular technique for the problem, ability to completely carry out the procedure, and availability of instrumentation, sutures, implants, and other items necessary for a successful outcome. Unfortunately, some practitioners are overaggressive in these areas, and the patient's problem is mismanaged. This is underscored by the numerous patients referred to specialists that have been misdiagnosed or mismanaged. This emphasizes the importance of close collaboration between practitioners and specialists.

When specialists present detailed instructions over the telephone to the practitioner about various aspects of managing a patient, it is appropriate for the specialist to charge the practitioner a fee. This is true when the practitioner sends radiographs to a specialist (board-certified radiologist or other clinical specialist). The practitioner should then pass the fee on to the client. The client fee should probably not exceed the fee charged by the specialist. It would be advisable for the specialist to provide the practitioner with a fee schedule outlining fees for various forms of consultation.

The practicing veterinarian may telephone the specialist to discuss a case. In one instance the call may be to set up a referral. In other instances the practitioner may specifically wish to glean information from the specialist on how to manage a disease that has been diagnosed or review details about how to perform a certain surgical procedure. In these latter instances, the practitioner should pay a fee for the specialist's help. The specialist, on the other hand, may feel reluctant to charge a fee because he does not want to create ill feelings with the general practitioner. To avoid this, the specialist should publish a schedule of his consultation fees and distribute it to the community veterinarians so that it is well understood that fees for consultations are expected. The specialist might waive the consultation fee when a direct referral takes place.

□
Office consultation

When the client and pet go directly to the specialist's office, several consultation settings my ensue. The client may be there to gain a diagnosis only. Once the specialist arrives at the diagnosis and relates this back to the veterinarian, the veterinarian may then proceed with the patient management. The important aspect in this situation rests in the practicing veterinarian being critical of his own ability and availability to properly carry out the best care for the patient. One should not choose to maintain a case merely for the preservation of income.

The client may arrive at the specialist's office for a second opinion. The client could do this either on his own or at the request of the family veterinarian. Although the first instance has the potential to create conflicts and negative feelings among all parties involved, the specialist should try to communicate with the family veterinarian to gain a position of collaboration. It is always in the best interest of the two veterinarians to be very understanding with each other, perhaps setting egos aside and trying to answer the problem for the client in the best possible way. This will set the stage for the utmost professionalism and avoid the loss of communication that often results in complaints to the local associations or state board of examiners. Direct and open communication is always the best policy.

Large-animal consultations may occur from diagnostic pathologists providing consultations in the field. Diagnostic necropsies may be performed by the pathologist with tissue collected for toxicological and histopathologic evaluations. Where reference laboratories exist, the associated board-certified pathologists provide this service for an established fee. Food-animal and equine board-certified specialists (surgery, internal medicine, and theriogenologists) consult with local veterinarians on the farm or ranch. These consultants may be employed by universities or private industry.

Consultation with commercial and state diagnostic laboratories takes place between veterinarians and the specialists (pathologist) at their laboratory. Rarely do clients consult directly with the laboratory. Their assistance is provided in interpretation of clinical pathology tests, histopathology, necropsy, and toxicology.

In states that have a college or school of veterinary medicine a wide variety of specialty services are available. Most professional schools have all clinical specialists represented in addition to diagnostic laboratory support. Telephone and in-hospital consultations may be arranged. In those states without colleges or schools of veterinary medicine, specialty-trained private practitioners are usually available for consultation and referral. The lack of an available specialist is no longer a viable excuse for poor case management.

□ Consultation as continuing education

Consultations take on a source of continuing education since information often provided in reports from the specialists back to the referring veterinarian relates the latest techniques, methods, and concepts of management for the problems presented. Comparing notes on related cases where electrocardiography and radiography are involved provides the practitioners with an educational experience. Additionally, performing surgery with a surgeon or necropsy with a pathologist can be very educational. The referring veterinarian can gain new insight through the case management or histopathology performed.

As veterinary medicine progresses and more knowledge about animal disease comes forth, it will be increasingly difficult for each veterinarian to have a full grasp of this body of knowledge. Specialization is part of a natural evolution that accompanies this explosion of knowledge. Communication between all sectors of the veterinary community will result in benefits to the client, patient, and profession.

Index

☐

Page numbers in italics denote figures.